WHAT YOU REALLY NEED TO KNOW ABOUT CANCER

Dr. Robert Buckman is Medical Oncologist and Associate Professor, University of Toronto, and Adjunct Associate Professor, Department of Clinical Investigation, M. D. Anderson Cancer Center.

What You Really Need to Know about Cancer

A Comprehensive Guide for Patients and Their Families

DR. ROBERT BUCKMAN
in collaboration with the specialists at M. D. Anderson Cancer Center

FOREWORD BY DR. ROBERT C. BAST JR.
M. D. Anderson Cancer Center

THE JOHNS HOPKINS UNIVERSITY PRESS
Baltimore and London

Note to the reader: This book is intended to provide information that will promote and facilitate the conversation between you and your doctor and your medical team. It is not intended to substitute for medical care, however, and treatment must not be based solely on the contents of this book.

 Published 1997

Printed in the United States of America on acid-free paper

9 8 7 6

The Johns Hopkins University Press
2715 North Charles Street
Baltimore, Maryland 21218-4363
www.press.jhu.edu

Library of Congress Cataloging-in-Publication Data will be found at the end of this book.

A catalog record of this book is available from the British Library.

ISBN 0-8018-5594-2
ISBN 0-8018-5593-4 (pbk.)

Illustrations by Martin Nichols

To the clearest thinker
I have ever known —
John Cleese

Contents

Foreword, by Robert C. Bast Jr., M.D. xiii

Acknowledgments xv

Introduction Why Are We *So* Afraid of Cancer? 1

Chapter 1 What This Book Is All About 5
Happy Endings 6
Who Should Read This Book? 6
What This Book Isn't 7
About the Style Used in This Book 7
How the Material in This Book Is Arranged 7

Chapter 2 What Is Cancer? 9
What's in This Chapter 9
What Cancer Is 9
How the Growth of Cells Is Usually Controlled 9
Uncontrolled Growth 11
The Primary Tumor: Size and Growth 12
How Cancer Cells Invade Neighboring Areas 14
Distant Spread: Secondary Tumors or Metastases 15
Other Effects of Cancer 18
The Definition of "Cure," "Remission," and Some Other Terms 19
Summary 19

Chapter 3 How Cancer Is Caused 21
What's in This Chapter 21
The Types of Factors That Cause Cancer 21
Tumor Biology: The Study of Cancer in the Laboratory 24
Oncogenes and Tumor-Suppressor Genes 25
Epidemiology: The Study of the Different Incidences of Cancer 27
Summary 30

Chapter 4 An Overview of the Most Common Cancers 31
How the Information in Chapter 4 Is Organized 31
Bladder 36
Bone (Osteosarcoma and Other Types) 41
Osteosarcoma 42
Ewing's Sarcoma 45
Chondrosarcoma 45
Bowel (Colon and Rectum) 46
Brain and Spinal Cord 56
Breast 63
Cancer with No Known Primary Site 77
Cervix 81
Choriocarcinoma and Hydatidiform Mole (Tumors of the Placenta) and Related Trophoblastic Tumors 89
Endometrium (Womb) 92
Esophagus 97
Hodgkin's Disease 101
Kaposi's Sarcoma and AIDS-Related Lymphoma 106
Kidney 109
Larynx (Voice Box) and Pharynx (Throat) 113
Leukemias 119
Chronic Lymphocytic Leukemia (CLL) 122
Chronic Myeloid (or Granulocytic) Leukemia (CML or CGL) 126
Acute Lymphoblastic Leukemia (ALL) 127
ALL in Childhood 127
ALL in Adulthood 129
Acute Myeloid Leukemia (AML) 129
Hairy-Cell Leukemia 132
Liver (Hepatocellular Cancer) 133
Lung 137
Non–Small-Cell Lung Cancer 138
Small-Cell Lung Cancer 140
Lymphoma (Non-Hodgkin's Lymphoma) 142
The Low-Grade Lymphomas 146
The Intermediate and High-Grade Lymphomas 147
Treatment of Extranodal Lymphomas 148
Treatment of Lymphoma If It Recurs 148
Melanoma Skin Cancer (Malignant Melanoma) 149
Mouth (Oral Cancer and Adjacent Areas) 157
Myeloma (Multiple Myeloma) 161
Ovary 165
Epithelial Cancer of the Ovary: The Most Common Type 165
Other Tumors of the Ovary 172

Pancreas 174
Prostate 177
Sarcomas of the Soft Tissues 183
Skin Cancers (Excluding Melanoma) 187
Stomach 190
Testicular Cancer 196
Thyroid 200
Rarer Cancers in Childhood 203
Wilms' Tumor of the Kidney 203
Neuroblastoma 204
Retinoblastoma 204
Rarer Cancers in Adulthood 205
Anus 205
Bile Duct 207
Carcinoid Tumors 208
Gallbladder 209
Mesothelioma 210
Vulva 211

Chapter 5 The Main Types of Conventional Treatment 213
What's in This Chapter 213
The Four Main Types of Conventional Therapy: A Brief History 213
Combining Types of Treatment: Multidisciplinary Care 214
Surgery 215
Radiotherapy 216
Chemotherapy 221
Biologic Therapy 231
What Is a "Clinical Trial"? 233
Why It's Worth Considering a Clinical Trial 234

Chapter 6 Complementary, Alternative, or Unconventional Treatments 235
What's in This Chapter 235
By Way of Definition 235
The Frontier 235
Advantages of Complementary Medicine 236
What We Want When We Are Ill 237
Possible Explanations of Inexplicable Miracles 238
Should You Try a Complementary Medicine Anyway? 243
Summary: Hopes and Facts 244

Chapter 7 Cancer, Attitudes, and the Mind 245
What's in This Chapter 245
Humankind's Attitude to Cancer 245
Historical Attitudes to Illness 246
Diseases and Longevity 246
Can the Mind Cause Cancer? 246

Individual Stories and Case Histories 247
Data from Large Studies 249
Can the Mind Change the Outcome? 249
Psychoneuroimmunology 253
Blaming the Patient 253
Summary: The Importance of Mind-Body Interactions 254

Chapter 8 Screening, Early Diagnosis, and Prevention 255
What's in This Chapter 255
Definitions 255
Why Is Cancer Detected So Late? 256
Screening 256
Early Diagnosis 258
Prevention 258
You Can Quit Smoking 260

Chapter 9 With So Many Breakthroughs, Why's There No Progress? 261
What's in This Chapter 261
A Near-Crisis of Confidence: Public Perception of Cancer Research 261
The Gap between Lab and Bedside 262
Early Victories 262
Advances in Understanding the Cancer Cell 263
Current Limitations of Laboratory Research in Cancer 264
Collaborative Optimism: How Research Is Reported 265
Research That Might Have Worked Out but Didn't 266
Research That Is Currently Interesting and Might or Might Not Work Out 269
Front-Page Stories 272
Too Many Breakthrough Headlines: A Personal View 273

Chapter 10 Living with Cancer 275
What's in This Chapter 275
Three Common Symptoms 275
Pain and How to Cope with It 276
Tiredness 283
Depression 284
Emergencies and When to Get Urgent Help 287
Sexuality 287
Colostomies and Other Stomas 291
- What Is a Stoma? 291
- How Stomas Work 292
- Care of a Colostomy 292
- Care of an Ileostomy 293
- Care of a Urostomy 293
- Living with a Stoma 294
- Effects on Your Sex Life 294

Communication Suggestions for the Patient: How to Talk with Other People 294
- What's in This Section 294
- Why It's So Difficult to Talk about Cancer 295
- Your Feelings 295
- Other People's (and Society's) Attitudes 296
- The Benefits of Talking 297
- Who Is the Best Person to Talk To? 298
- How to Ask for What You Need or Want 298
- How to Talk about Your Feelings 300
- How to Respond to Other People's Reactions 301
- How to Tell Other People 302
- Talking with Doctors and Other Health Care Professionals 303
- Talking with Children 305
- Hints for Resolving Conflict 306
- Conclusion 307

Communication Suggestions for Friends and Family Members: How to Listen to and Talk with a Person with Cancer 307
- Not Knowing What to Say 307
- Why Talk, Why Listen? 308
- Obstacles to Talking 309
- How to Be a Good Listener 309
- Understanding What Your Friend Is Facing 313
- How to Help: A Practical Checklist 315
- Conclusion 316

Spiritual Aspects 316

When Things Are Going Badly 317

Issues and Decisions about Dying 318

For Friends and Family Members: How to Give Help and Support 321

What Dying Means: A Personal View 323

Conclusion 325

Appendix A Some Commonly Used Medical Terms and What They Mean 327

Appendix B Commonly Asked Questions 333

Appendix C Further Readings and References 337

Appendix D Other Sources of Help 341

Index 347

FOREWORD

So many people are affected by cancer that very few families exist who haven't been touched by this disease. In fact, one U.S. citizen in three will develop cancer at some time in his or her life. The good news is that the rate of cure has increased in recent years. Several forms of advanced cancer can be cured with chemotherapy alone. Combinations of surgery, radiotherapy, and chemotherapy have increased the number of lives saved with the more commonly occurring cancers of the breast and colon. Multidisciplinary treatment with chemotherapy and radiotherapy has reduced the need for radical surgery for several forms of cancer.

Just as important is the fact that many people are living longer, fuller lives, even when cancer cannot be completely eliminated. Methods for controlling pain have improved dramatically, and new drugs have been developed to neutralize the toxic effects of chemotherapy. Even more promising for the twenty-first century are advances in preventing and detecting cancer before it has spread. The revolution of our understanding of cancer at the level of individual genes has made it possible for us to identify persons at increased risk for developing cancer at specific sites.

Despite these advances, the diagnosis of cancer causes great anxiety and raises a number of questions. This book begins to answer many of those questions. Dr. Robert Buckman has a remarkable talent for translating complex medical concepts into terms that have meaning for all readers. The physicians at the University of Texas M. D. Anderson Cancer Center, who carefully reviewed all of the material in this book, share Dr. Buckman's belief that the more a patient and family understand, the better they are able to cope with an illness. Increasingly, well-informed people are taking a greater role in deciding what treatment is best for them. Empowered with a better understanding of cancer and armed with knowledge of the technical language, they can ask more specific questions and have greater confidence that they understand the significance of the answers they receive.

In *What You Really Need to Know about Cancer,* Dr. Buckman explains what cancer is and what causes cancer. He then provides a clear description of cancers that occur in many different sites in the body. He describes the main types of conventional treatment, discusses the attraction of so-called alternative treatments, explores the possible interaction of cancer and the mind, and supplies a good deal of practical advice about living with cancer. This book should prove enormously valuable to people with cancer, their families, and their friends. It is also a useful introduction for any concerned person who seeks an overview of cancer in understandable prose.

For patients who want to become better informed about their illness, in addition to Dr. Buckman's book and the other literature cited in Appendix C, the Cancer Information Service hotline can be reached by calling 1-800-4-CANCER; this hotline, sponsored by the National Cancer Institute, provides a great deal of valuable information.

Sometimes all of the available information and advice can seem overwhelming, especially to a person with an illness who is facing difficult decisions. At these times, your primary oncologist, family doctor, nurse, or physician's assistant can help to identify what is relevant for you and help to sort out alternatives for treatment and care. There are times when getting a second opinion at a major cancer center can be very helpful, too. Although this book cannot replace a health care professional, it is a useful place to begin.

Robert C. Bast Jr., M.D.
Head, Division of Medicine
The University of Texas M. D. Anderson Cancer Center

Acknowledgments

No book like this can be written without help from many colleagues and friends. In particular, I would like to thank Anna Porter for persuading me at the outset that I ought to write this book when I was certain that I shouldn't, and my invaluable assistant Susan Mawhood for continuing to believe that I could write it, when at various stages I was certain that I couldn't. In addition, special thanks are due to several people with whom I had valuable discussions early in the development of the book: Ken Holland, Dr. John Bailar, Professor Edward Shorter, Dr. Bernard Fox, Dr. Donna Stewart, and also the wonderful members of the focus group in London, Ontario, kindly organized by Shelly Markland, Director, and Gale Carew, Project Coordinator, of the Community Cancer Program at the London Regional Cancer Centre (of the Ontario Cancer Treatment and Research Foundation), and guests at Thameswood Lodge, and also to three people who kindly read the entire manuscript: Dr. Carol Sawka, Dr. Robert Mackenzie, and Ms. Sandy Naiman. Special thanks also to the illustrator, Martin Nichols, whose work I have known and admired for many years. The mathematics in Chapter 2 was kindly checked for me by the wonderful Mike Gallop of Microsoft (a company that produced an auto-correcting word-processor program just in time for this book).

The following people were kind enough to read a section or several sections of the text and to give me valuable and detailed feedback:

Ida Ackerman, M.D., FRCPC, Radiation Oncologist, Toronto-Sunnybrook Regional Cancer Centre, Assistant Professor, Department of Radiation Oncology, University of Toronto

*Frederick D. Ashbury, Ph.D., Associate Director, NCIC, Centre for Behavioural Research and Program Evaluation, Assistant Professor, Department of Behavioural Science, University of Toronto

*J. David Beatty, M.D., FRCSC, FACS, Executive Director, NCIC, Professor, Department of Surgery, University of Toronto

Robert S. Bell, M.D., FRCSC, Director, University Musculoskeletal Oncology Unit, Mount Sinai Hospital, Associate Professor, University of Toronto

Georg A. Bjarnason, M.D., FRCPC, Medical Oncologist, Toronto-Sunnybrook Regional Cancer Centre/Sunnybrook Health Science Centre

*Jacques Cantin, M.D., FRCSC, FACS, Surgical Oncologist, Hôtel-Dieu Hospital, Montréal, Associate Professor of Surgery, University of Montreal

Wayne E. Chapman, Chair of Psychiatric Oncology, Professor and Vice-Chairman, Department of Psychiatry, Cornell University Medical College

Flay Charbonneau, B.Sc. (Pharm), Supervisor, Toronto-Sunnybrook Regional Cancer Centre Pharmacy

Pamela Chart, M.D., CM, Toronto-Sunnybrook Regional Cancer Centre, Medical Director, Preventive Oncology Program, Medical Coordinator, Ontario Breast Cancer Screening Program

Allan Covens, M.D., FRCSC, Head, Division of Gynecologic Oncology, Toronto-Sunnybrook Regional Cancer Centre, Assistant Professor, Department of Obstetrics and Gynaecology, University of Toronto

*Donald Cowan, M.D., FRCPC, Vice-President and Director, Treatment Services, O.C.T.R.F., Professor, Department of Medicine, University of Toronto

Cyril Danjoux, M.D., FRCPC, Radiation Oncologist, Toronto-Sunnybrook Regional Cancer Centre, Assistant Professor, Department of Radiation Oncology, University of Toronto

Phillip Davey, M.B., FRCPC, Radiation Oncologist, Toronto-Sunnybrook Regional Cancer Centre, Assistant Professor, Department of Radiation Oncology, University of Toronto

*A. L. A. (Tony) Fields, M.D., FRCPC, FACP, Director, Cross Cancer Institute, Associate Professor and Acting Chair, Department of Oncology, University of Alberta

Lynn From, M.D., FRCPC, Professor of Medicine and Pathology, University of Toronto, Head, Division of Dermatology, Department of Medicine, Women's College Hospital

Ralph W. Gilbert, M.D., FRCSC, Director of Surgical Oncology, Toronto-Sunnybrook Regional Cancer Centre, Associate Professor, Department of Otolaryngology, University of Toronto

*Neil Hagen, M.D., FRCPC, Head, Cancer Pain Clinic, Tom Baker Cancer Centre, Associate Professor, Departments of Clinical Neurosciences, Oncology, and Medicine, University of Calgary

Sherif Hanna, M.D., FRCSC, FACS, General Surgeon, Gastrointestinal and Hepatobiliary and Pancreatic Cancer, Head of Division of General Surgery, Toronto-Sunnybrook Regional Cancer Centre, Assistant Professor, Department of Surgery, University of Toronto

Jimmie Holland, Psycho-oncologist, Memorial Sloan-Kettering Cancer Center, Chief, Psychiatry Service

*Neill A. Iscoe, M.D., FRCPC, Medical Oncologist, Toronto-Sunnybrook Regional Cancer Centre, Assistant Professor, Department of Medicine, University of Toronto

*Elizabeth Kaegi, MBChB, M.Sc., Director, Medical Affairs and Cancer Control, CCS and NCIC

Robert Kerbel, Ph.D., Director, Division of Cancer Biology Research, Sunnybrook Health Science Centre, John and Elizabeth Tory Professor of Experimental Oncology, Department of Medical Biophysics, University of Toronto

Ian G. Kerr, M.D., FRCPC, Medical Oncologist, Toronto-Sunnybrook Regional Cancer Centre, Assistant Professor, Department of Medicine and Pharmacology, University of Toronto

Laurence H. Klotz, M.D., FRCSC, Uro-oncologist, Sunnybrook Health Science Centre, Associate Professor, Department of Surgery, University of Toronto

*Isra Levy, MBBCh, M.Sc., FRCPC, Medical Consultant, Laboratory Centre for Disease Control, Health Canada, Adjunct Professor, Department of Epidemiology and Community Medicine, University of Ottawa, Clinical Assistant, Department of Radiation Oncology, Ottawa Regional Cancer Centre

Robert Mackenzie, M.D., FRCPC, Radiation Oncologist, Toronto-Sunnybrook Regional Cancer Centre, Assistant Professor, Department of Radiation Oncology, University of Toronto

*Charlotte McLeod, Chair, Patient Services Committee, CCS PEI Division

Anthony B. Miller, M.B., FRCP, Professor and Chairman, Department of Preventive Medicine and Biostatistics, University of Toronto

Doreen Millman-Wilson, Manager, Library Services, Toronto-Sunnybrook Regional Cancer Centre

*Christina Mills, M.D., FRCPC, Chief, Disease Control Division, Bureau of Chronic Disease Epidemiology, Adjunct Professor, Department of Epidemiology and Community Medicine, University of Ottawa

*Robin Moore-Orr, M.D., Chair, Patient Services Committee, CCS Newfoundland and Labrador Division

Balfour Mount, M.D., CM, FRCSC, Eric M. Flanders Professor of Palliative Medicine, McGill University, Director of Palliative Care, Royal Victoria Hospital, Montreal

*Eleanor Nielsen, Director, Patient Services and Public Education, CCS National Office

*Raymond Osborne, M.D., Gynecologic Oncologist, Toronto-Sunnybrook Regional Cancer Centre, Assistant Professor, University of Toronto

*Brian O'Sullivan, MBBCh., FRCPC, FRCPI, Radiation Oncologist, Princess Margaret Hospital, Associate Professor, Department of Radiation Oncology, University of Toronto

*Eleanor G. Pask, R.N., MSc.N., EdD., Executive Director, Candlelighters Childhood Cancer Foundation Canada

Peeter A. Poldre, M.D., M.Ed., FRCPC, Haematologist, Sunnybrook Health Science Centre

Kathleen I. Pritchard, M.D., FRCPC, Medical Oncologist, Head, Division of Medical Oncology/Haematology, Toronto-Sunnybrook Regional Cancer Centre, Professor, Faculty of Medicine, Department of Medicine, University of Toronto

*Paul-E. Raymond, M.D., D.M.R.T., FRCPC, Radiation Oncologist, Pavillon Carlton-Auger, L'Hôtel-Dieu de Québèc, Professor of Radiation Oncology, Laval University, President, Quebec Division

*Susan Russell, R.N., E.T., M.N., St. Elizabeth Healthcare

Carol Sawka, M.D., FRCPC, Medical Oncologist, Toronto-Sunnybrook Regional Cancer Centre, Assistant Professor, Department of Medicine, University of Toronto

Patricia A. Shaw, M.D., FRCPC, Anatomical Pathologist, Sunnybrook Health Science Centre, Assistant Professor, Department of Pathology, University of Toronto

Donald Sutherland, M.D., FRCPC, Ph.D., Medical Oncologist, Toronto-Sunnybrook Regional Cancer Centre, Associate Professor of Medicine, University of Toronto

Ian F. Tannock, M.D., Ph.D., Medical Oncologist, Princess Margaret Hospital, Professor, Department of Medicine, University of Toronto

*Brian Taylor, former Patient Services Coordinator, CCS Nova Scotia Division

Glen A. Taylor, M.D., FRCSC, General and Thoracic Surgeon, Sunnybrook Health Science Centre, Toronto-Sunnybrook Regional Cancer Centre, Associate Professor, Department of Surgery, University of Toronto

Gillian M. Thomas, B.Sc., M.D., FRCPC, Radiation Oncologist, Toronto-Sunnybrook Regional Cancer Centre, Professor, Department of Radiation Oncology and Department of Obstetrics and Gynaecology, University of Toronto

*Donald Wigle, M.D., Ph.D., MPH, Director, Bureau of Chronic Diseases, Health Canada, Adjunct Professor, Department of Epidemiology and Community Medicine, University of Ottawa.

In collaboration with specialists at The University of Texas M. D. Anderson Cancer Center:

Robert C. Bast Jr., M.D., Head, Division of Medicine; Chairman, Department of Clinical Investigation (ad interim); Professor of Medicine; Harry Carothers Wiess Chair for Cancer Research

James L. Abbruzzese, M.D., FACP, Deputy Head, Division of Medicine; Chairman, Department of Gastrointestinal Medical Oncology and Digestive Diseases; Associate Professor

Raymond Alexanian, M.D., Deputy Chairman, Department of Hematology; Professor of Medicine

Joann L. Ater, M.D., Chief, Section of Neural Tumors, Department of Pediatrics; Associate Professor of Pediatrics

Alberto G. Ayala, M.D., Head, Division of Pathology (ad interim); Chairman, Department of Anatomic Pathology; Professor of Pathology; Ashbel Smith Professor

Robert S. Benjamin, M.D., Chairman, Department of Melanoma/Sarcoma Medical Oncology; Medical Director, Sarcoma Center; Professor of Medicine

Archie W. Bleyer, M.D., Head, Division of Pediatrics; Chairman, Department of Pediatrics; Professor of Pediatrics; Mosbacher Pediatrics Chair

Antonio C. Buzzaid, M.D., Medical Director, Melanoma Skin Center; Associate Professor of Medicine

Fernando F. Cabanillas, M.D., Chief, Section of Lymphoma; Department of Hematology; Professor of Medicine; Ashbel Smith Professor

Donna R. Copeland, Ph.D., Chief, Section of Behavioral Medicine, Department of Pediatrics; Professor of Pediatrics

James D. Cox, M.D., Head, Division of Radiation Oncology; Professor of Radiation Oncology; Hubert L. and Oliver Stringer Chair in honor of Sue Gribble Stringer

Madeline Duvic, M.D., Chief, Section of Dermatology, Department of Medical Specialties; Professor of Medicine

James L. Gajewski, M.D., Associate Medical Director, Hematology Disease Center; Associate Medical Director of Blood and Marrow Transplantation; Laboratory Director, Allogeneic Blood and Marrow Processing Facility; Associate Professor of Medicine

David M. Gershenson, M.D., Deputy Chairman, Department of Gynecologic Oncology; Director, Sandra G. Davis Ovarian Cancer Research Program; Professor of Gynecologic Oncology; Anderson Clinical Faculty Chair for Cancer Treatment and Research

Helmuth Goepfert, M.D., Head, Division of Surgery and Anesthesiology (ad interim); Chairman, Department of Head and Neck Surgery; Professor of Surgery; M. G. and Lillie A. Johnson Chair for Cancer Treatment and Research

Waun Ki Hong, M.D., Chairman, Department of Thoracic/Head and Neck Medical Oncology; Professor of Medicine; Charles A. LeMaistre Chair in Thoracic Oncology; American Cancer Society Clinical Research Professor

Gabriel N. Hortobagyi, M.D., FACP, Chairman, Department of Breast and Gynecologic Medical Oncology; Professor of Medicine; Nylene Eckles Professor in Breast Cancer Research

Hagop M. Kantarjian, M.D., Chief, Leukemia Section, Department of Hematology; Professor of Medicine

John J. Kavanagh, M.D., Chief, Section of Gynecologic Medical Oncology, Department of Clinical Investigation; Professor of Medicine

John F. Kuttesch, Ph.D., M.D., Assistant Professor of Pediatrics, Department of Clinical Pediatrics

Bernard Levin, M.D., Vice President for Cancer Prevention; Professor of Medicine; Betty B. Marcus Chair in Cancer Prevention

Victor A. Levin, M.D., Chairman, Department of Neuro-Oncology; Professor of Medicine; Bernard W. Biedenham Chair in Cancer Research

Christopher J. Logothetis, M.D., Chairman, Department of Genitourinary Medical Oncology; Professor of Medicine; Bessie McGoldrick Professor in Clinical Cancer Research

Gordon B. Mills, M.D., Ph.D., Chairman, Department of Molecular Oncology; Professor of Medicine

Rebecca D. Pentz, Ph.D., Clinical Ethicist and Associate Professor of Clinical Ethics

R. Beverly Raney, M.D., Chief, Section of Non-Neural Solid Tumors, Department of Pediatrics; Professor of Pediatrics

Stephen C. Stuyck, B.J., Associate Vice President for Public Affairs

Theodore F. Zipf, Ph.D., M.D., Chief, Leukemia Section, Department of Pediatrics; Professor of Pediatrics

I also wish to thank the following individuals for their contributions from a lay person's perspective:

Mrs. Naomi Stearns and Mrs. Ina Bond.

All of the people mentioned above, as well as several other experts and advisers to whom sections of the manuscript were sent, helped me by detecting any factual errors or major omissions. The responsibility for the opinions expressed in this book (particularly on controversial issues) and for the emphasis or any prejudice or bias is mine and mine alone.

* These individuals are dedicated volunteers or staff members of the Canadian Cancer Society/National Cancer Institute of Canada.

WHAT YOU REALLY NEED TO KNOW ABOUT CANCER

INTRODUCTION

Why Are We *So* Afraid of Cancer?

We are all afraid of cancer. In fact we usually feel more frightened of cancer than of any other equally serious (or equally curable) medical condition. Often a diagnosis of cancer seems to produce in our minds a particular and deep feeling of helplessness, sometimes verging on terror or paralysis. It is as if those mental strategies that we could use coping with a diagnosis of, say, a heart attack or multiple sclerosis disappear and are no use to us when the diagnosis is a cancer.

Because that fear seems to be so closely linked to the two hundred or more diseases that make up "the cancers" and because it is so particular, and is so deep and so widespread, I have written this book to try and give clear factual explanations of the various cancers and how they are treated. But before I go into the specific details, I think it is worth spending a moment or two looking at our attitudes to cancer, to try and find out why we are *so* afraid of it—so much more afraid of it than we are of other medical diseases, even ones that have just the same potential for harm and the same chance of treatment or cure. There seem to be four major elements to our fears of cancer.

Cancer Is Thought of as a Single Disease

The first component of our fear is that we tend to think of cancer as a single disease. I shall explain in a moment why that perception makes the word and the diagnosis of cancer seem so terrible and frightening, but first let me explain clearly that cancer is not a single disease. In fact, *cancer is not a disease at all but a process* that happens to be shared by more than two hundred different diseases (the cancers) which have some other features in common.

As I explain in more detail in Chapter 2 of this book, cancer is what happens when a group of cells grows and multiplies in a disorderly and uncontrollable way and some of those cells are then able to invade into neighboring tissues. But apart from that process which they have in common—uncontrolled growth and then invasion—cancers vary enormously in their potential for causing harm or threatening life. Some cancers, for example, in addition to growing and invading, also have a high tendency to spread to distant parts of the body, and it is this that makes them dangerous and potentially lethal. Other cancers—in fact many of them—have a *low* tendency to do that and are much more likely to be cured at the first surgical operation. Some cancers (such as the two commonest types of skin cancer) almost never spread to distant areas of the body and are therefore never life threatening.

So the cancers are not one disease but a group of more than two hundred different diseases, each of which has its own behavior pattern and therefore its own chance of spreading to distant parts of the body and therefore threatening health and life. To lump them all together and think of them as one disease called "cancer" is not only inaccurate but is also very frightening because it makes this supposed single disease "cancer" appear to be infinitely variable and therefore entirely unpredictable and lethal. Here's a useful comparison. Suppose we had only one word to describe these infectious illnesses: *the common cold, flu, tuberculosis, measles, hepatitis, AIDS.* Suppose we had just the one word, *infection,* to describe all of those different illnesses. Wouldn't that *infection* be a frightening illness? You would probably think of it as an illness that might give you a runny nose for a few days or might cause a red rash or might give you weakness and nausea for a few weeks—or might kill you in a few years. If you thought that all of those different infectious illnesses were actually different manifestations of a single "infection" disease, then the word *infection* would appear to you as a very frightening, unpredictable, and always dangerous disease. If you had a friend with a cold or flu, you would wonder—as would they—whether the "infection" illness might suddenly and unpredictably turn into the deadly kind of infection and cause rapid deterioration. The diagnosis of *infection* would be very likely to cause deep and widespread feelings of terror and helplessness.

And that is what has happened to our understanding of *cancer.* Because we say *cancer* instead of *the cancers,* it appears to us that we are dealing with a single dangerous, unpredictable disease that at any moment might suddenly change its track and threaten our life. Whereas once we understand the facts—that the cancers are a group of some two hundred diseases, some of which are potentially very serious, some of which are never life threatening, and most of which are in between—the whole picture becomes more intelligible and less frightening.

Cancer Is Perceived as If It Were an Alien Invasion

Another important component of our fear is the feeling that somehow cancer is a condition that has its own intelligence, almost like an invasion from outer space. This fear is probably a basic and primeval fear built into the human species. Some centuries ago, the kinds of medical conditions that caused something to grow inside and burst out were usually infectious abscesses (for example, in the chest, abdomen, or skin). Nowadays, with antibiotic treatment, abscesses are very rare, and this basic fear of something growing inside fits our perceived image of the cancers. So a diagnosis of cancer "buys into" a basic human fear. In fact, of course, cancer cells are normal cells that have gone slightly wrong in their behavior—they are not alien at all (unlike, for example, viruses, which some scientists believe *might* have originated on other planets!). Yet even though the cancer process is caused by our own cells escaping growth control mechanisms, that image of an alien, animal-like intelligence lurking inside, growing, and doing damage is a powerful one and an important and deep-seated component of our feelings about cancer.

Cancer Seems to Be Inevitably Mysterious

Another feature that seems to make cancer unusual among other chronic or potentially serious diseases is that it seems to have acquired a label of inevitable mystery. As in "they'll never really understand cancer." Of course, there are millions of questions that we cannot answer about the cancer process, but the same is true of almost every other condition you can think of. We don't understand why some people get multiple sclerosis and others don't, what causes ALS (Lou Gehrig's disease), what triggers ulcerative colitis, and so on. Yet somehow as a society we accept these areas of mystery relatively calmly, and we believe (I'm sure correctly) that some of the important questions about these conditions will be answered in the future. Yet with cancer there is a public perception that the major mysteries will *never* be unraveled and *can* never be. Of course, that too is true. Still, we are beginning to learn a great deal about the pathways that lead to the cancer process (including, for example, the role of some genetic fragments called oncogenes and the role of control mechanisms called tumor-suppressor genes; see Chapter 3) and some of the methods by which cancers keep themselves growing (such as growth factors, the process of angiogenesis, and so on; see Chapter 9). Yet the aura of "inevitable mystery" seems to cling to cancer, perhaps partly because there have been so many stories of major breakthroughs in the press and on TV—when these seem to have failed to produce eradication of cancer, the myth of inevitable mystery gets another boost. So this, too, adds to the fear of cancer as an unknown and unknowable condition.

Cancer Is Often Perceived as Some Sort of Manifestation or Metaphor of Personality or Psychological Problems

Of all the reactions that cancer patients and their families experience, perhaps the most damaging and crushing is the idea that somehow the cancer patient might have brought the condition on himself or herself by having the wrong attitudes, thoughts, or personality. I deal with this in detail in Chapter 7, but let me stress right away that humankind has always had a tendency to blame the patient for the disease, and there has been a recent upsurge of this in cancer. As I shall show, there are very many carefully conducted studies that show that attitudes, personality, life events, grief, and depression do not cause cancer at all (as opposed to behavior patterns such as smoking, which does cause cancer). Furthermore, there are also important studies that show that changing your attitude and your thinking undoubtedly has a positive effect on your quality of life but does not change the behavior of cancer. Even so, the belief that somehow a diagnosis of cancer is a metaphor for some undefined "wrongness" of the person is a very subtle and powerful part of many people's reactions.

So, for all those reasons, the word *cancer* produces particular and deep-seated feelings of fear and dread. That is why a book like this is needed—to explain and demystify cancer and its treatment and so reduce as far as possible those feelings of fear and helplessness. As has often been said, "understanding what's going on always makes things better," and that's especially true of cancer. A clear understanding will always help you feel more in control of your own situation, and by doing that it will really help you cope.

1

What This Book Is All About

As I said in the Introduction, we are all afraid of cancer. The reasons for that particularly deep, almost ingrained fear may be complex, and I talked about the main reasons in that introductory section. For the reasons discussed there, we all have a tendency to think of cancer as if it were a single disease, some sort of alien invasion that is inevitably mysterious and unknowable, and in some way deserved by the type of person who develops it. Of course, all these things are untrue, yet they almost always produce that particular feeling of helplessness in so many people. And that, of course, is why there is a real and urgent need for a book like this to offer clear and simple explanations of the facts—a process of genuine demystifying.

Obviously, knowledge of the available facts about cancers and their treatment cannot suddenly change the nature of the disease—cancer will not disappear from our species simply because we understand it. But even though a clear understanding of the facts cannot in itself alter those facts, it can certainly help everyone (patients, friends, family members, health care workers, and anyone who is interested or involved) cope with the disease. That is why I felt this book was needed in the first place: the more you understand about what is happening and why, the better you will be able to deal with the disease and the treatment. Furthermore, when you come to make decisions about treatment choices, the more likely it is that those choices will represent what you really want.

Of course, many of the most important questions about cancer are still unanswered. Some of those central issues may even prove to be unanswerable. In other areas, we do not even know the right questions to ask yet, nor how to frame them, let alone begin to look for answers. On the other hand, in some areas we now do have clear factual answers to the important questions, and in other areas there are at least a few beginnings, hints, and glimmerings of answers. As is always the way in science and medicine, the moment you answer one question you raise dozens of others. Yet even if more questions are created than are answered, there is still a lot to be gained from the process of defining that frontier between the known and the unknown. Which is what this book does. It explains what is known about cancer, however insufficient that may seem, as almost all answers are not complete enough to satisfy us—patients, doctors, or anyone else. It also defines the areas we do *not* know about. In the process I try to summarize those hints and glimmerings of knowledge and theory that at least allow us to speculate about what we might know one day. That process of explaining the known and defining the unknown may in itself help you think about cancer as a disease process (or rather as a group of more than two hundred diseases sharing several important features and processes). And that may in turn help to overcome the feelings of helplessness and dread that tend to appear when the diagnosis is cancer.

Happy Endings

Shortly after I started preparing this book, I called together a focus group—a dozen people of different backgrounds and different experiences, each of whom was suffering from cancer. I wanted to find out specifically what it was that cancer patients would want to know—what they would expect and hope for from a book like this. In the group, the first person to speak was Juliette, an intelligent and articulate woman in her late forties who had just completed chemotherapy after surgery for breast cancer. She knew exactly what she wanted from this book: *"A happy ending,"* she said. She wanted to know that her cancer had been cured and that it would never bother her again, and she wanted the same for everybody with cancer. Juliette immediately identified one of the most unpleasant aspects that all people with cancer face—uncertainty. Of all the daunting and frightening aspects of cancer, perhaps the worst is the uncertainty: uncertainty about the disease, the cause, the treatment, the symptoms, and most of all the future.

Of course, this book cannot abolish uncertainty and promise happy endings for everybody. That simply isn't possible with the current state of our knowledge about cancer and its treatment. But at least it can help you see what we are all uncertain about. Even more important, it can help you understand the ways in which uncertainty is (or will be) diminished. Nowadays some cancers are curable, and most sufferers from these cancers will be treated successfully and will never have to worry about that cancer again. For people who have been diagnosed with those particular cancers, there *is* a genuinely happy ending. Unfortunately, for other people (as Juliette herself said at that first meeting), the happy ending of a cure or long-term remission is uncertain and may not be guaranteed at the outset. But even if no one can guarantee the delivery of a happy ending, at least this book can help you—patients, friends, family, and supporters—to make some sense of what is going on and why things happen the way they do. To quote Frank, another member of the focus group, this book will provide "the big picture . . . the context that cancer is in. A map of the forest, not just a catalogue of all the trees."

Who Should Read This Book?

This book is primarily for people with cancer and their families and friends. For those people, I try to explain and demystify cancer and its treatment so that you may be able to discern some logic underlying events that at first seem random and chaotic. The book will also be of some interest to the general reader, to people who want to understand the basics of cancer and its treatment even though they have not been affected by it personally or through their friends. I hope that this book *will* be read by the general reader, but I should stress that the *primary* aim of this book is to help people with cancer to deal with their illness. If it helps anyone else as well, that's a bonus; but I am assuming that this book will be read mainly by people to whom cancer is not merely an interesting concept or a fascinating mistake of biology but a fact of life and a threat *to* life. So whenever I say "you" in this book, those are the people I am talking to. That brings me to another few points that need clarifying.

"You," "We," and "We All"

This book is written for people who have cancer and for their friends and family. That's the "you." But when I need to indicate that I'm talking solely about the person who has cancer (not to friends or family members), then I use the word "patient." Because the word sounds rather impersonal, I use it as little as possible. In using "patient," however, I'm not trying to remove the personal element from what is a very personal situation, but simply to indicate clearly whom I am talking about.

Similarly, I use "we" to indicate people in the health care disciplines: doctors, nurses, scientists, and the many other groups of people who contribute to cancer treatment and research. I cannot get away from the fact that I'm able to write this book because I've been working in the medical profession. And I've grown accustomed to saying "we" when I mean the health care professions as a whole. But when I want to talk about experiences or feelings or reactions that *all* human beings have in common, I use the phrase "we all" (as in *"We all fear pain"* or *"We are all afraid of cancer"*). Of course, the context will likely make that clear anyway, but there is no harm in underlining my intentions.

What This Book Isn't

This book is not a step-by-step best-buy guide to the current treatment of cancer. It will not tell you which treatment specifically is the best choice if you have, let's say, early-stage cancer of the breast or cancer of the esophagus. There is a good reason why that kind of information is *not* in this book. That kind of advice should not be in any book because if you have a complex treatment decision to make or to share in, that kind of specific information should come from the consultation between you and your doctor. It is the central element of the relationship between the two of you. In addition, of course, some of the information about the current treatment of cancer will be out of date even before the book is printed. That means that this book gives you the background, not the foreground. It will help you understand the terms in which your doctor talks about your diagnosis and treatment and why some things are known about the disease and so many aren't. It gives you the basic facts about cancer, so that when you spend time with your doctor you can concentrate on the fine details of your own personal case and use your time to discuss individual aspects and decisions rather than going over the basics. In other words, this book gives you the foundation so that you can use the time you spend with your doctor more effectively to get specific information about your own individual case.

About the Style Used in This Book

I have tried hard to make this book as easy to read and understand as possible. I have therefore deliberately written it in a rather conversational way. I think most readers of this book will welcome explanations in the language that they use every day, not in medical jargon or legalese. In addition, I have used **bold** letters to emphasize certain phrases and words. I have done this where a new topic or a new idea is introduced, and also where there is some general rule or principle that really needs emphasis. I use *italics* to indicate quotations—things that other people have said or written—and also sometimes for emphasis within a sentence. I realize that some people may find that this makes the text look a little busy, but in my experience when you are feeling anxious, you need all the assistance you can get to make sense of what you read.

How the Material in This Book Is Arranged

Because this book is written primarily for the person (and family) coping with cancer, I begin in Chapter 2 with an overview of what cancer is and how it is able to grow and spread. I also define what is meant by the words "cure" and "remission." In Chapter 3, I look at what we know about the causes of cancer: what it is that makes cells turn cancerous in the first place and what is currently known about the various mechanisms involved in that process. In Chapter 4, I discuss the most common sites of cancer and give you an overall understanding of how each particular cancer behaves and how treatment can be used to try to control it. With a few small variations, all the sections that make up Chapter 4 follow the same organizational pattern, which I outline in the first section of Chapter 4. I then move on to deal with other issues in cancer. The four types of conventional treatment are explained in Chapter 5. Some of the most important topics in complementary medicine are covered in Chapter 6. The controversies over the role of the mind are discussed in Chapter 7. Screening, early diagnosis, and prevention are covered in Chapter 8. In Chapter 9, I look at why cancer research does not appear to be changing the situation for the cancer patient at the moment, and in Chapter 10, I deal with a number of questions related to living with cancer: how to control pain, how to manage some of the other common symptoms, how to live with a colostomy or ileostomy, how to recognize a medical emergency, how to communicate with friends and family (or the cancer patient) and the medical team.

What Is Cancer?

2

What's in This Chapter

In this chapter I give an overview of how cancer cells differ from normal cells and how they go on growing and multiplying in an uncontrolled way to form a tumor or lump (the primary tumor). I then discuss the two processes that make cancer so damaging: the ability to invade into neighboring areas and the ability to spread to distant areas of the body (forming secondary tumors or metastases) via lymph vessels, blood vessels, and other means.

What Cancer Is

Cancer is what happens when a part of your body grows in an uncontrollable way and damages healthy parts. In other words, cancer results when one group of cells (cells are the basic components of our bodies) grows and multiplies in a disorderly and uncontrolled way. By various means, one type of cell becomes able to disobey or escape from the control mechanisms that usually keep cells growing in their normal, orderly way. The key to understanding the nature of cancer is to find out what normally keeps our cells in order and how some cells are able to escape from that regimentation. If we knew that, we would know what causes cancer, and that might, perhaps, help us work out how to treat it and how to prevent it.

So in order to look at the ways in which cancer creates problems, we need a summary of how cancer cells grow in their abnormal way. (Chapter 3 discusses this process in more detail.)

How the Growth of Cells Is Usually Controlled

Repair of Daily Wear and Tear Even though we are not usually aware of it, cells in virtually every part of our body are growing all the time. We may be aware that some parts of our body are growing—our fingernails and hair, for example. Other areas are not growing bigger, but the cells within them are multiplying. Such growth is necessary because almost all parts of the body are subjected to daily wear and tear that kills cells, or damages them, or makes them fall off. For instance, every day we lose many millions of cells from the skin, the lining of our mouth, and the rest of the digestive tract. The cells that are lost are replaced daily by new cells created by growth and multiplication. That process goes on in almost all areas of the body—including, for example, the bone marrow where blood cells are manufactured—so that as daily wear and tear takes its toll, there is always an appropriate supply of new cells ready to replace the damaged and lost ones. Without that continuous process, the human body would literally wear out and fall apart in a few days.

Response to Injury As well as growing simply to keep pace with daily living, the body occasionally has to respond to trauma or injury. In the event of an injury or any trauma, cell growth has to accelerate in order to repair the damage and to produce what we recognize as healing. For example, after a surgical operation, within (on average) a week or ten days, the cut in the skin (the incision) will have healed, and the skin in that area will be almost at normal strength. To achieve that, the skin cells will have accelerated their growth rate dramatically (although in an orderly way) and will have produced several billions of cells in a few days.

Control of Growth The important point is that when the growing skin cells have filled in the gap created by the incision, they stop growing. The growth continues until the cells growing in from each side of the gap meet. At that point, the accelerated growth slows down to the normal (replacement) rate (this process is sometimes called **contact inhibition**). There must, therefore, be a set of control mechanisms that can encourage cell growth to go on at a very fast rate for as long as needed, and then, when the gap is filled in and the skin is back to its accustomed contour, can stop the accelerated growth, instead of continuing indefinitely and making a large mound of skin.

Very occasionally, skin cells are not quite as good at stopping their growth as they should be. In some cases, they may go on growing and heaping up for a while and produce a thick, piled-up scar, say a centimeter or so thick (see illustration). Even then, however, the cells do not continue growing at this rate for very long: overgrown scars may be a centimeter or so thick, but they do not grow forever.

At present, we do not completely understand this behavior, although we believe there are at least two processes going on. One process involves substances called **growth factors**. These are substances that stimulate cells to grow and multiply. They are produced all the time to keep daily repair going, and in larger amounts when there has been

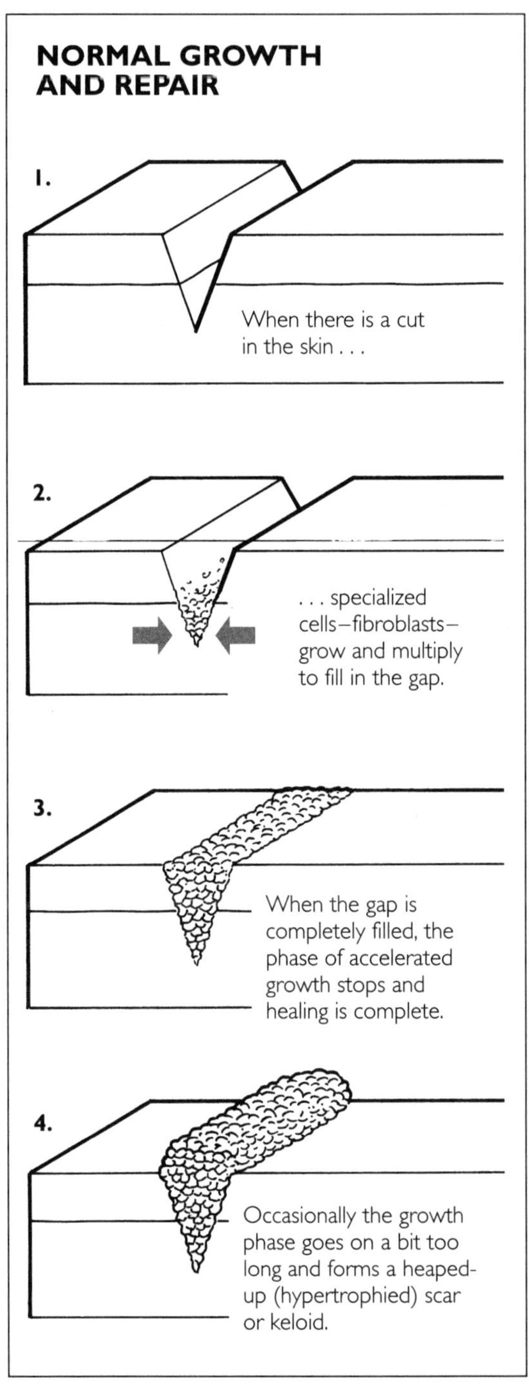

trauma, as in the healing of the surgical incision, for example.

In normal daily life, we know that cells stop growing when they are supposed to. Probably this is because the increased production of growth factors returns to normal levels when the trauma has been repaired. We do not know exactly how that happens, but it involves substances that *inhibit* the growth of cells (**inhibitory growth factors**). When there is an injury, we think, the normal production of these inhibitory factors *decreases,* while the production of growth factors *increases,* and growth occurs. When normality is restored, the inhibitory factors are switched on again and the phase of accelerated growth is over.

There is a second, built-in control process affecting the way in which normal cells die. This process, called **apoptosis**, allows a single cell to die within a group of cells. Thus the group can stay the same size as new cells are formed by multiplication. The signal for this type of "single cell death" seems to come from within. This is sometimes called "programmed cell death" and is clearly of great importance in making sure that cells do not go on accumulating. We are only just beginning to learn more about apoptosis, but it seems that cancer cells have found a way of avoiding it.

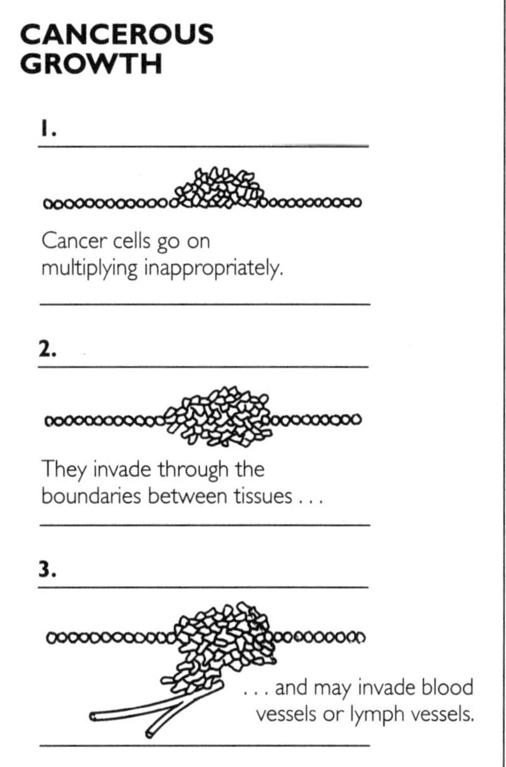

Uncontrolled Growth

So cancer is what happens when cells "refuse" to obey the body's control mechanisms and ignore the messages that would normally tell them when to stop growing and multiplying. Uncontrolled growth alone does not produce a cancer, however. After all, cells heap up when you have a wart on your skin or if you have one of those heaped-up scars mentioned earlier. Cancer cells do other things as well as heaping up. There are five basic properties of cancer cells that account for nearly all of the things that they do.

- **Cancer cells** go on growing and multiplying when they should not.
- **Cancer cells are capable of crossing the normal boundaries** of the tissue they start in. In other words, they invade surrounding areas.
- **Cancer cells can get into the bloodstream** or other channels or routes, such as lymph vessels, and can travel to areas distant from their starting place.
- **Cancer cells can establish secondary tumors** at those distant areas.
- **Some cancer cells may produce substances** that interfere with the control of various body functions, and may affect nerves, muscles, salt regulation, and other systems.

It is possible to sum up the problem of cancer cells under two headings. First, cancer cells have the ability to invade normal tissues in the neighborhood. Second, they have the ability to **spread** to distant areas. If cancer cells did not do these two things, cancers would be no more trouble than warts. They could simply be removed and would never cause any further difficulty.

We can look at the behavior of cancer under three headings: first, the uncontrolled growth itself wherever it begins, that is, the primary tumor; second, the invasion of surrounding normal tissues; and third, the spread to distant parts of the body, that is, the establishing of secondary tumors or metastases.

The Primary Tumor: Size and Growth

The place where the cancer begins is called the **primary site**, and as the cancer begins to form a mass of cells, that is the **primary tumor**. Most types of cancers begin with a primary tumor in one place—for example, the breast, lung, or bowel—then invade neighboring tissues and later on form secondary tumors in other places. Some types of cancer, however, seem to begin in several places at once: for example, the leukemias, some lymphomas, and myeloma each begin inside the bone marrow or in the lymph nodes and often appear to start in several areas almost simultaneously.

It is important to understand how much growing and multiplying usually goes on before a cancer is detectable. Almost all human cells are very small. The average cell may be about 20- or 30-thousandths of a millimeter across, that is, about one-twentieth of the width of an average human hair. This means that even if there are 100,000 cells in a clump, the clump is only just visible to the naked eye. Even ten times more than that—a million cells—is only about the size of a slightly swollen pinhead.

As a rough guide, cancer cells reproduce themselves every two to six weeks on average (depending on the type of the cancer and how aggressive it is). Suppose, for example, that a cancer cell divides once a month. If a single cancer cell starts off (and most cancers do begin from a single cell), say, on January 1 and reproduces every month, then by February 1 there will be two cells, by March 1 there will be four cells, in April there will be eight, and so on. After a year there will be 4,000 cells, and after twenty months—by September of the second year—there will be a million cells. As I have said, you could just see a million cells if they were set alone on a microscope slide (they would be about the size of a large pinhead), but if they were inside any part of the body, they would be totally undetectable.

With most cancers, therefore, you could only begin to detect a lump when the number of cancer cells reached approximately a billion cells—a tumor approximately the size of a small grape. If the cancer cells are dividing every month, then it will be two and a half years before they produce a billion cells—in our example, by July of the third year. Once there are about a billion cells, each doubling will produce an enlargement that is noticeable, so that about seven months later (at some time during February of the fourth year) there would be more than 100 billion cells, which would produce a mass weighing around 125 grams (about four ounces). By about forty months—around May of the fourth year—the cancer cells would produce about a kilogram of cells (about two and a quarter pounds). The human body cannot usually tolerate more than two or three kilograms of tumor, so that (again, on average) by three and a half years after the first cancer cell developed (if growth proceeded at a steady pace and was not checked by any treatment), one cancer cell will have produced enough cancer to be lethal.

The important point is that the number of times a cancer cell needs to reproduce itself to reach lethal proportions is actually quite small—about forty-two doublings. And for approximately thirty of those doublings, the mass of accumulated cancer cells will be too small to be detected. In other words, at present we are unfortunately unable to detect cancer until it has proceeded nearly three-quarters of the way along the road to being a potentially life-threatening condition. In some cancers, as we shall see, we can still cure the patient at that

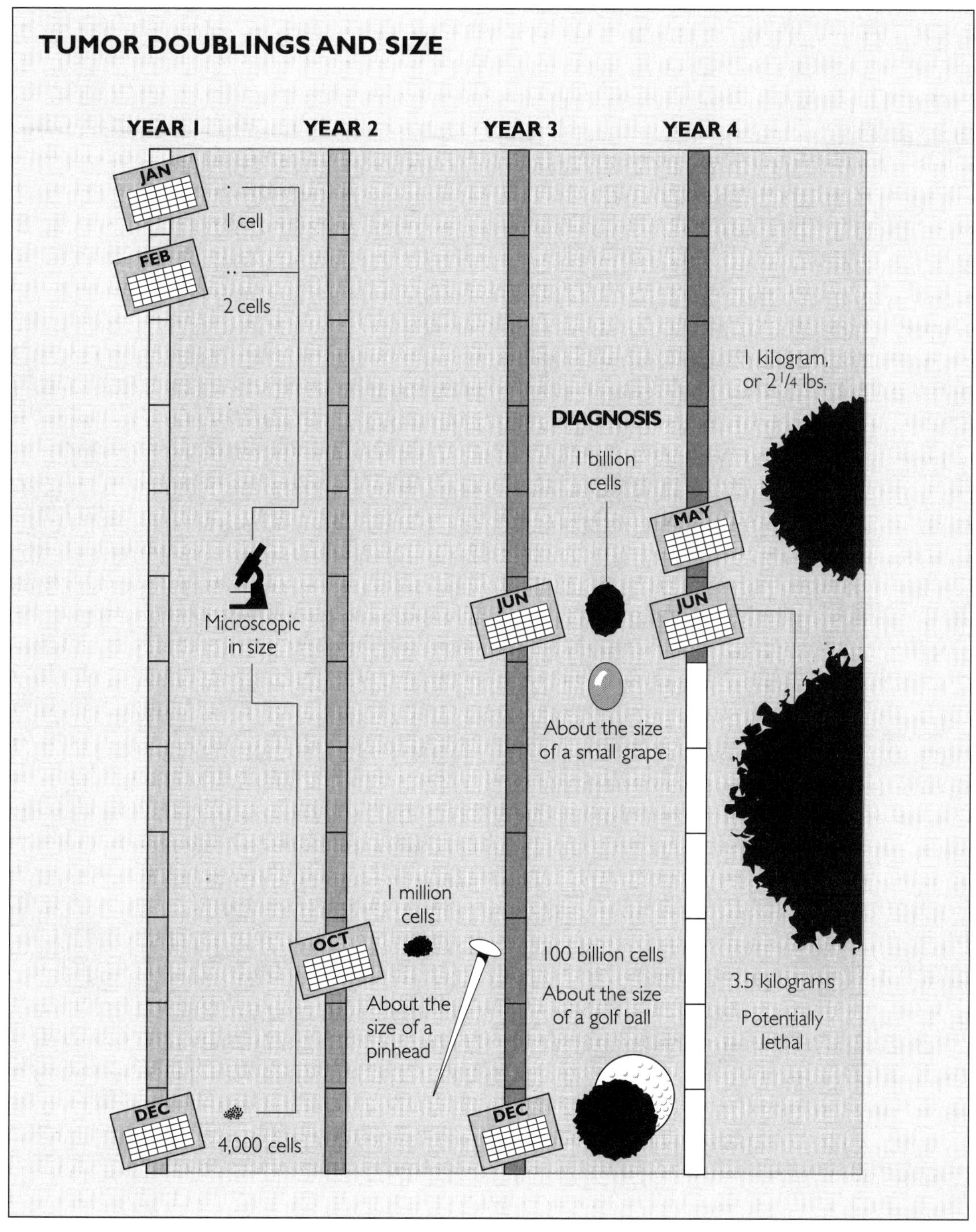
TUMOR DOUBLINGS AND SIZE
YEAR 1
YEAR 2
YEAR 3
YEAR 4
JAN
FEB
1 cell
2 cells
Microscopic in size
DEC
4,000 cells
OCT
1 million cells
About the size of a pinhead
DIAGNOSIS
1 billion cells
JUN
About the size of a small grape
100 billion cells
About the size of a golf ball
DEC
1 kilogram, or 2 1/4 lbs.
MAY
JUN
3.5 kilograms
Potentially lethal

point, no matter how many cancer cells there are. In many cancers, however, that is not possible, and the fact that cancer cells can do so much of their growth and multiplication before we can detect them poses a very serious problem.

There are, as well, many areas of the body where even a mass the size of, let's say, a small grape may cause no symptoms. For example, a grape-sized lump in the wall of the bowel may cause no symptoms at all, and may cause only a partial blockage when it is much bigger. The same is true in the prostate gland—the patient might have no idea that a tumor the size of a grape was there. Even in a part of the body such as the breast that can be assessed by the patient, depending on how large the breast is and exactly where the mass is, it is quite possible that a grape-sized mass might not be easily detected. It is relatively common, therefore, for primary tumors to achieve that sort of size before they are detected.

How Cancer Cells Invade Neighboring Areas

As the cancer cells grow and form the enlarging clump or tumor, they also invade the neighboring normal areas. They do this by breaking down the normal barriers or frontiers that keep the body's cells in order. Often the frontier or boundary that separates one group of normal cells from the next is quite easy to see when the tissue is examined under a microscope: when it can be identified easily it is called a **basement membrane**. For example, there is a basement membrane in the skin, the gut, the lung, the linings of the ducts of the breast, the kidney, and so on. One of the hallmarks of a cancer is that under the microscope it can be seen to be penetrating through the basement membrane. We do not know all the mechanisms that cancers are able to use to penetrate membranes, but we do know a few of them. For example, cancers can produce substances that attack constituents of the "glue" that binds cells together (the technical term is **intercellular matrix**). This matrix contains many different components, such as a substance called **collagen**, which gives strength to many tissues. Cancers may produce a type of substance called **collagenase** (the ending *-ase* usually refers to an enzyme that attacks and breaks down the substance in the first part of the word: so lactase is an enzyme that breaks down lactic acid, collagenase does the same to collagen, and so on). Cancer cells can also produce other substances such as **hyaluronidase**, a group of substances called **proteases**, and probably dozens of others that allow the growing cancer cells to push through normal tissue boundaries.

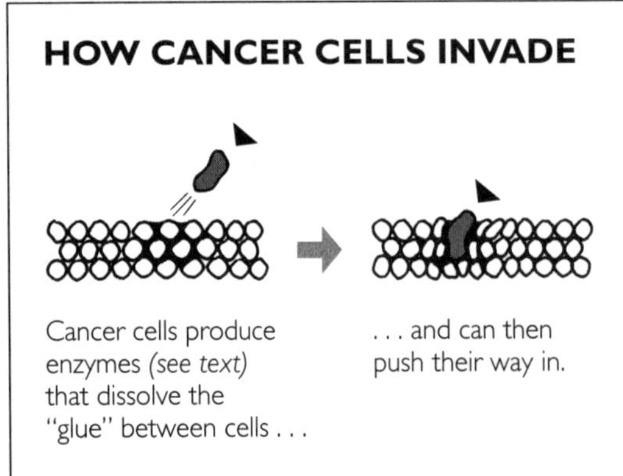

HOW CANCER CELLS INVADE

Cancer cells produce enzymes *(see text)* that dissolve the "glue" between cells . . .

. . . and can then push their way in.

FUZZY BORDERS

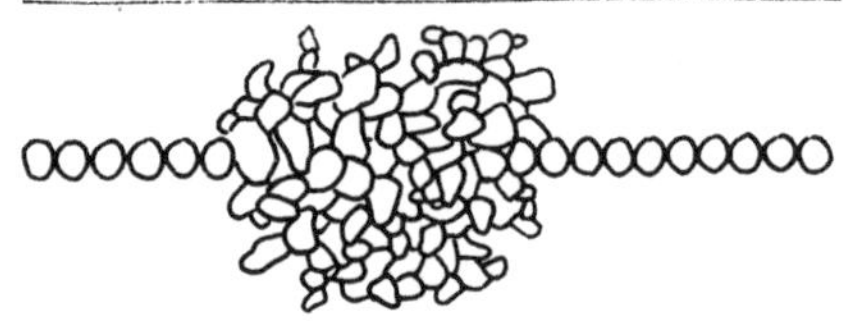

Cancerous tumors often have indistinct and irregular borders.

As a result, cancers often have a very ragged, irregular, and indistinct border—a feature that is often important in distinguishing a cancer from a nonmalignant lesion, as nonmalignant areas (such as warts, benign tumors, or cysts) have a border that is clearly visible and quite distinct.

The process of invasion allows cancer cells to interfere with neighboring structures. As we will see in Chapter 10, usually a mass of cancer cells does not in itself cause pain, but if that clump invades nearby nerves or stretches the covering of a bone or of the liver, it may cause pain by irritating pain-carrying nerve fibers in that area.

The characteristics of a growing primary tumor, therefore, are an increase in size, invasion of neighboring structures, and possible pain (or other problems) if it happens to be close to sensitive areas.

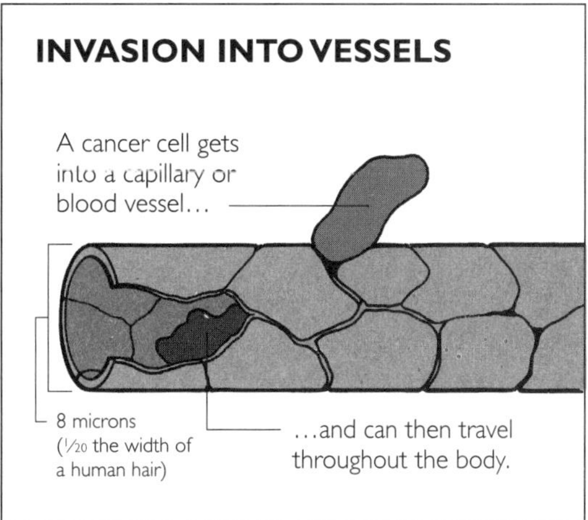

Distant Spread: Secondary Tumors or Metastases

If cancers were able to invade only adjacent tissues, they would be curable (by surgery) in the vast majority of cases. What makes cancers so dangerous is that they are able to spread to distant parts of the body and form **secondary cancers** there. The correct term for secondary cancers is **metastases**, and the process by which a cancer does that is called **metastasizing**.

There are many steps involved in the process of metastasizing, and we do not yet understand any of them completely. In general, however, we can identify four major components of the process.

1. Entry into a Blood Vessel, Lymph Vessel, or Some Other Channel Cancer cells can spread to distant parts of the body by various means. Probably the most common route is by channels that exist in every part of the body called **lymph channels** or lymphatic vessels (or **lymphatics** for short). These make up a very fine network of vessels that carry the liquid portion of the blood (that is, *not* the red cells, white cells, and platelets) from every part of every tissue in the body. Every tissue (with very few exceptions), therefore, has a fine network of these vessels all the way through it, and these very small vessels collect into bigger and bigger lymphatics as they exit from the tissue. On the way back to the bloodstream, the lymph running through the lymphatics is filtered in the filtering stations that we call **lymph nodes** (such as those in the armpit, neck, or groin), and thereafter the lymph (now containing many wandering lymphocyte cells) returns to the circulation via a large lymph vessel near the heart.

If a cancer develops, let's say, in the bowel, cancer cells may gain entry to the nearby lymphatics (probably using a variety of enzymes and other mechanisms). They can then travel to the local lymph nodes and then on into bigger lymph vessels and finally into the bloodstream. Many types of cancer, including cancer of the bowel and cancer of the cervix, probably use the lymphatics as their first and most important method of spreading. Other cancers, such as cancer of the breast, probably use lymphatics and blood vessels equally; and some cancers, such as sarcomas, seem to use blood vessels first. Yet other types of cancer, such as cancer of the ovary, use the abdominal cavity as their most immediate method of spread.

2. Travel of Clumps of Cancer Cells along the Channel Whatever the route, clumps of cancer cells detach themselves from the primary tumor and float along the channel that they have invaded.

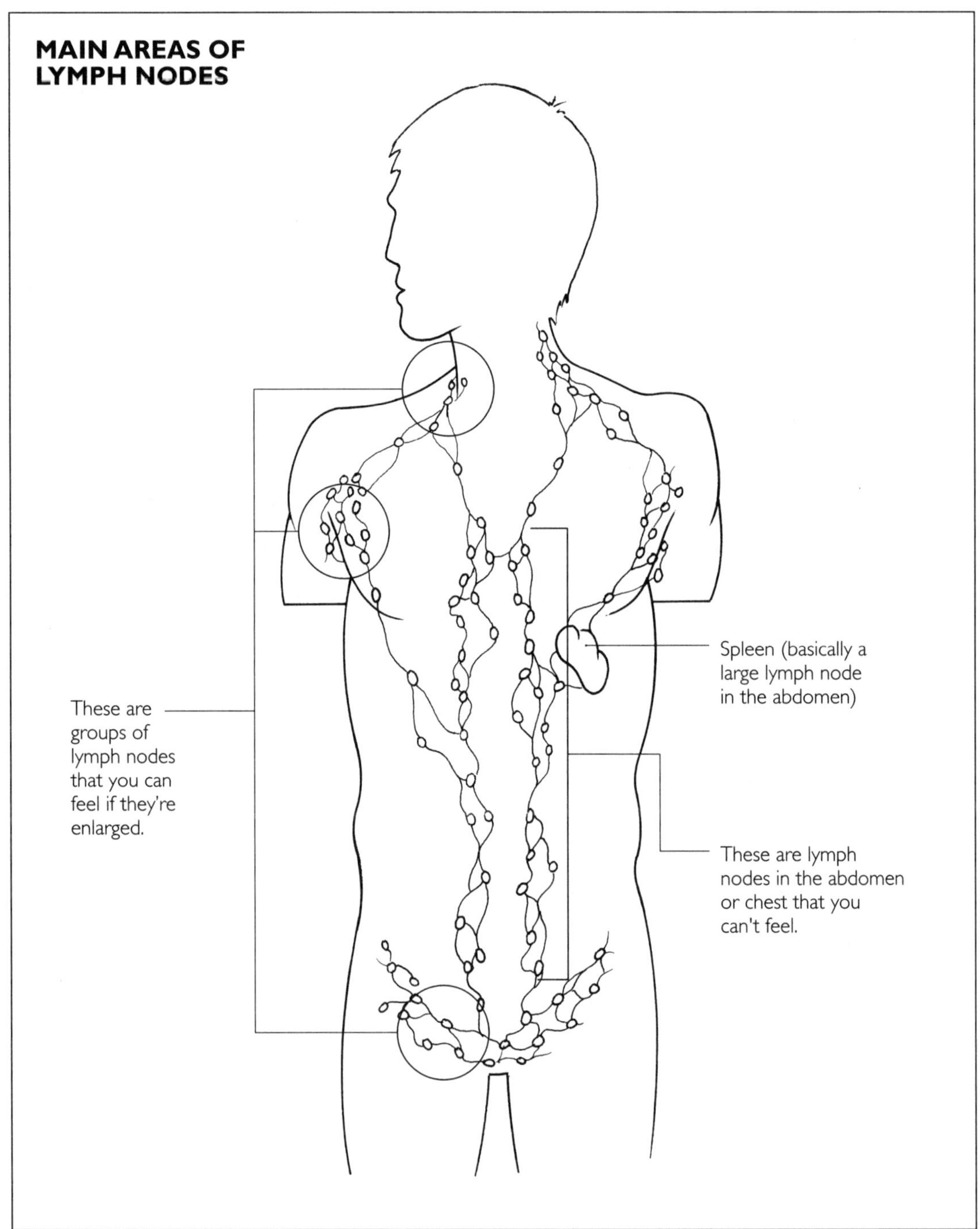
MAIN AREAS OF
LYMPH NODES
Spleen (basically a
large lymph node
in the abdomen)
These are
groups of
lymph nodes
that you can
feel if they're
enlarged.
These are lymph
nodes in the abdomen
or chest that you
can't feel.

Occasionally, these clumps can actually be seen while they are doing that (for example, in blood samples taken in a certain way during operations for cancer of the bowel). Because cancer cells are not foreign substances, they usually manage to elude the body's reactions to them and are therefore not entrapped in a web of blood clot or something similar.

3. Arrival of Cancer Cells at a Distant Site and Formation of a Tumor This third step in the process of metastasizing is also one we know little about. Somehow, the cancer cells end in very narrow vessels (capillaries) and, we assume, become lodged there. By a process we do not fully understand (but that may resemble the way the cancer cells initially got into the lymphatics or blood vessels), the clumps somehow get out of the capillaries and into the tissue itself—the lung or the bone, for example.

4. Building a Blood Supply and Obtaining Other Essentials for Growth Having arrived inside the tissue of a distant part of the body such as lung or bone, the tumor cells then establish their own territory. Because cancer cells are basically normal cells gone wrong, they are not recognized by the immune system as foreign invaders, and therefore there is usually no immune reaction that we can detect. There probably *is* some minor type of immune reaction, but by various mechanisms, the cancer cells manage not to be affected by it. For example, researchers have taken metastases removed at surgery and have then separated the lymphocytes in the metastases from those cancer cells in them. They have been able to show that when on their own and kept by themselves in a dish, those lymphocytes are later capable of killing the cancer cells. Yet when they are adjacent to cancer cells in the secondary tumor inside the body, somehow they are prevented or blocked from killing those cancer cells. In other words, cancer cells as they grow and establish a metastasis can somehow paralyze or neutralize the cancer-killing abilities of the neighboring lymphocytes.

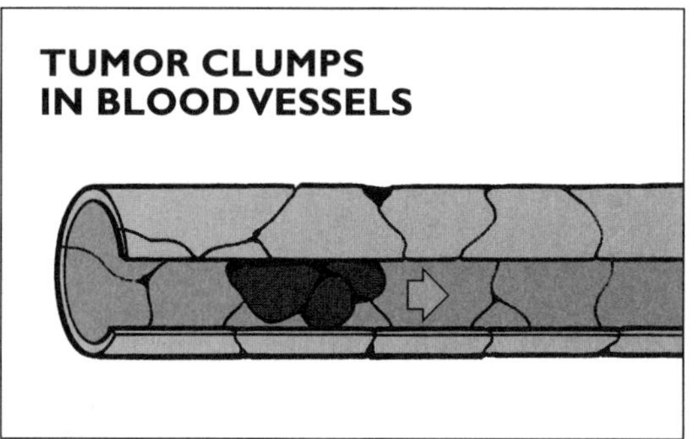

Furthermore, as the tumor establishes itself, it manages to persuade adjacent tissues to form new blood vessels and bring a blood supply into the tumor, providing it with a plentiful supply of nutrients and oxygen and allowing the disposal of waste products. To give you an analogy: it is almost as if a vagrant moved into a residential neighborhood and managed to persuade the local water and sewerage services to lay down illegal pipes to his or her shack. This process of developing a blood supply, called **angiogenesis**, is of exceptional importance to the growing tumor, and without it no cancer would be able to grow larger than a pinhead.

In addition to growing and developing a blood supply, some cancers can do other things to help themselves establish a secondary tumor. For example, several different cancers can do damage to bone and are capable of dissolving away areas of bone around them. Different cancers probably do this in different ways, and we are just beginning to be able to identify some of the substances that various cancers may manufacture to help them do this.

These, then, are the four major steps by which a primary cancer is able to produce secondary cancers at distant parts of the body. One point should be emphasized, however: **a secondary tumor is basically the same material as the primary**. If a cancer begins in the breast, for example, and then creates metastases in the liver, the tumors in the liver

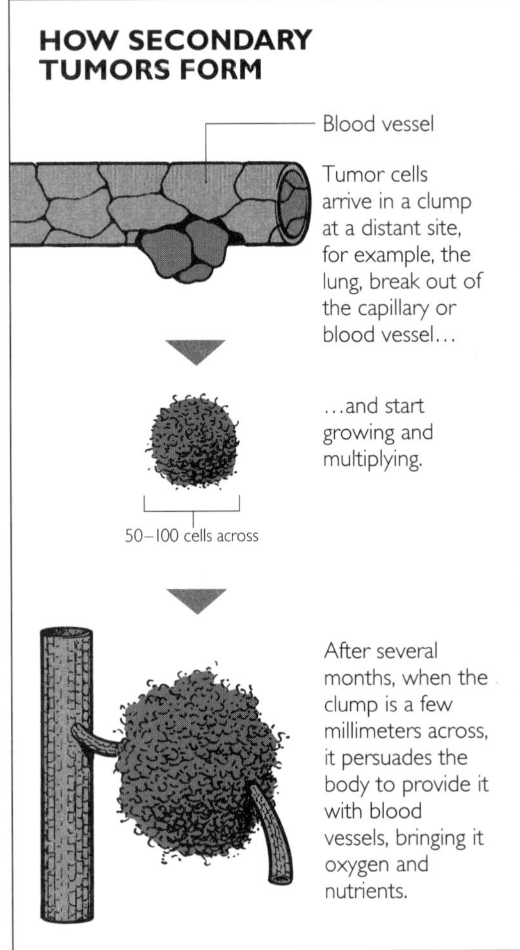

are *secondary cancers of the breast.* In other words, the cancers that are seen in the liver are offspring, as it were, of the primary breast cancer and will (in most circumstances) behave like breast cancer. This is a very important point, as we will see in Chapter 4, and makes a great deal of difference to the kind of treatment that is used.

One final point: sometimes secondary cancers may grow faster and be more obvious than the primary tumor from which they have developed. In fact, occasionally a person may notice the first symptoms or problems not from the primary but from a secondary tumor. In a few patients, the primary may be so small that it is never detected at all, and the person only ever has detectable secondary cancers. This is not very common, but it does happen (see page 77).

Other Effects of Cancer

As well as developing into a primary tumor, invading into adjacent areas, and spreading into distant ones, some cancers may cause a variety of types of problems.

Cachexia or Weight Loss Many types of cancer can cause you to lose weight. The correct medical term for weight loss (when it is not deliberate) is **cachexia**, and cancers are able to cause cachexia by different methods. They can make you lose your appetite, and, if they are in or near the digestive tract, they may also interfere with the body's ability to digest and absorb food. Also, some cancers seem able to interfere with the body's ability to make muscle and may cause loss of fat and muscle by several different means.

Production of Hormones Several types of cancer are able to manufacture their own variations of the body's hormones (see page 330) and release these into the bloodstream. These substances may interfere with several body functions, for example, regulation of the body's calcium, or the amount of urine produced, or the balance of the body's own steroid hormones.

Effects on Nerves and Muscles Some cancers seem to be able to produce substances (which we cannot yet identify) that cause certain types of damage to parts of the brain or spinal cord. Thus, although there may be no cancer present in the brain, parts of the brain may start functioning badly, causing (for example) difficulty in balancing or walking steadily.

The Definition of "Cure," "Remission," and Some Other Terms

A **cure** means that all evidence of the cancer has been eliminated and there is **no chance of the cancer coming back**. In order to define what a cure is, therefore, you must know what the chances are that the cancer will come back. A **recurrence** occurs when some cells from the primary tumor have been able to hide and remain undetected in some part of the body. Depending on the type of cancer, they may later start growing and produce a detectable recurrence of cancer. That may happen within a few months or a year or so of the primary tumors being removed, or it may happen much later. For example, suppose you have been successfully treated for cancer of the cervix or the endometrium of the womb or of the testicle. With all of those cancers, any recurrence will almost certainly happen in the first five years (actually in the first two or three years in the case of cancer of the testicle). Thus, if you are clear of all evidence of cancer of the cervix, endometrium, or testicle after five years, then you are cured. The situation is different with, say, cancer of the breast. With that disease, recurrences can occur up to twenty years after the event. You cannot be called cured of breast cancer, therefore, for at least fifteen or twenty years (depending on your individual case). In brief, then, a cure means that there is no chance that the cancer will come back, and that depends on the type of cancer.

Remission means that the **cancer gets smaller**. For example, if the treatment is successful so that there is **no detectable evidence** of cancer, we call that **complete remission**. Unfortunately, a complete remission is not always the same as a cure, because there may be microscopic clumps of tumor cells that have survived the treatment (and may be resistant to it) that are too small to be detected. For example, in cancer of the lung, complete remissions are quite common, but in most cases, unfortunately, the chance that the cancer will return remains high. Some people who have a complete remission will *not* get a recurrence, and once the relevant time has passed (again, depending on the type of the cancer), they may well be considered cured. If the cancer shrinks to **less than half** of its original size (as measured, say, on scans or X rays), that is usually called a **partial remission**.

Summary

This chapter discussed how cancer cells are able to grow into a primary tumor and how they may then invade and spread to other parts of the body. The next chapter deals with what triggers this process in the first place: what happens to turn cells malignant and cause a cancer to develop.

How Cancer Is Caused

3

What's in This Chapter

In Chapter 2 I defined cancer as what happens when a group of cells escapes from the body's normal growth-control mechanisms and multiplies in a disordered and uncontrollable way. Here in Chapter 3 I explain what is known about the factors that cause or allow those cells to escape from the body's control.

There are basically two types of causes: a **tendency** to grow abnormally that is inherent in those cells and that is probably (in various ways) inherited; and the **triggers** that push those particular cells into turning cancerous. Most common cancers require, we believe, a combination of both types of causes. For example, if you are a nonsmoker, your chances of getting lung cancer are very low; yet even with a lifelong heavy exposure to cigarettes, not every smoker will develop lung cancer: presumably, therefore, some people's lung cells are less ready to turn cancerous than others'. Although most cancers seem to develop when there is a combination of triggers and tendency, a few cancers — such as the rare cancer of the eye in childhood, retinoblastoma — seem to be purely inherited.

If we can learn more of the details of this process and predict which people have the greatest tendency to develop a particular cancer, we may in future be able to give much more specific and valuable advice than at present about who should try to avoid which triggers (for example, which people should not smoke even occasionally or which should avoid even a mild suntan). This could be an important way of reducing the incidence and the impact of cancer in the future.

The Types of Factors That Cause Cancer

Damage to the Genetic Material It is probable that almost any growing human cell is capable of turning malignant if it is insulted — chemically or biologically — badly enough (and in a certain way) and for long enough. In other words, in order to develop into cancer, most cells have to be damaged over a long period of time, or rather, their genetic material has to be damaged. It is worth stressing that the type of damage that causes cancer has to affect the genetic material of the cell, its DNA inside its nucleus. For example, if I spill acid on my hand, the acid will kill some skin cells and will damage others. Eventually, the dead cells fall off my skin, some of the damaged cells die, and, if the acid burn was bad enough, I develop a blister and then a raw area that will eventually heal. Acid merely kills or injures the cells themselves by damaging the outer surface or membrane of the cell, however; it does not affect the genetic material of

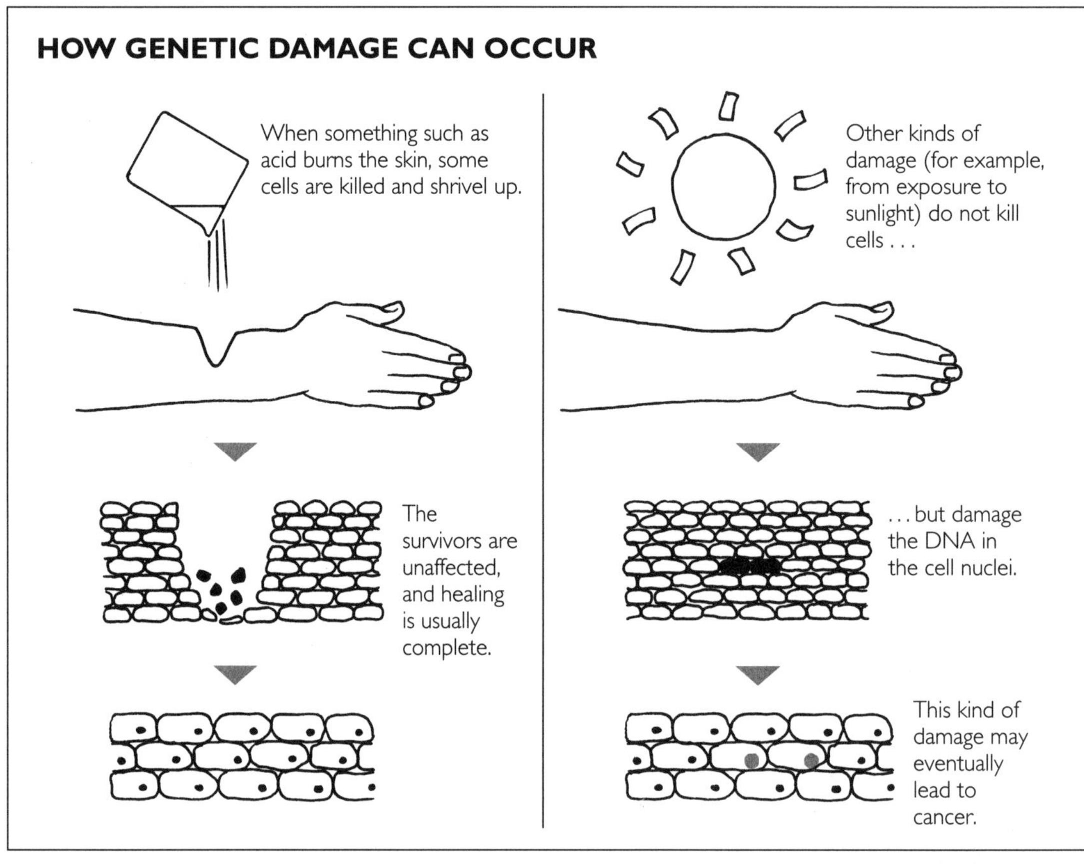

the cells. By contrast, if every day I expose my hand to strong sunlight (perhaps along with the rest of my body), there will be steadily increasing damage to the genetic material of some of my skin cells. That is because sunlight contains several types of rays, some of which (the ultraviolet rays) have the ability to cause chemical changes *in the nucleus* of human cells. Over a long period of time, they contribute to the chance that my skin will develop cancer. Similarly, there are chemicals in cigarette smoke that damage the *genetic material* of lung cells, which is why cigarettes can cause lung cancer. Of course, not all the harmful chemicals in cigarette smoke cause cancers. The substances that cause chronic bronchitis and emphysema, for instance, are similar to the acid I might have spilled on my hand: they cause damage but not cancer. Substances such as the carbon monoxide in the smoke cause heart damage, but again, not cancer. The damage that causes cancer (as opposed to other diseases) is damage to the nucleus of the cell, in fact, to the DNA within the nucleus.

Tendencies and Triggers Some cells (or rather their nuclei) seem to require less damage than others to turn malignant. Some cells are almost designed or preprogrammed to become cancerous with little (or even no) damage from the outside world. Others seem to be highly resistant.

This brings us back to the two types of causes:

the underlying **tendency** to become malignant—that is, the inherent **predisposition** to become malignant—and the **triggers** that cause the actual genetic damage and push cells into becoming malignant. If a cell or group of cells has a *high* predisposition to become cancerous, it will require less damage or insult to become malignant: if that predisposition is low, it will require a greater degree of insult or for a longer time. Cancer can be thought of, therefore, as the result of a combination of adverse factors: a lot of predisposition requires little in the way of triggers; a lot of damage from triggers and a cancer will develop even if there is little predisposition. As you can see from the illustration, it is a bit like a diving board balanced by a pile of heavy weights (representing growth-control mechanisms). If there is a big pile of weights, it will take a lot of external damage (represented by pebbles falling on the board) to topple it over. If there are only a few weights, a much smaller quantity will cause the board to topple.

We do not fully understand the factors that control the tendency to develop a cancer or the triggers that precipitate it. We do know some of the factors that influence a cell's tendency to become malignant; and for some cancers, we know some of the important triggers. For instance, we know that sunlight in the case of skin cancers and cigarettes in the case of lung cancer are certainly triggers. In other cancers, we know that certain viruses are triggers for cancer of the cervix and perhaps a low-fiber, high-fat diet is a trigger for cancer of the bowel. In many cancers, however, we cannot yet identify the triggers.

Understanding what goes on in any particular type of cancer is difficult. So let's look first at the ways in which we can try to find out what causes cancer—the types of research that are done into the causes of cancer. There are two main types.

In one approach, scientists look at cells growing in the laboratory and try to find out what causes them to turn cancerous and why, how they behave, how they influence other cells, and so on. This is the science of **tumor biology**.

CANCER AS A FAILURE OF GROWTH CONTROL

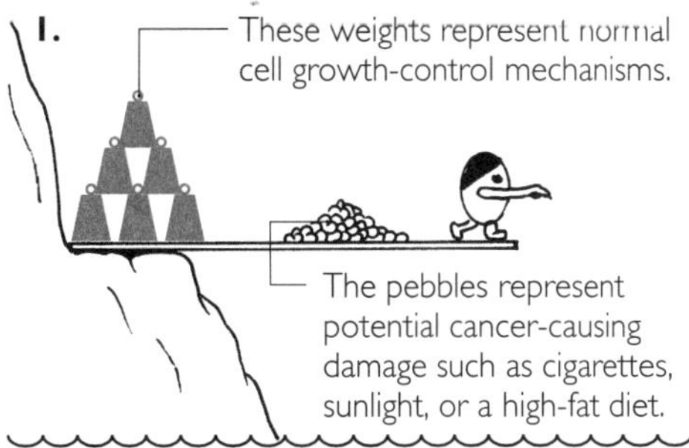

2. Most cancers are caused when the amount of damage exceeds the regulatory capacity of the growth-control mechanisms.

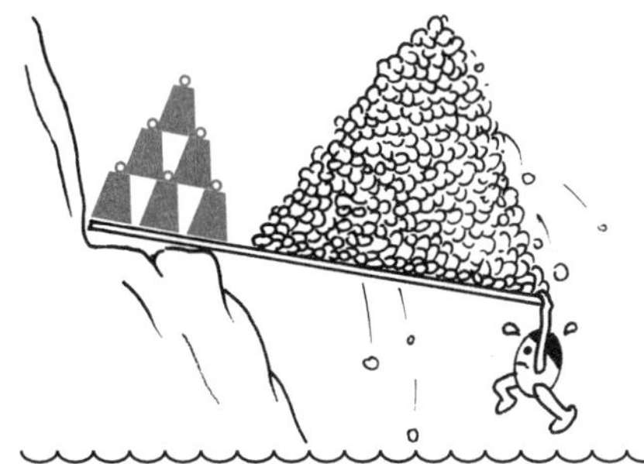

3. In rare cases, some cells have very poor growth-control mechanisms. Then very little damage will be needed to create cancer.

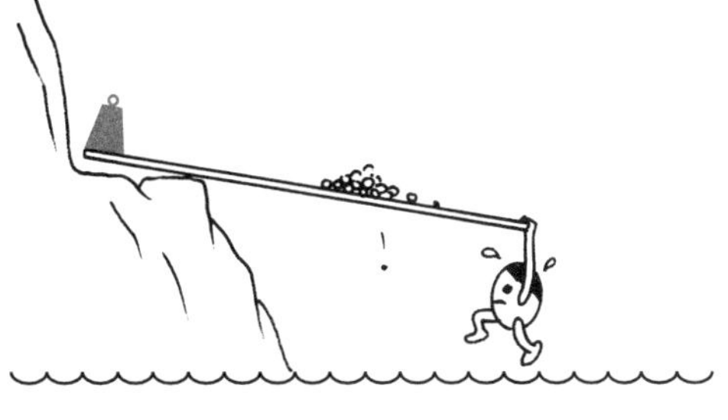

Another approach is to look at the rates at which different people all over the world develop various cancers. For instance, you may decide to look at the different rates for bowel cancer. As it happens, bowel cancer is quite common in North America but rare among the Bantu tribes of South Africa and among older Japanese people. Researchers might therefore look at cancer of the bowel among people who were born in Japan but who immigrated to America. They would then find that two decades or so after they immigrated, those migrants had a risk of getting bowel cancer almost the same as that of Americans born in the United States. This is good evidence that bowel cancer is caused by something in the lifestyle that is associated with America. This type of research—comparing the rates of cancer in different peoples—is called **epidemiology**.

Both methods of research are essential in discovering what causes cancers to develop. Some of the most significant achievements of each type of research are summarized below.

Tumor Biology: The Study of Cancer in the Laboratory

A Brief Caution about Interpretation of Results Most human cells will grow in the laboratory for a short time only, perhaps a few days or so. Then they will stop growing and die. Because there is little time to study the effects of anything, there are only a few things that you can try out on human cells. About fifty years ago, scientists found ways of keeping cells derived from cancer alive and growing continuously. Nowadays there are literally thousands of different types of cancer cells derived from human tumors growing in laboratories. But these cells (growing in laboratories all over the world) can only *partially* represent what cancer cells are like in human beings. There is a certain artificiality about cells grown continuously in the laboratory, so that what researchers discover about these cells may not necessarily represent what happens in real life. Thus, as you read about the results of research (here and in the media), you should bear in mind that not all the features that can be analyzed in the laboratory will necessarily be the same in human beings. Some results will be directly applicable to human cancer and some will not. And at present we do not know which are which. Please keep that in mind during the following survey of some of the most significant findings in tumor biology.

Malignant Transformation In the laboratory, normal—that is, noncancerous—cells have certain characteristics: they usually grow for a few days only; they tend to form orderly layers; they do not heap up on top of each other (in other words, they show contact inhibition); their nuclei look tidy and round and are quite small, and so on. Cancer cells, on the other hand, grow faster than normal cells and for long periods of time; the cells themselves are usually bigger than their normal counterparts; they heap up on top of each other (they have lost contact inhibition); their nuclei are big and often irregular, and so on. There are many things that can be done to normal cells in the laboratory that turn them into what are apparently cancer cells. As further proof of this, cells that have been turned apparently cancerous may be injected into laboratory-bred animals and may produce tumors in the animals as they grow (something that normal cells will not do). Thus the visible changes in the cells are associated with the acquired ability of those cells to grow as a cancerous tumor. The technical name for the process by which normal cells turn into cells that are apparently cancerous is **malignant transformation**, or **transformation** for short.

It has been known for more than two hundred years that it is possible to cause cancers in certain tissues such as the skin. This type of research began when a British physician, Sir Percival Pott, noticed that chimney sweeps' apprentices who had to crawl into chimneys had a high incidence of cancer of the scrotum. He proved that this was due to the carcinogenic effect of soot and could be prevented by regular bathing—a revolutionary idea at the time in both epidemiology and personal hygiene. Years later, scientists were able to identify some of the carcinogens in soot, and in cigarette smoke, and show that these chemicals could cause cancer in the skin of animals. Eventually, scientists showed that those chemicals could also cause malignant transformation when tested on cells growing in a dish. Clearly, then, the ways in which cells change in a dish represent at least a partial model of the development of cancer. We therefore believe that the process of transformation (and the various factors that affect it) may tell us something about how cancer develops in humans. It is an imperfect model but an important one nonetheless.

APPEARANCE OF NORMAL AND CANCEROUS CELLS

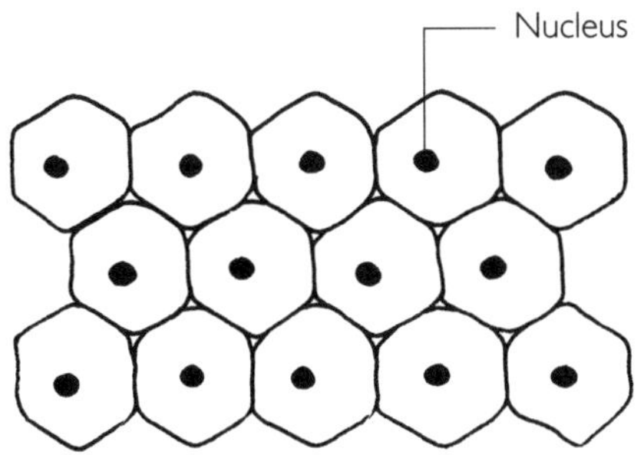

Normal cells are mostly the same size as each other in the same tissue. Nuclei are small and in the same position in each cell. They grow in an orderly way and don't heap on top of each other. Normally, few of the cells are multiplying at any one time.

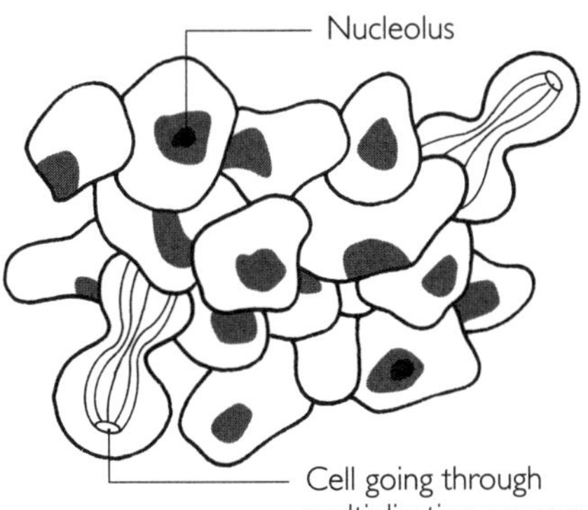

Cancer cells tend to be of different sizes and shapes from each other. The nuclei are large and may have prominent nucleoli. They heap up on top of each other, and many of them are multiplying at any one time.

Triggers of Transformation Many things will cause normal cells to undergo malignant transformation in the laboratory. The complete list of substances that will do this is very long, and many of those chemicals need to be given in immense doses. Thus a substance might be found to be carcinogenic in the laboratory but only in doses equivalent to, say, what an average human would receive from eating two or three kilograms (six pounds) of that substance daily for forty years.

It gradually became clear that research was needed not only into *"What can cause cancer?"* but also into *"How do carcinogens cause cancer?"* As a result of research accumulated over decades by thousands of workers all over the world, the focus began to shift to the genetic material of human cells and how it was that some substances could cause cancerous changes. The answer—or rather part of the answer—was surprising.

Oncogenes and Tumor-Suppressor Genes

We are beginning to understand two of the many genetic factors that seem to play an important part in the development of cancer. One of these is a group of genes called **oncogenes**, which seem to be involved in several different cancers and can play a role in carcinogenesis in several different ways. The other is a group of genes—of which we have begun to identify only a few—called **tumor-suppressor genes**, which function to prevent cells from becoming malignant and which, when lost, removed, or damaged, may allow a cancer to develop.

Oncogenes Oncogenes may be one of the most important ways in which various types of genetic damage—chemical or biological—can cause cells to become malignant. Oncogenes are short segments of DNA or genetic code: that is, they are genes. And like most genes (of which every cell has about 100,000, arranged on its forty-six chromosomes), they can and do control several major functions of the cell, including cell-to-cell signaling, certain aspects of growth, and certain types of importing and exporting across the cell membrane. We have now identified at least forty oncogenes, which, because of the way they behave under certain conditions, are different from all other genes. When certain events occur—such as damage to neighboring areas on the chromosome, or the switching of one area on a chromosome with another (a process called **translocation**, which happens in certain cancers)—an oncogene may become part of the problem instead of part of the solution. It appears that under certain carcinogenic conditions, oncogenes may be altered and, after that alteration, may play a part in the development of the cancer.

We now understand some of the steps by which this happens; and we are able, in certain laboratories, to test for some oncogenes to determine whether they are involved in a particular cancer or not. This particular branch of tumor biology is developing very rapidly, and it may be possible in the future to use the presence or absence of a particular oncogene to help predict the behavior of a particular cancer or perhaps to predict which individuals are at a particularly high risk of developing a certain cancer.

Thus oncogenes may be part of the process in which some normal cells become cancerous. It seems, however, that some cancers develop *without* any oncogenes that we can detect at present (though, of course, we may find others). So it is quite likely that oncogenes are only part of the answer and do not explain carcinogenesis in all situations.

Tumor-Suppressor Genes In a few situations, other genetic processes may be very important. In some cases, genetic factors by themselves may be sufficient to cause the cancer without any identifiable outside stimulus at all. In some circumstances, the cause may involve the loss of a controlling mechanism. We know that some genes are tumor-suppressor genes and behave almost as genetic policemen. Their main function is to control abnormal or disorderly growth, in other words, they prevent a particular cell from becoming malignant. In certain tumors we know that the loss of tumor-suppressor genes is important in the development of cancer.

In a small number of human cancers, the role of tumor-suppressor genes has been clearly established. One of the best examples is a type of very rare tumor of the eye in childhood called retinoblastoma (which is fortunately curable in most cases). Some detailed research into the genetic material of the retinoblastoma cells has shown that a proportion of cases of this cancer are caused by the loss of tumor-suppressor genes. Most of us have two of these genes—called RB1 (for "retinoblastoma")—which ensure that, as we develop, the retina of the eye develops normally. If one of those RB1 genes happens to be missing or damaged, then there is the potential for trouble. The potential for trouble increases if something happens to the other RB1 gene. Cells that have two damaged or incomplete RB1 genes have a greater than 95 percent chance of developing a retinoblastoma tumor. This condition is probably the first instance we have identified in humans in which we know for certain that the cause of a cancer is directly related to the fate of a single pair of genes.

Other types of genetic factors may be important in some cases. Some recent work has suggested that there may be a genetic factor involved in a few cases—probably about 5 percent or fewer—of cancer of the ovary and cancer of the breast. A gene called the BRCA1 gene has been identified (another called the BRCA2 may also be important). If you have this gene, your chance of developing a particular form of breast or ovary cancer is very high. If you do not have it, your chance of developing these cancers is the same as any woman's. Further research is seeking to discover whether this gene plays a part in the development of other types of breast or ovary cancer (that is, the nonfamilial types) or any other cancers.

These examples show that all cells have a threshold for turning into cancer. If the dice are heavily loaded (for example, by one damaged, lost, or incomplete RB1 gene), then the threshold is low, and the cells will become cancerous if spontaneous mutation damages the other RB1 gene. In other cancers, we suspect that there are lesser (but still important) predisposing factors present in the genetic material, although as yet we have little idea of what they are. If the predisposing factors are present, outside stimuli may trigger the development of cancer relatively easily. We still do not know what those triggers are for many types of cancer, however, and that is where epidemiology may help.

Epidemiology: The Study of the Different Incidences of Cancer

Looking for Clues The first step in trying to identify the triggers that cause cancer is to look at one particular cancer and how the chance of getting that tumor varies around the world. Let's take a theoretical example. Suppose there is a Cancer X that happens to be very rare in, say, New York. In fact, let's suppose that New York is the place where the incidence of this cancer is the lowest in the world, and that in New York one in 1,000,000 people get it. Then suppose that studies from all over the world also show that this Cancer X happens to be very common in Seattle where, let's say, one in 1,000 people get it. One way of thinking about the meaning of these figures is to postulate, first, that Cancer X has a minimum incidence of one in 1,000,000 (the New York incidence) and, second, that of the cases detected in Seattle (say, 2,000 cases in all), two cases would have happened anyway—the "inevitable" number of cases. All the rest—in this example a total of 1,998 cases—have therefore been caused by something that people in Seattle do that people in New York do not do. The epidemiology of Cancer X tells you only that there is a difference between New York and Seattle. It does not tell you which differences between the two cities are important. For example, the fact that Seattle has much more rainfall per year than New York does not necessarily mean that Cancer X is caused by rain; the fact that traffic is much noisier in New York does not mean that traffic noise protects people against getting Cancer X. Thus, in order to find out what it is that causes Cancer X in Seattle (or protects against it in New York), we think of a possible explanation and then test it.

Supporting Evidence: Finding Out Whether a Theory Is True The second step in finding out what causes cancer is to look for any other evidence that confirms or disproves your original idea. That may come from work in the laboratory or from more epidemiological work. If, for example, somebody had done some experiments showing that rainwater could indeed cause cancer in the laboratory, this would be supporting data that your theory about Cancer X was valid.

As well as—or instead of—evidence from tumor biology, you might also look for support from other types of epidemiological research. Let's look for a moment at how additional epidemiological research can be used to test and support (or refute) a theory.

In the example of Cancer X, the goal is to establish whether or not a particular candidate (such as rainwater or traffic noise) truly contributes to causing cancer (or protecting against it) in human beings. In order to test the theory that it is caused by rainwater, you would look at other cities all over the world and arrange them in a table of increasing rainfall. If you find that New York was the lowest (not very likely!) and that Seattle was the highest, and that all the figures in between showed that the more rainwater you had, the greater your chance of getting Cancer X, then you would have strong evidence suggesting that Cancer X is caused by rainwater. Similarly, with the theory that traffic noise protects against cancer, you would arrange the cities of the world according to levels of traffic noise. If Seattle happened to be the lowest and New York the highest, and if there appeared to be a correlation between traffic noise and a low chance of getting Cancer X, then you would have evidence that traffic noise protects against Cancer X.

These two examples are, of course, frivolous, but the method is not. Using this method, figures from cancer incidences all over the world can be used to generate and test ideas about what causes cancer. Particularly important are studies on different populations in the same area. For example, studies of people of the Mormon faith show that they have a lower chance of getting cancer of the bowel, lung, and breast (among others) than their non-Mormon neighbors in the same regions of the United States. Geography appears to be less important with these cancers than lifestyle—in other words, it is not where you live that matters with these cancers, it is what you do. Mormons have a diet different from that of the average American: certain foods and other substances are forbidden, while others are encouraged. Epidemiological data suggest, therefore, that some elements of the Mormon lifestyle (for example, diet and avoidance of both alcohol and cigarettes) protect against cancers of the bowel, lung, breast, and so on. The fact that other data suggest that high dietary fats can contribute to cancer of the bowel (and possibly breast and prostate) strengthens the possibility that it may be the fat in the diet (and the reduction of fat in the Mormon diet) that counts.

Although such data may strengthen your belief in your theory, it could still be that your theory is incorrect. What else can you do to determine which theories are correct and which are not?

How Step One Might Lead You Astray It is possible that the relationship you imagined between the cancer and a particular factor is not a true causal relationship. What you find from your research data depends on what you are looking for. If in your research you did not ask a group of people about their smoking habits, for example, you will not find a relationship between smoking and lung cancer. If you ask the "wrong" questions, not only will you miss the right answer, you might actually come to the wrong conclusion.

Imagine, for example, that a large group of people have emigrated from Scotland to northern Idaho. And suppose that this particular group of Scottish people smoke more heavily than the natives of the area to which they have immigrated. If you do research in that area and you fail to ask the people about their smoking habits, you might find that cancer of the lung is much more common among people whose family names begin with M (the *Mac* and *Mc* prefixes). You might conclude that simply having a family name that begins with M is a primary contributing cause of lung cancer! (This type of argument was actually used by tobacco companies until it was refuted by further research.)

Despite the possibility for error, this kind of research is a very useful and important way to develop a theory, or hypothesis, about the cause of a cancer. In itself, however, it can only suggest a theory. Two further steps are needed in order to find out whether the theory is valid or not.

In the second step, you test your theory by applying it to a *different* group of people. If you had your original idea based on a study of people in northern Idaho, you would have to test it by applying the same theory to studies of people in, say, Alaska. There are several different ways of doing this, and each way has its own advantages and disadvantages. If you find as a result of these further studies that in Alaska cancer is *not* common in people whose family names begin with M, then there are two possible explanations. The first possibility is that the M name does not cause cancer in itself, but that in northern Idaho something else was causing the difference, of which the M name was simply a marker. The other possibility is that having an M name does cause cancer, but only in northern Idaho. This would not be a very worthwhile theory and would probably not stimulate further research unless there were data from some other source showing that family names did affect the incidence of cancer. (In practice, tobacco companies used the argument that the desire to smoke and lung cancer were both caused by an inherited trait, that is, smoking was merely a sign or a marker of the presence of something that caused lung cancer and not the true cause. This was disproved by research involving identical twins, who have the same genetic makeup. The twins who smoked had a high risk of cancer, whereas their identical siblings who didn't smoke had a low risk. It was not inherited characteristics that caused the lung cancer, therefore, but smoking.)

Step Two—Further Testing The second step is absolutely essential in the testing of any scientific theory, particularly when that theory proposes the cause of a disease. If the second step confirms the findings of the first step, then the theory begins to

TABLE 3.1: CONTRIBUTING CAUSES OF SOME CANCERS

FACTOR	CONTRIBUTES TO CANCER OF THE	DEFINITELY OR POSSIBLY?
Smoking	lung, mouth, larynx, bladder, pancreas, kidney	definitely
Sunburn and excess exposure to sun	skin (all types of skin cancers)	definitely
Human papilloma virus	cervix	definitely
HIV	Kaposi's sarcoma, AIDS-related lymphoma	definitely
Chronic liver damage	liver	definitely
High-fat, low-fiber diet	bowel	almost definitely
High-fat, low-fiber diet	breast, prostate	possibly
The presence of an abnormal form of the BRCA1 or BRCA2 gene (applies to 5 percent of all breast and ovarian cancers)	breast or ovary	definitely
Mother taking stilbestrol during pregnancy	cancer of the vagina in the daughter	definitely

look as if it may be of some importance. The real test is then to do a quite different type of research in order to test the idea in a different way.

Step Three—Prospective Studies If the second step genuinely confirms the hypothesis raised by data from the first step, the definitive test is what are called **prospective studies**. The word "prospective" means looking forward in time, and a prospective study (in cancer, let's say) is one in which you identify something that you think may be the cause of cancer in a group of people who do not have cancer at that time. Then you check on the same people every few years, making repeated observations to see whether those with the possible risk factor (say, the smokers) develop cancer (lung cancer) more often than those in the low-risk group (the nonsmokers). This kind of study is difficult to do. It requires a detailed study of a large number of people at the start and follow-up observations over many years. Because prospective studies are difficult and costly, they are done only when step one and step two studies have suggested that a very important factor (such as cigarette smoking or sunlight) might be at work.

Some Causes of Cancer That We Know About
The epidemiology of cancer, using these rigorous procedures, is only just beginning to help us sort out what is important. Even so, several factors have been identified as important contributing causes of some cancers. The most important of these are summarized in Table 3.1.

Summary

At present, there is much more that we do *not* know about the causes of cancer than that we do know. Even the clearest, most firmly established facts have been the subject of bitter debate. (For example, tobacco manufacturers have used the law courts to fight claims that smoking causes lung cancer.) Nevertheless, our understanding of the basic process of carcinogenesis is proceeding rapidly, and in twenty years we could have a clear picture of how many or most cancers develop. Such knowledge will be an important tool in changing our behavior to reduce the risk of cancer, although it may not necessarily help people who already have cancer. Research into causation may well be the means by which the impact of cancer on our species is most dramatically reduced.

An Overview of the Most Common Cancers

4

HOW THE INFORMATION IN CHAPTER 4 IS ORGANIZED

In this part of the book, I explain the most important aspects of each of the most common types or sites of cancer. As I said in Chapter 1, it would be wrong for me to try to give all the minute details of current treatment, first, because those change very rapidly as research continues, and second (and even more important), because the exact details of your treatment are things you should discuss with your doctor. My own experience suggests that the most difficult thing for people to understand is how the cancer behaves: what it has done to cause the symptoms that they are experiencing, what it is likely to do next, and what treatment options are available to try to stop or control it. Chapter 4 will give you a general idea of what matters most with each tumor. In order to make the information easier for you to assimilate, for each type or site of cancer I set out the information under the following headings.

Summary of the Key Facts in This Section

This box will contain the "headlines" only. It is difficult at the best of times to read medical books—doubly so if you are a patient. The purpose of the headlines is simply to give you a quick overview so that you can put the details that follow into their overall context.

The Most Important Features of the Tumor

This section will summarize how this particular cancer behaves, what problems it may cause, and the basic plan of diagnosis and treatment. Each of the points in this section will be discussed in more detail in subsequent sections.

In some tumors, such as cancer of the lung or cancer of the testicle, there are two or more different types of cancer that behave and are treated differently. Where that is the case, I explain in this section what the main types are and then deal with each of the types separately. So, for example, I distinguish between small-cell cancer of the lung and non–small-cell cancer of the lung in this first section, and then deal with them individually. I follow the same procedure with the seminomatous types of testicular cancer, which are quite different from the nonseminomatous types.

Age and Incidence

Cancer (or rather the cancers) are not rare. In the United States, there will be more than 1,250,000 new cases this year. The word "incidence," although it sounds rather forbidding, simply means the number of new cases of any disease that are diagnosed each year. For all types of cancer the overall incidence is more than 1,250,000, while for breast cancer, in the United States, it is 185,700 (that is, based on estimates for 1995, approximately 185,700 women will have a new diagnosis of breast cancer during the year). For lung cancer the incidence is nearly 180,000. Under this heading, I also include information about whether the chance of getting that cancer increases or decreases as you get older and in what age group this particular tumor is most common. In general, most cancers become more common as one gets older, and some (such as multiple myeloma) are actually quite rare in people who are in their thirties or younger. A few cancers are somewhat more common in early adulthood (such as testicular cancer and germ-cell tumors of the ovary), and some (such as acute lymphoblastic leukemia of childhood and neuroblastoma) are quite rare in later life.

Causes

For most of the common cancers we simply do not know all the causes, and often we are not even sure about the main ones. For some cancers (brain tumors and Hodgkin's disease, for example), we have hardly any clues as to their cause(s). In other cases (breast cancer, for example), although we don't know the actual cause, we do know some of the things that increase a woman's likelihood of getting the cancer. The things that make a person more likely to get the cancer are called **risk factors**, and in some cancers we have an idea of what risk factors there are. If they are known (or if there is some evidence about them), I list them in this section.

How the Cancer Tends to Spread

A large number of people will be diagnosed with a cancer that has *not* spread, and that is good news. Even so, it may be useful for you to know how the cancer *might* spread, to help you make sense of why certain tests are being recommended, why certain precautions are being taken, and sometimes (as in cancer of the breast, for example) why a certain treatment is recommended. The information in this section is not meant to alarm you if your cancer has not spread, but to explain what the cancer *may* do in some cases. Since understanding and predicting the way a cancer may behave is the basis of much of the medical approach to the cancer, the information in this section can be useful to all patients with the cancer.

Symptoms or Problems That You May Notice

This section will describe the most common types of problems or symptoms that the cancer may cause. It should be emphasized, however, that many of the symptoms that are caused by a cancer *can* be caused—and often are caused—by a variety of other medical problems that are far less serious than cancer. In fact, *most* of the symptoms that cancers can cause are actually far more likely to originate from less serious problems. Headaches are more likely to be due to stress or migraine than to brain tumors, for example. Rectal bleeding is far more likely to be due to hemorrhoids or an anal fissure (or crack) than to rectal cancer. Pain in the upper abdomen is more likely to be due to dyspepsia or an ulcer than to stomach cancer. Back pain is more commonly caused by strain or disc problems than by cancer in the vertebrae. Do not, therefore, immediately assume that you have cancer if you have some of the symptoms or problems mentioned in this section.

At the same time, remember that where a problem or symptom *might* be due to cancer, you should see your doctor about it. If you have bleeding from the rectum (or blood on the toilet paper when you wipe), for instance, you must see your doctor so that she or he can tell you if the problem is only a hemorrhoid or whether some additional tests would be useful. In many cases, after listening to your story and examining you, your doctor may be able to reassure you that the symptom is not cancer-related. In some cases, additional tests may be needed, often simply to confirm that there is no serious problem. Although having tests done and waiting for the results may cause you some anxiety, the information from tests can be genuinely helpful. So try to be patient for the sake of the useful information that tests can yield.

Diagnosis and Tests

This section will explain (with a small amount of detail) how your doctor decides whether it is cancer that is causing your problems or not. In every case, your doctor will go over your story in some detail and then examine you. In medical terms that is called a "clinical history and physical examination" or "history and examination." In some cases, it may be very easy to rule out cancer. For example, you may be worried about a lump in or on your skin, and your doctor may be able to tell you right away that you have an ordinary wart or a fatty lump that is an ordinary, benign lipoma and not serious at all. In other cases, tests may be needed, and this section will set out the most useful kinds of tests in each category. This does not mean that your doctor *must* do these tests; but, depending on the circumstances, these are the tests that your doctor *may* recommend for you.

The Main Types of the Cancer

In some cancers, the appearance of the tumor under the microscope makes a considerable difference to what happens next. Where that is the case, I explain the main types in this section. Where major differences between the main types mean that they require different treatment, I say so in the first section ("The Most Important Features of the Tumor") and then treat the different types separately.

Factors That Influence the Treatment and Prognosis

This section will explain which aspects of the cancer are important in deciding whether the cancer is likely to recur and what type of treatment is most likely to be effective (if any). In some cancers, the appearance of the tumor under the microscope—the **grade** of the cancer—is very important, and cancers that look more aggressive require different treatment. In other cancers, it is not the grade but the **stage** of the cancer (whether it has spread to lymph nodes or other structures) that is most important. In some cancers both the grade and the stage are important. Since estimating the risk of recurrence is a major part of your doctor's recommendations in your case, I explain what factors are most important in forming that decision.

The Main Objectives of Treatment

This section will explain briefly what the main aim of treatment is. In many cases, the primary aim of the treatment is to cure the patient. In some cases, cure is very unlikely and the main aim of treatment is to control the disease for as long as possible, or, if that later becomes impossible, to control the major symptoms.

Types of Treatment

This section will explain what types of treatment are generally used with this cancer and how and why. The three main types of treatment are **surgery** (removing the cancer by means of an operation), **radiotherapy** (using specialized machines to direct high-dose X rays, or other types of rays similar to X rays, at one part of the body in order to kill tumor cells), and **chemotherapy** (using drugs to kill tumor cells). A newer form of therapy is now developing in which the body's response to cancer is altered. This is called **biologic therapy**, and it is currently being actively investigated. In Chapter 5, I explain in greater detail the principles of these types of treatment and set out the details of some of the more common side effects. In Chapter 4, I mention only the types of therapy that are most often used. Readers wishing more information should therefore also look up the relevant section or sections of Chapter 5.

Screening and Early Diagnosis

With some cancers, it is possible to detect early stages of the cancer or occasionally the precancerous changes that happen before a true cancer develops. Tests that do this may be recommended to entire groups of the population. (For example, mammograms are commonly given to women over fifty, Pap tests to all sexually active women, and perhaps rectal examinations to men over forty, and so on.) Where tests have proven useful in detecting early signs of trouble and are therefore recommended for screening, I discuss them. There is more about screening in Chapter 8.

Prevention

Prevention is also very important with some types of cancer. Of course, to make effective recommendations, we have to know the factors that cause or are associated with that type of cancer (such as cigarettes for cancers of the lung, bladder, pancreas, mouth, and kidney). Where factors such as these are known, I set them out in this section and explain the current recommendations for prevention.

Information about Survival

Throughout this book, I deliberately do *not* set out the statistics concerning survival. For example, there are no sentences such as *"With cancer of the X, 32 percent of patients will be alive at five years."* There are good reasons for not giving bald percentages like that.

Global Figures Are Not Helpful With most cancers, several factors are important for determining the future, and to be accurate, a prognosis should take into account a separate figure for each of those factors. For example, suppose there is a Cancer Y that responds to chemotherapy in 75 percent of cases, and when it does, the average survival period is more than five years. For the 25 percent who do not respond to chemotherapy, however, the average survival period may be less than eighteen months. Which figure accurately expresses the prognosis for Cancer Y? I think the answer is neither. Thus, instead of giving a single figure that may be misleading, I explain the main factors that determine the future and then specify in general terms for each type of treatment what the chances of success are. That will give you an idea about the most important features of your own situation so that you can discuss them with your doctor.

The Prognosis Is an Important Part of Your Relationship with Your Doctor Even if accurate statistics could be given for every factor in every type of every cancer, it is still important for you to get such information from your own doctor rather than from a book. The information is extremely important to you. It will affect how you arrange your life. You should not get such information from an impersonal source. You need to receive it from someone who can explain to you what the statistical information means in *your* case. Personal communication is a fundamental part of the relationship between you and your doctor, and in some respects the most important part of your treatment. Every patient needs someone to help him or her make sense of the situation, and that is what doctors are for.

Figures Can Be Misleading Statistics are very perplexing—for doctors and medical students as well as for patients. For example, you may read in a newspaper that Treatment Z has a 34 percent success rate in Cancer Y. You may read elsewhere that the usual treatment of Cancer Y (which has been Treatment X) has a less than 30 percent chance of success. And so you may conclude that Treatment Z is better than Treatment X, and that you should be getting Treatment Z immediately. Often, however, such figures are misleading. The research that you read in the newspaper may have been based on the results from a small group of patients, say twenty or thirty patients. With such a small number of patients, the stated figure of 34 percent may be what we call statistically "soft," that is, in future trials the figure may turn out to be 18 percent or 26 percent. This type of uncertainty can be expressed mathematically (it includes calculations of factors such as a mathematical term called the "standard deviation"), but the uncertainty factors are rarely mentioned in newspaper articles. You have no way of knowing that one study with a 34 percent success rate was based on data from twenty patients and is less reliable than another study with a 30 percent success rate based on data from 200 patients.

It can also be the case that patients used in one particular research study differ significantly in some way from the average person. For example, it might be that Cancer Y usually affects people over the age of sixty, but is known to be easier to treat in patients who are younger than that. In one study cited in a newspaper, perhaps more than half of the patients were under fifty-five years of age. This difference may account for an apparently better than usual outcome for that study. In short, when all factors are carefully analyzed, an apparently superior result for a new type of treatment may not represent any genuine improvement over the current types of treatment.

Reports Can Be Misunderstood It is quite easy to misunderstand some reports of results. For example, if an article says *"Drug A has a 75 percent response rate in Cancer B,"* many people will get the impression that Drug A works in every case but only causes the cancer to shrink by 75 percent of its original size. In fact, this is not what a 75 percent response rate means. It actually means that in 75 percent of cases of Cancer B, there is shrinkage of the cancer (either partial or complete), but in 25 percent of cases there is no response at all. It is easy to be misled unless you know how to interpret the words used accurately.

For all these reasons, then, I discuss the future only in terms of likelihoods, using phrases such as *"in the majority of cases," "in a few cases,"* or *"this is rare,"* rather than offering potentially misleading figures. By doing so, I hope to support and reinforce the relationship between you and your doctor rather than undermine it with misleading or controversial information.

REMINDER!
The object of this book is to support the information that is given to you by your doctor and your medical team. If there appears to be any conflict between information in this book and what you are told by your medical adviser, you should accept what your medical advisers recommend in your individual case.

BLADDER

Number of new cases diagnosed per year in the United States: 52,900

> **SUMMARY OF THE KEY FACTS IN THIS SECTION**
>
> - Bladder cancer is quite common. It affects men twice as frequently as women and is often caused in part by cigarette smoking.
> - There are two important types of bladder cancer: the superficial type that quite often recurs but does not usually invade the bladder wall; and the invasive type that does.
> - The superficial type can be controlled by regular cystoscopies. Cystoscopy is a procedure during which the inside of the bladder is examined and tumors can be removed.
> - The invasive type often requires surgery, which involves removing the bladder or a part of it.

The Most Important Features of the Tumor

Cancer of the bladder is a common cancer, which, in this country, is partly caused by smoking and affects twice as many men as women. The substances that cause the cancer to develop affect the entire lining of the bladder, so that after one tumor is removed another tumor may develop in another area of the bladder. There are two basic forms of the cancer: the superficial form, which recurs quite frequently but does not usually invade into the bladder wall; and the other type, which begins invading into the bladder wall at an early stage. With the superficial type, the only treatment needed for much of the time may be regular surveillance with cystoscopy (described below) and removal of the problem areas. Sometimes putting medications into the bladder may be recommended. If there is invasion of the bladder wall, then surgical removal may be recommended as curative therapy with or without chemotherapy, and in certain circumstances radiotherapy may also be curative.

What You Really Need to Know about the Bladder

The bladder acts as a reservoir for urine, allowing us to pass urine every few hours. Urine is produced by the kidneys continuously at the rate of about a half or quarter of a cupful every hour. The urine passes down slender tubes called ureters leading from each kidney to the bladder. The bladder itself is really a bag with a muscular wall which can expand as it fills with urine. As the volume of urine reaches about a third to a half of the bladder's maximum capacity, we experience the desire to pass urine. The action of passing urine is started under voluntary control but is basically a reflex action that involves relaxing the muscles that control the exit from the bladder. The urine then passes down the **urethra**. In the male, the urethra is a few inches long and takes the urine through the prostate gland and then through the penis. In the female, the urethra is about an inch long and is located in front of the vagina with its exit between the labia.

Age and Incidence

Bladder cancer is predominantly a disease of late adulthood—the fifties, sixties, and older. It affects men twice as frequently as women because of patterns of cigarette smoking. As smoking habits change, the patterns of bladder cancer change two decades or so later.

Causes

Cigarette Smoke Bladder cancer is predominantly caused by substances in the urine that remain in contact with the bladder wall while there is urine in the bladder, which is most of the time. The known substances most likely to cause bladder cancer in this country are derived from cigarette smoke. It may seem peculiar that smoking, an activity that appar-

THE KIDNEYS AND BLADDER (URINARY SYSTEM)

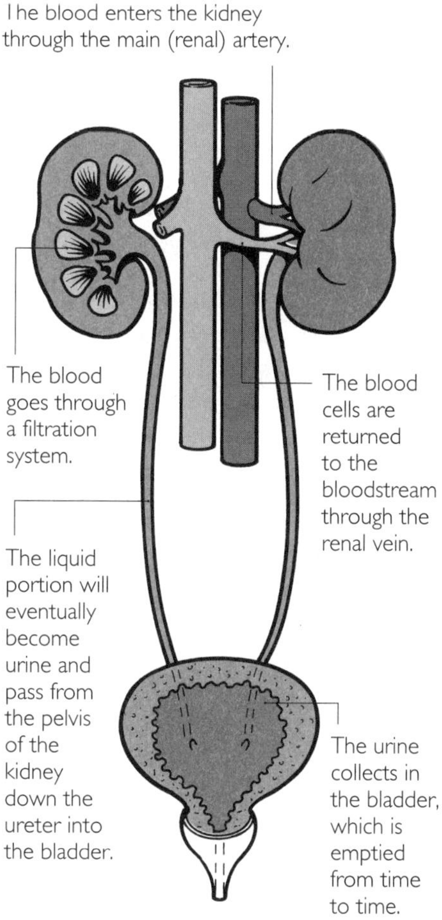

ently involves only the lungs, should have other effects. In fact, cigarette smoke contains a variety of tars and other chemical substances, some of which are highly carcinogenic and disposed to cause cancer in any area with which they come into contact. The tars and other chemical substances in cigarette smoke pass quite rapidly and easily from the lungs into the bloodstream and then into the urine, and accumulate in the bladder in quite high concentrations. Although the lining of the bladder is designed to withstand many chemical insults, it often cannot withstand decades of contact with these particular substances. Hence the high incidence of bladder cancer in smokers.

Other Cancer-Causing Factors Cigarette smoke is not the only source of substances that may promote bladder cancer, although it is by far the most common in this country. In other parts of the world, bladder diseases can set up irritation in the bladder wall that may eventually lead to cancer. The most common of these is a parasitic worm called Schistosoma.

A number of chemicals may also promote the condition. Most if not all of these have now been identified, and regulations of employment in this country ensure that the chance of exposure to potential carcinogens is reduced to a minimum. Up to fifty years ago, however, exposure was a problem in certain occupations and is still a problem in some less well regulated areas of the world.

How the Cancer Tends to Spread

The pattern of spread varies with the type of the cancer. See "The Main Types of the Cancer" below.

Symptoms or Problems That You May Notice

The most common symptom caused by bladder cancer is blood in the urine, for which the medical term is **hematuria**. Hematuria is a very common symptom and can be caused by many less serious problems, such as infections in the urine, prostate enlargement, and so on. Nevertheless, because blood in the urine might be a symptom of bladder cancer, it is imperative for anybody with this problem to see his or her doctor.

There is usually **no pain** with hematuria caused by bladder cancer. Thus it is even more important to check blood in the urine if it is painless.

In some cases a patient may want to pass urine

more often (a symptom called **urinary frequency**) and may experience **pain or discomfort** on passing urine. Usually, though, these symptoms occur in the later stages of the condition after there has been bleeding for some time.

Diagnosis and Tests

Your doctor will first take your history in detail (including any history of cigarette smoking) and examine you. The examination will include a rectal examination and, in addition, a pelvic examination for women. Then some or all of the following tests may be recommended to you.

Urine Tests Samples of urine are sent for testing to check for the presence of red blood cells. These may be present even if the urine looks clear. In some circumstances the laboratory may examine the urine for the presence of cancer cells. This may not be done in all cases because it is not a very reliable guide to the presence of bladder cancer, and because in many cases your doctor may recommend that a cystoscopy be done anyway.

Examination under Anesthetic Sometimes, depending on your body shape and your level of discomfort during examination, it may be preferable for your specialist to examine the bladder while you are under a short general anesthetic. Anesthesia allows the extent of any involvement of the bladder wall by the tumor to be assessed without anxiety about causing you undue discomfort. This procedure may be done at the same time as the cystoscopy.

Cystoscopy Cystoscopy simply means looking inside the bladder, and it is done with a **cystoscope**, a thin instrument that works like a telescope, which is passed along the urethra into the bladder. The procedure usually requires a general anesthetic. Looking through the cystoscope, the specialist can easily examine the whole of the bladder lining and take biopsies of any suspicious areas. For many types of lesions, the specialist can also use **cautery** to remove the suspicious areas or visible tumors. The procedure usually lasts from ten to forty minutes or so, depending on what needs to be done. Afterwards you may feel some soreness or discomfort in the urethra, particularly when you pass urine. There is very often some blood in the urine after cystoscopy, but this clears up in a day or so.

IVP An IVP is an X ray of the kidneys and ureters that can also give some information about the bladder. In the test, you will be given an injection of a dye that passes through the kidneys and shows up white on an X ray. An IVP may be needed because there are sometimes other problems, even other tumors, in the kidneys or ureters.

Other Tests It may also be useful for you to have a CT scan (an X-ray scan that gives very detailed cross-section views of the inside of the body) of the abdomen and pelvis, or an ultrasound or an MRI scan (a scan that uses magnetic waves to produce very detailed views of the inside of the body).

The Main Types of the Cancer

There are two important types of bladder cancer. One is a rather frondlike type of tumor and looks (during cystoscopy) almost like seaweed growing from the bladder wall. This is the **papillary** type of cancer. It is usually superficial (limited to the surface of the bladder wall) and does not invade deeply into the wall. The other type of bladder cancer looks more like a plate of tumor stuck to the bladder wall, and it tends to grow deeply into the wall. This type is sometimes called the **solid** or **non-papillary** or **invasive** type. There are other types as well, but by far the most important feature is whether or not the tumor is invading.

If the tumor does invade the wall of the bladder, it may subsequently spread into the lymph nodes. It may later also spread to other areas of the body, particularly the lungs, liver, or bones.

TYPES OF BLADDER CANCER

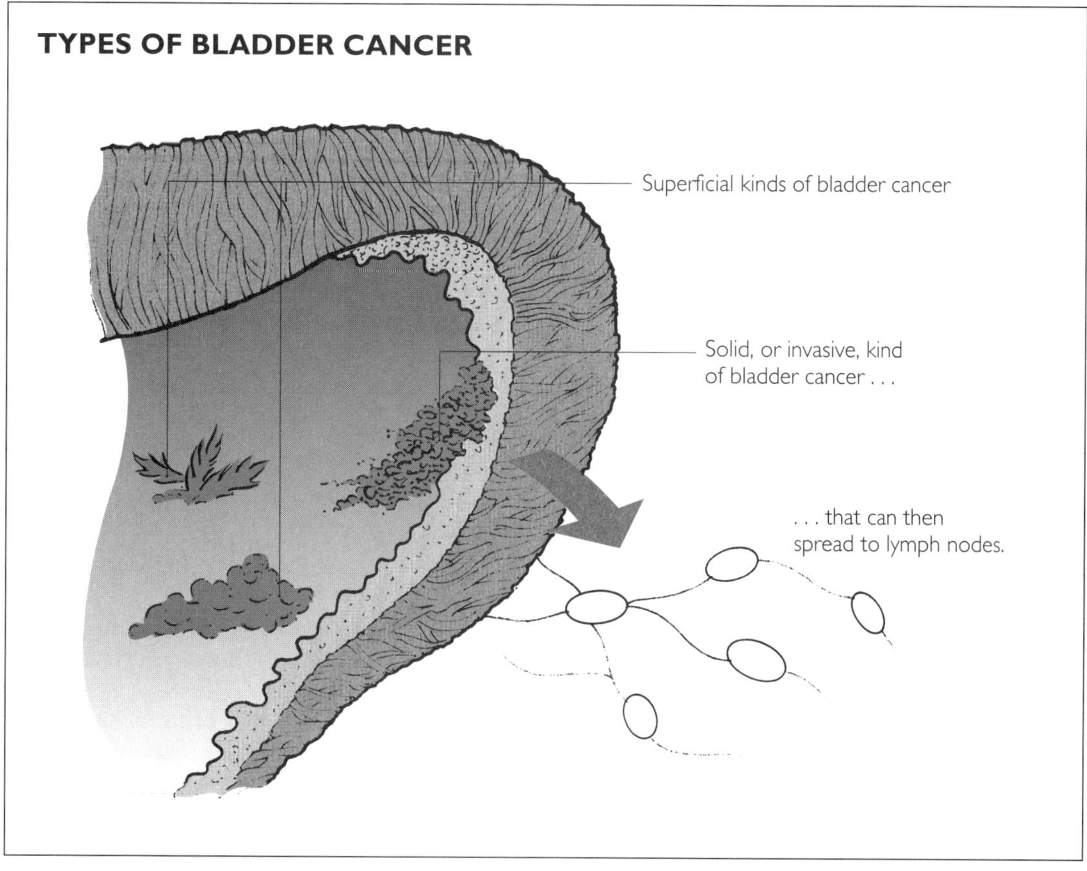

Factors That Influence the Treatment and Prognosis

As mentioned in previous sections, the most important consideration is the **stage** of the tumor—whether the tumor is invading into the bladder wall. The **grade** of the tumor (whether the tumor's appearance under the microscope suggests aggressive behavior or not) may also provide some information. Studies have shown that, by and large, the low-grade tumors are less likely to invade through the bladder wall and may often be treated with less extensive therapy, whereas the high-grade tumors are more likely to invade and may require more extensive therapy.

The Main Objectives of Treatment

The superficial types of tumor recur in about half of all cases, and the objective of treatment is to keep the tumors under control and prevent recurrence. This usually means regular cystoscopies. If the tumors are of the invasive type and are limited to the bladder, the objective is cure, and that is most likely to be achieved by surgery.

Types of Treatment

Cystoscopy and Removal of Superficial Tumors

If the tumor is of the superficial type, then you will probably be advised to have regular cystoscopies, perhaps every few months or so. At each cystoscopy your specialist can look for any tumors and can remove them using cautery or a laser. In addition to this regular surveillance-and-removal program, your specialist may also recommend instillation of a drug into the bladder. When the tumor is superficial, the great majority of patients—approximately nine out of ten—will be alive five years after diagnosis, and the chance that the condition will progress and become invasive is low.

Intravesical or Instillation Treatment instillation simply means "putting material in." With bladder tumors this means putting a drug solution into the bladder by means of a catheter inserted along the urethra. Usually this is done without a general anesthetic, though the urethra itself may be numbed using a jelly with a local anesthetic in it. The drug is put into the bladder through the catheter, the catheter is removed, and you are usually asked not to pass urine for a few hours. Discomfort is minimal. There are several different drugs that may be used in these circumstances. One of them is a preparation of BCG (the tuberculosis vaccine). There may be some irritation of the bladder after the treatment, sometimes with temporary bleeding. If one of these treatments is recommended, your specialist will discuss the potential benefits and risks with you.

Surgery If the tumor is of the invasive type, then the treatment required is more extensive. The mainstay of therapy for invasive bladder cancer is surgery, and this means removal of the entire bladder, a **total cystectomy**. In a few cases, only part of the bladder may be removed (**partial cystectomy**). The exact nature and extent of surgery depends on several factors. It depends on the position and size of the bladder tumor, on your general medical condition, and on how you will be able to cope with looking after yourself following the surgery (see below). You and your surgeon will discuss the specifics of the type of operation and the care you will need after it. Usually the whole bladder has to be removed. In that case your surgeon will divert the urine stream. There are several different ways of achieving this. One is called the **ileal neobladder**. In this operation the surgeon attaches both ureters to a length of bowel (which he or she separates from the rest of the bowel). That length of bowel may function as a reservoir to hold the urine, and therefore act as a replacement for your bladder, and may be connected to the urethra. In other circumstances, a length of bowel may carry the urine from the ureters to a stoma on the skin. (There is more on urinary stomas in Chapter 10.) There the urine is collected in a bag that you can empty yourself. In addition, there are some ways of performing surgery so that you have control of the urine flow yourself (emptying the collected urine by using a catheter introduced into the stoma). These are called **continent diversions**, meaning that you are not incontinent as a result. There are several different ways of doing these operations, and if one of them is suitable in your case, your surgeon will discuss it with you.

A total cystectomy will bring about quite a major change in your lifestyle, and it is important that you are prepared as well as possible for it. In particular, it is worth meeting with a clinical nurse specialist (usually called a **stoma therapist**) before or shortly after the operation to help you with all the details. At first, you may feel daunted by the various procedures, but in a fairly short time you will find that you can incorporate it all into a routine that you will soon be able to do relatively automatically.

Radiotherapy Radiotherapy is sometimes used in addition to surgery, sometimes after, sometimes before. It can also occasionally be used instead of surgery, if, for example, for some reason surgery is not feasible, or if the patient will be unable to cope with the aftereffects of surgery. The long-term effects of radiotherapy are generally not as good as with surgery, however, and therefore it should not be regarded as an alternative to surgery in every case.

Chemotherapy Chemotherapy drugs show some results in bladder cancer. In some circumstances, chemotherapy using agents such as **methotrexate**, **vinblastine**, **Adriamycin**, and **cis-platinum** may be recommended before surgery, radiotherapy, or both. Before making a decision about any form of chemotherapy for bladder cancer, make sure that you understand the potential benefits—and the chance of a remission—and the potential side effects of the particular therapy that is being proposed.

Phototherapy An interesting method of treating certain tumors has recently been investigated that may be useful in a few cases of bladder cancer. It involves giving the patient substances called **porphyrins**, which happen to be taken up particularly by cancer cells. The porphyrins render the cells very sensitive to damage by laser light. After the drugs have been given, the tumor is then exposed to laser light via a cystoscope for some minutes. The exact role of this type of therapy is not yet fully established, but it may be useful in certain cases.

BONE (OSTEOSARCOMA AND OTHER TYPES)

Number of new cases diagnosed per year in the United States: 2,500

SUMMARY OF THE KEY FACTS IN THIS SECTION

- Primary cancers of the bone (as opposed to secondary cancers from a primary tumor elsewhere in the body) are not very common.
- Generally they occur in adolescents and young adults and are usually found in the area around the knee joint, although they can occur in almost any bone.
- They are often aggressive and have a high tendency to spread to distant areas.
- If they are treated appropriately with surgery and additional chemotherapy, they are curable in many cases.
- With the latest surgical techniques, and radiotherapy when needed, it is possible to avoid amputation of the affected leg or arm in many cases.

The Most Important Features of the Tumor

Cancers that begin in the bone—*primary* cancers of the bone—are quite uncommon. By contrast, many cancers that begin in other areas of the body—such as the breast, prostate, or lung—may spread to bone and may cause *secondary* tumors there. This section will therefore deal only with the rarer primary tumors of the bone, and secondary cancers in bone will be discussed with the relevant primary cancer. (For example, cancer of the breast that has spread to bone is discussed in the section on cancer of the breast.)

Among the *primary* cancers of the bone, the commonest type is **osteosarcoma** (formerly called osteogenic sarcoma). This is a cancer that tends to develop in growing bones and so occurs most commonly in adolescents and young adults. It is usually found in the area of the knee joint (in the lower part of the upper leg or the upper part of the lower leg), though it can occur in the arm or the back or, less commonly, in any other bone. The main danger of osteosarcomas is that they have a high tendency to spread to distant areas of the body, particularly the lungs.

Treatment is designed with two important objectives: (a) to cure the patient, which almost always means chemotherapy after surgery and usually before surgery as well; and (b) to produce the minimum amount of interference with the appearance and function of the part of the body affected. This means that if it is safe and technically possible, the tumor should be removed without amputating the whole limb.

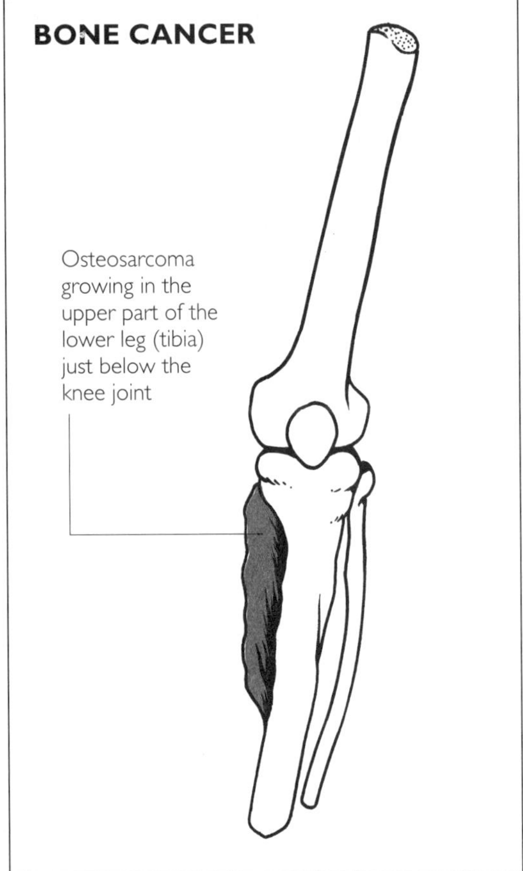

Other types of bone cancer include a rarer cancer called **Ewing's sarcoma**, which occurs in childhood and adolescence, and a cancer that begins in cartilage called **chondrosarcoma**, which is usually very slow growing and rarely spreads to distant areas of the body.

Because these three types of bone cancer are somewhat different, I discuss osteosarcoma first and deal with Ewing's sarcoma and chondrosarcoma separately, pointing out the ways in which the tumors and the treatments are different.

OSTEOSARCOMA

Age and Incidence

Osteosarcomas are cancers that occur almost exclusively in older children, adolescents, and young adults. They are slightly more common in males than in females. They are rare in the forties or beyond, except those osteosarcomas that develop in an area of bone that has been affected by Paget's disease for many years (see below).

Causes

In the great majority of cases, the cause of an osteosarcoma is unknown. Because the cancer occurs in adolescence at a time of great growth, and because the cancers are most common around the knee—in which area the bones are growing most rapidly—we assume that somehow osteosarcoma is associated with rapid growth of bone. This is a reasonable assumption since, as discussed in Chapter 2, cancers represent a failure of normal growth-control mechanisms, and the chance that a failure will occur is higher when growth is proceeding very rapidly. These are speculative assumptions only, however. In a few cases the factors contributing to osteosarcoma are known; these are Paget's disease and radiation.

Paget's Disease In Paget's disease, for unknown reasons, parts of the skeleton become overactive and dismantle and simultaneously rebuild themselves at an abnormally fast rate. This condition occurs in the elderly and can be so mild that it is unnoticeable, although in other cases it can affect the legs or the back, causing pain and deformity. Areas or parts of bones that are badly affected by Paget's disease may, after several years, develop an osteosarcoma. This is further supporting evidence that osteosarcoma is associated with rapid bone growth.

Radiation Radiation is associated with the onset of osteosarcoma in a very few cases. It has been shown that sarcomas of all types, including bone, occur more often than expected in people who have received high doses of X rays or nuclear radiation, and then only in the part of the body that has actually received radiation. Such (rare) cases include survivors of nuclear bombs or accidents and patients who received radiotherapy several decades ago when less was known about radiation safety.

Note: Osteosarcoma Is Not Caused by Injury In many cases, an osteosarcoma will first be diagnosed shortly after an injury. Typically the patient is playing football or some other sport and falls or injures a leg. There may be a fracture or severe pain that does not go away. This may be the first clue that there is an underlying problem. There is no evidence that previous injuries are associated with a higher chance of osteosarcoma, but it is very common for a small injury to be the circumstance that reveals the presence of the cancer.

How the Cancer Tends to Spread

Osteosarcoma has a high tendency to spread, which it does by means of the bloodstream. As a result, secondary tumors are most likely to appear first in the lungs (which is where the small blood vessels — the capillaries — filter the cancer cells from the bloodstream). Because osteosarcomas may grow for some time before they cause pain or tenderness, and so may have time to spread before they are removed, about 15 percent of patients also have secondaries in the lungs at the time of diagnosis. The cancer may also spread to other bones and very occasionally to other parts of the body.

Symptoms or Problems That You May Notice

Pain Some osteosarcomas may be painless, but most commonly cause an **ache** or **pain** in a limb or in the back. Of course, aches and pains in the limbs are common in adolescents; they used to be called "growing pains" (which they probably are). However, pain in a bone, particularly if it comes on **at rest** or **at night**, requires medical assessment if it is **severe** and has **no explanation**, if it is localized to **one place** and stays there for **more than a couple of days**. Fleeting pains that last a few minutes or an hour or so and pains that move from place to place are not usually a sign of a bone cancer.

Other Symptoms In addition to pain in the area involved, the area may also be **tender** when you touch it or press it, there may be some **swelling** over the area, and it may feel **warm** to the touch. These are all features that can also accompany an ordinary bruise or injury. With a bruise or injury, the symptoms should settle down and almost disappear in two or three days; if there is a tumor in the bone, however, the problems will get worse over several days or weeks. Hence **medical assessment is important if the problem shows no sign of improving** after a few days.

Diagnosis and Tests

With any suspected problem in the bone, your doctor (or your child's doctor, if you are the parent) will take a detailed history and perform an examination.

These are both very important, so please be patient. Then the following tests are likely to be done.

X Rays X rays of the area can give important clues about the presence of a bone tumor. Sometimes the X ray may be highly suggestive of a tumor, sometimes it may confirm that there is nothing wrong at all, and occasionally there may be a slight change that needs further investigation. If there is evidence of a cancer or anything suspicious on the X ray, then almost always the next investigation is a CT scan.

CT and MRI Scans A CT scan is most important in showing the exact extent of the tumor and how much bone is involved. Often an MRI scan is also important to show the extent of the tumor inside and outside the bone.

Biopsy A biopsy is usually done under a brief general anesthetic (and whenever possible it should be done by the surgeon who will do the later surgery). It is a very important procedure in bone tumors, because the type of treatment and the prognosis are affected by the type of tumor (whether it is an osteosarcoma or a Ewing's sarcoma, for example) and also to some extent by the grade of the tumor.

Other Tests In some circumstances, other tests may include a bone scan, chest X ray, and CT scans of the chest to see if there has been any spread.

Factors That Influence the Treatment and Prognosis

The most important feature that determines the future is whether there has been **spread** to distant areas of the body, particularly the lungs. However—and this is an important and encouraging point—unlike most cancers, some cases of osteosarcoma can be cured even when there has been spread to the lungs. In the approximately 85 percent of cases where there is no spread, the next most important features are the **position and type** of the tumor. Generally speaking, the tumors that begin in the legs or the arms have a more favorable prognosis than those that begin in the spine or in the more central areas of the skeleton. The variant or subtype of osteosarcoma, if any, is also important. One type, the **parosteal** osteosarcoma, is usually slow growing, and treatment often does not require chemotherapy. Another type, the **periosteal** osteosarcoma, seems to be slightly more aggressive than the parosteal type. If you have (or your child has) one of these types, you may find that some of the general points that I make below do not apply in your individual case.

Two other factors may be important. One is the **grade** of the tumor (how aggressive it appears when seen under the microscope). The other is whether or not the tumor **responds to chemotherapy** given before surgery. If it is sensitive to drug therapy, the chance of cure is increased when those drugs are given as adjuvant therapy after surgery.

The Main Objectives of Treatment

The main objective is cure, and this can be achieved only with a combination of the appropriate surgery and chemotherapy.

Types of Treatment

Two types of therapy are used in order to maximize the chance of cure and minimize the effect of treatment on the function of the limb or part of the body.

Treatment to Prevent Spread—Chemotherapy Because of osteosarcoma's tendency to spread, treatment is needed both to prevent spread and to kill any cancer cells that may have spread. Nowadays many cancer centers give some chemotherapy before the cancer is removed (called **neoadjuvant chemotherapy**). Doing so enables them to see whether the cancer responds to the chemotherapy. For example, it may shrink, or appear smaller on the CT scan. Or it may be found at the time of surgery that much of the cancer has died when seen under the microscope. If that has happened, the cancer is sensitive to those particular chemotherapy drugs, and they will be used for several more courses after the surgery. The drugs that are used most commonly nowadays include **methotrexate** (given in high doses usually), **Adriamycin**, **platinum**, **ifosfamide**, and others.

Treatment of the Primary Cancer—Surgery and/or Radiotherapy The exact type of surgery is extremely important, and your surgeon (or your child's surgeon) will be trying to do two things: remove the primary cancer as completely and safely as possible in order to reduce the chance of recurrence or spread; and also minimize the impact of the operation on the function and appearance of the affected part of the body. This will require some very detailed discussion between you and the surgeon. With cancer in a limb, it used to be routine practice to amputate the limb up to the joint above the tumor. That may sometimes still be necessary, but in some cases a less extensive operation can be done using various kinds of prostheses (artificial bones and/or joints). Sometimes, too, these can be adjusted to accommodate changes in the patient's height. Such operations are usually called limb-preserving or limb-sparing operations. In general, radiotherapy is not used unless surgery to remove the tumor is not possible.

Whatever the type of surgery, rehabilitation after the operation is very important. That means careful planning for physiotherapy, prosthetic limb fitting (if required), and other forms of assistance. Most adolescents have a remarkable ability to adapt to the new situation and show great energy and determination in regaining function of the limb. Quite often, patients are able to continue previous activities in sports and to learn new ones as well.

Later Treatment In a few cases, a single metastasis (or a few metastases) may later appear in the lungs (or one may still be present at the end of therapy). It may be appropriate to remove that lesion or those lesions surgically. If that treatment is being considered, you and the surgeon will need to discuss it in some detail.

EWING'S SARCOMA

Ewing's sarcoma looks different under the microscope from osteosarcoma, and used to be regarded as a more aggressive type of bone cancer. Fortunately, it is often responsive to both radiotherapy and chemotherapy and can be cured in many cases.

Ewing's sarcoma usually occurs in the same age group as osteosarcomas (teenagers and young adults) and most often in the leg or pelvis. Like osteosarcoma, it has a high tendency to spread. Treatment usually consists of chemotherapy, of which several courses are needed, and surgery, radiotherapy, or both.

CHONDROSARCOMA

Chondrosarcomas are rare tumors that start in cartilage (as opposed to bone). They are usually very slow growing and have a low tendency to spread. The prognosis is better than that of osteosarcomas or Ewing's sarcomas, and usually surgery is the only treatment required.

Other Bone Tumors

There are other tumors that can begin in bone, although they are less common. For example, some **lymphomas** can begin in bone. For further information, see the section on lymphomas later in this chapter. Other tumors of bone include conditions such as **myeloma** (discussed in detail later in this chapter).

BOWEL (COLON AND RECTUM)

Number of new cases diagnosed per year in the United States: 133,500

SUMMARY OF THE KEY FACTS IN THIS SECTION

- Cancer of the bowel (of the colon or the rectum) is very common and is caused by a variety of factors mostly associated with the Western style of living.
- Bowel cancer is relatively slow growing and progresses in a methodical, predictable way.
- In the large majority of cases, the early stages of bowel cancer are curable by surgery.
- In some cases of more advanced cancer, therapy after surgery with drugs may improve the outlook and increase the number of people who are cured.
- Although many studies have been done, an effective screening method that detects bowel cancer in the early stages is still under research and investigation.
- There is good evidence that certain kinds of dietary changes and changes in bowel habit may prevent some, perhaps most, cancer of the bowel in this country.

The Most Important Features of the Tumor

Cancer of the bowel (that is, of the colon or the rectum) is a very common tumor that grows and progresses fairly slowly and in a predictable way. It starts on the inner lining of the bowel wall and then grows deeper into the wall, until it spreads through the wall and to the lymph nodes in the abdomen. Further spread usually goes to the liver. If removed before it has spread deeply into the bowel wall, it is cured in nearly three-quarters of cases. Unfortunately, it is very difficult to diagnose bowel cancer in the early stages because it may not produce any symptoms. Although we do not know precisely what causes a particular person to develop bowel cancer, we do know a good deal about the risk factors, including the kinds of diet and bowel habit that put a person at higher risk. For this reason, certain specific changes in lifestyle (see below) may well reduce a person's risk of developing bowel cancer in the first place. In other words, prevention is to some extent feasible.

What You Really Need to Know about the Colon and the Rectum

The colon and the rectum are the two components that make up the large bowel, the last part of the digestive tract through which food passes before reaching the anus. The rectum is the name for the last six inches (fifteen centimeters) or so of bowel, the straight portion that leads to the anus. The colon, which is about three feet (ninety centimeters) in length, leads from the small bowel to the rectum.

How does the digestive tract work, and how do the colon and the rectum function as parts of it? Briefly, food is digested in the stomach and duodenum, and nutrients are extracted from it as it passes onward through the **small bowel** (so called because it is rather small in diameter). After passage through the small bowel, the contents are basically liquid. They then pass through the **large bowel** (which is noticeably larger in diameter), which consists of the colon and rectum. It is the function of the colon and the rectum to **absorb water** from the bowel contents so that the liquid contents of the small bowel are converted into the semisolid material recognizable as stool or feces. Other processes besides water absorption also occur as the bowel contents travel along the colon and the rectum, among them the breakdown of certain materials (such as salts from the bile) in the stool into simpler substances some of which can be reabsorbed and reused by the body. A number of these processes depend on **bacteria**— called the **bowel**

THE DIGESTIVE TRACT SHOWING THE COLON

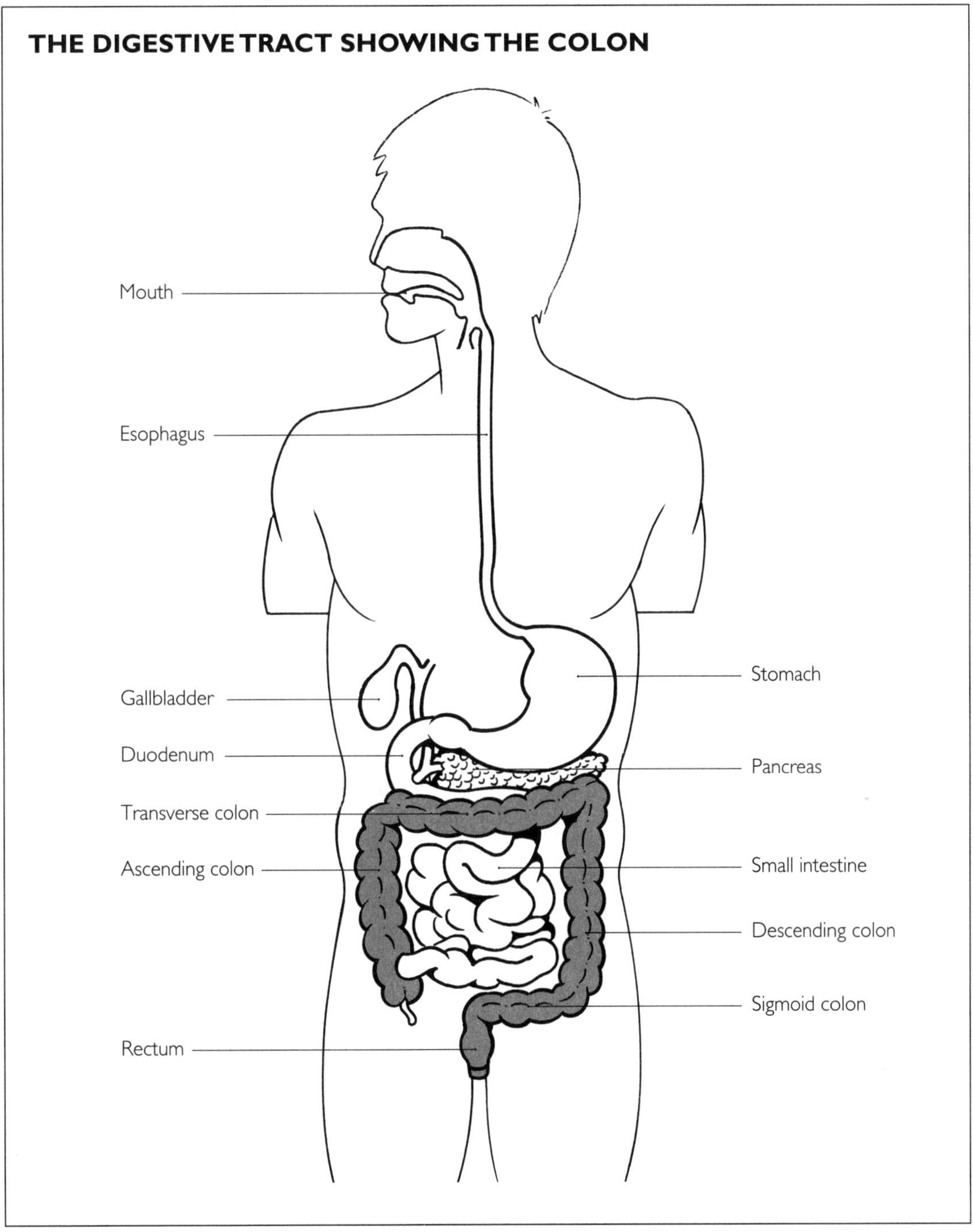

flora— that live in the colon and the rectum. They live only in the colon and rectum and do not normally inhabit the small bowel. Bowel flora give the distinctive odor to feces and, as discussed below, may contribute to the development of cancer in certain susceptible individuals.

Age and Incidence

Bowel cancer is predominantly a condition of middle age and beyond. The peak incidence of the disease occurs in the early sixties. It can occur in the thirties or slightly earlier, but is very rare in that age group unless there is some specific predisposing reason or cause (see below). It occurs in men and women equally.

Causes

Cancer of the colon is predominantly a condition caused by aspects of our "Western" lifestyle (a term frequently used for the kind of lifestyle that is common in the so-called developed countries). This cancer is very rare among people living in rural areas of developing countries and among people in the developed countries who have adopted dietary habits that resemble those of developing nations in certain respects (for example, members of certain faiths). We do not yet know all the factors involved, but we can identify some of them. For convenience, the following summary of risk factors is divided into those that everybody should be aware of—the *general* risk factors—and those that affect a small proportion of people—the rarer *specific* conditions that increase the risk of bowel cancer. Although it is always useful to know the risk factors, **many people who have bowel cancer have no identifiable risk factors at all**. In other words, in many cases bowel cancer happens apparently of its own accord.

General Factors That Contribute to Bowel Cancer

Diet It is likely that something in the Western diet contributes to the development of bowel cancer, and the probable culprits are (a) **too much fat** in the diet and (b) **too little fiber** in the diet. The saturated fats are identified by many researchers as the major contributory factor. In general, these are animal fats (as opposed to vegetable fats). It also seems that eating a good amount of fiber helps your body to deal with the fat that you do eat. If you combine too much fat in your diet with too little fiber, therefore, you may be increasing your risk considerably.

Substances That Protect against Bowel Cancer Some substances have been identified as possibly decreasing the risk of cancer, and insufficient amounts in the diet may increase the risk. Among these potential protectors are substances found in the brassicae group of vegetables (such as broccoli), as well as beta-carotene (found in carrots and colored vegetables), calcium, and perhaps vitamin C and selenium.

The standard recommended maximum amount of fat and minimum amounts of fiber and other protective ingredients are given in the last part of this section, "Prevention."

Bowel Habit Diet is clearly not the sole cause of bowel cancer, because not everyone who eats a Western-type diet will develop bowel cancer. Among the other factors that increase an individual's risk is bowel habit. Cancer of the bowel seems to be more common among people who are constipated most of the time. The exact definition of constipation is controversial, but, in general, you are not constipated if you have your bowels open at least once a day, the stool is soft (but not liquid), and no real effort is required in passing it. People whose bowel habits do not meet those criteria are at a higher risk of getting bowel cancer. We suspect that this is because the stool in constipated people spends a longer time in the bowel, particularly in the colon and rectum. The standard medical term for this is a **slow transit time**. We think that a slow transit time with prolonged contact between the stool and the wall of the large bowel can produce cancer if the stool contains high amounts of residues of fat.

Another factor may also be relevant, although at present we do not have definite evidence one way or the other. Some people have bacteria in their bowel flora that are capable of converting some substances in the stools (probably derived from fats) into chemicals that may be carcinogenic to the bowel wall. Thus, if you eat a high-fat diet, *and* are constipated with a slow transit time, *and* have these bacteria-producing chemicals in the large bowel, *and* have a diet deficient in substances that protect the bowel wall against carcinogens, *and* (perhaps) have an inherited susceptibility to bowel cancer (see below), you may be at particularly high risk of developing bowel cancer. The story seems to fit together convincingly, but we do not yet have definite proof that all the apparent links in the chain have been identified correctly. There is, however, no doubt that a **good diet and a good bowel habit do definitely decrease the chance that a person will develop bowel cancer**.

Many people wonder why there is so little discussion of cancer of the small bowel. The answer is that cancer of the small bowel is very rare indeed, probably because all of the factors mentioned above do not apply to the small bowel, where the bowel contents are liquid, are not metabolized by bacteria, and do not spend a long time in contact with the bowel wall. That is why when we say "cancer of the bowel," we almost always mean "cancer of the large bowel (colon or rectum)."

Family History Another factor that plays a part in causing bowel cancer, though again we don't know why, is family history. If a first-degree relative of yours (parent, sibling, or child) has had bowel cancer, then your chance of developing bowel cancer is increased, compared to the general population. Although we do not, at present, understand the mechanism by which this risk is transmitted, we assume that in some people there is an inherited susceptibility or vulnerability of the bowel wall to carcinogens, and that if you have inherited that vulnerability, a bowel cancer may develop with less prompting and less stimulus than average.

Polyps Polyps are benign growths that develop in the linings of certain organs, particularly where the lining is responsible for producing mucus. For example, polyps are very common in the back of the nose and may contribute to the symptoms of nasal catarrh. Polyps are also found in the colon. There are many different types of these polyps, but nearly all of them represent some increase in the risk of developing bowel cancer. We know this because when polyps are removed from the bowel, many of them (at least a third of the larger ones) show some signs of developing a very small cancer. Some types represent more risk than others, and the larger the polyp the greater the risk. This does not mean that *all* cancers of the bowel start out as polyps. Some cancers probably develop in the wall of the bowel without any previous benign changes, such as a polyp. It does mean, however, that polyps are one potential route by which cancer may develop. This in turn means that if all polyps in the bowel could be removed as soon as they developed, the amount of bowel cancer in the world would decrease dramatically.

The difficulty is that polyps in themselves do not commonly cause symptoms until they are quite large, and it is not yet technically possible to screen the general population for polyps. As techniques advance, we may one day be able to identify particular individuals who are at especially high risk for both polyps and cancer and screen them, say, annually. At present, however, we do not have the right methods available for identifying them or for screening the general population.

Specific (Rarer) Conditions That Contribute to Bowel Cancer The factors mentioned above apply to the general population. In addition, one or two rarer conditions can occur that make the risk of bowel cancer particularly high. If you have one of these conditions, your doctor has probably already discussed the risk with you. For the sake of completeness, however, they are the following.

Ulcerative Colitis Ulcerative colitis is a condition in which the colon becomes inflamed for no known reason. If the condition involves much or most of the colon, the evidence suggests that after many years (ten or more) the chance of cancer is increased. For this reason, people with ulcerative colitis are usually recommended to have a colonoscopy regularly (once a year or so) and may require surgery to remove the colon if there are signs that cancer may be developing.

Familial Polyposis Coli This is a very rare condition in which the bowel is studded with polyps. The polyps themselves are not unusual, but there are so many of them and they grow so large that the chance that a cancer will develop becomes extremely high. Recently another genetic problem has been found in which families without multiple polyps have a higher risk of bowel cancer at an earlier age. This is called hereditary nonpolyposis coli (HNPC), and there is likely to be more information about the basic genetic defect in the near future.

Other Conditions In some other very rare syndromes, affecting a few families only, bowel cancers (and some other cancers) are particularly likely to develop.

How the Cancer Tends to Spread

Bowel cancer is among the slower-growing cancers, and it tends to progress predictably in the great majority of cases. It starts on the inside of the

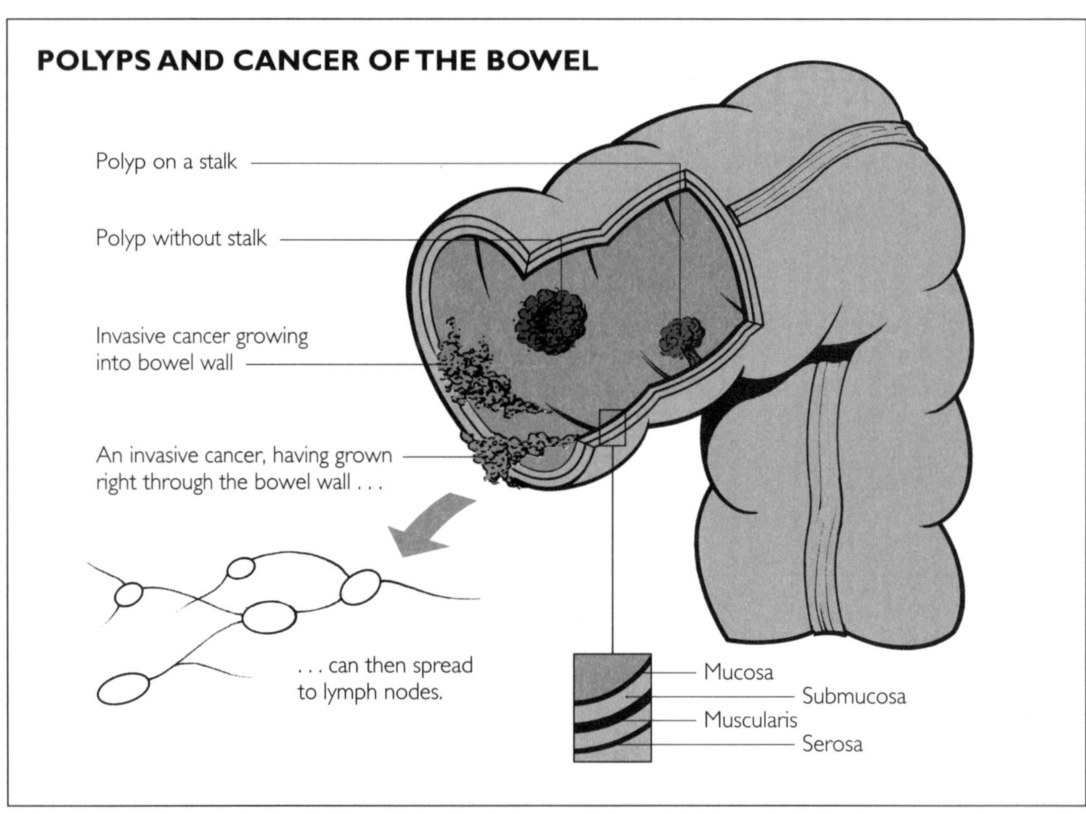

bowel wall (the mucosa) and grows deeper into the wall. In time, it will grow through the wall of the bowel and spread to the lymph nodes in the area. After that, bowel cancer tends to spread to other distant parts of the body—often other organs in the abdomen, particularly the liver, sometimes to the lungs, and rarely to other areas.

Symptoms or Problems That You May Notice

Cancer of the colon or the rectum can cause symptoms in several ways: it may affect the bowel habit; it may irritate the wall of the bowel, causing it to produce too much **mucus**; it may cause **bleeding**; or it may **block** the bowel, making it difficult for stool to get past.

The early stages of cancer of the bowel often cause **no symptoms** at all, which is what makes early detection so difficult. One of the most common early symptoms from bowel cancer (particularly rectal) is that the tumor might cause some **bleeding**. Usually that will be seen as a red streak of blood on the surface of the stool. There are many other causes for blood on the stool, however, the most common being hemorrhoids or a tear in the wall of the anus (an anal fissure). However, because blood in the stool *may* be a sign of cancer, **it is very important for anyone noticing blood in or on the stool to see her or his doctor**. One further point: sometimes the amount of blood from the cancer is too small to be seen. Tests on the stool will show that there is blood there, called **occult blood** (blood that is not visible). Hence you may be told that there has been blood in your stool after testing, but that does not necessarily mean that you should feel guilty for not having seen it.

Another possible symptom is a **change in bowel habit**. This is not an easy problem to define, as everybody's bowel habit varies from time to time anyway. However, a marked and prolonged change with no obvious explanation—along the lines of a definite change for, say, two weeks or so—is a possible symptom of bowel cancer and should prompt you to consult your doctor. If, for example, you normally have your bowels open daily, but this changes for no reason to once every three days, check with your doctor. You may notice **constipation** or **diarrhea**, sometimes alternating **diarrhea and constipation** or mucus mixed with the stool or on the surface so that it becomes somewhat slimy in appearance.

Depending on the position and the shape and size of the cancer, it may also cause blockage to the bowel and interfere with the passage of bowel contents. That may cause **colicky pain** in the abdomen (pain that comes and goes in waves), and sudden or marked **swelling** or distension of the abdomen. If it is very severe, there may be **vomiting** or the patient may be unable to pass stool or wind.

If the tumor is large enough to interfere with the ability of the bowel to absorb nutrition, then it may also cause **loss of weight**.

Diagnosis and Tests

Your doctor will first take your history and then give you a full physical examination, including a rectal examination (see page 180) or a pelvic examination or both. Routine blood tests will almost certainly be recommended. These are important since, if the cancer is causing blood loss, you can become slightly anemic.

In addition, some or all of the following tests will be recommended.

Occult Blood Testing Testing for occult blood simply means testing the stool to find out if there is blood in it that is not visible. Preparations for the test may require you to avoid eating meat for a day or so before the test. After that, all you need do is to give a specimen of your stool to the laboratory.

Sigmoidoscopy and Colonoscopy Depending on the circumstances, your doctor may recommend that the rectum be examined (sigmoidoscopy) or the whole colon (colonoscopy). If any suspicious lesion is seen, the specialist may take a biopsy of it for detailed analysis. The full details of these procedures will be explained to you if one or both of them are recommended.

Barium Enema Again depending on the particular case, a special X ray of the large bowel may be needed. In this procedure, a liquid containing barium, which shows up white on X rays, is given into the bowel in the form of an enema and X-ray pictures are taken. Usually the procedure requires you to prepare your bowel for a day or two beforehand so that it is relatively empty and any suspicious lesions can be seen clearly. The procedure is, it is true, somewhat uncomfortable, and as many patients say, not very dignified. Nevertheless, the information it provides may be extremely important.

CT Scan and Liver Ultrasound If a cancer of the bowel is detected, further tests will almost certainly be recommended to see if there is any evidence that the tumor has spread. Usually these consist of a CT scan of the abdomen, an ultrasound of the liver, or both.

Other Tests Several other tests can also be useful. Among them is a blood test called the **CEA**. CEA (or carcinoembryonic antigen) is a substance produced by many types of cancer, including most cancers of the bowel. CEA can be used as a **marker**, that is, a test that can be repeated to show whether the tumor is getting bigger. Or (sometimes) it is used after the tumor has been removed to alert your medical team to the possibility of a recurrence. There are a variety of tests similar to the CEA test, some of which show promise of being useful, but none of them has so far been established as routine.

Factors That Influence the Treatment and Prognosis

The most important factor in determining the treatment of bowel cancer is how far it has spread, that is, the **stage** of the cancer. If the cancer is limited to the mucosa, it is curable in the great majority of cases (and in certain circumstances that may mean almost all cases). If the cancer has grown through the muscular layer of the bowel wall, the chance of cure is decreased. If it has spread to the lymph nodes, the chance of cure is lower still (though the fewer lymph nodes involved the better), and if it has spread to distant organs the chance of cure is very small indeed.

Treatment will also depend to some extent on the **grade** of the cancer, that is, whether it appears under the microscope to be more aggressive or less so.

In some centers, various investigational tests can also be done to see if any other features of the cancer indicate a particularly bad or good outlook. It may be a few years before we know the real value of the information from such additional tests.

Bowel cancer is unlike almost all other cancers in one important respect: the size of the cancer does not affect the prognosis. Although it is not known why this is the case, we do know that it is the stage that largely determines the outlook, not the size.

The Main Objectives of Treatment

The objective of the treatments for bowel cancer is to cure whenever possible. In practical terms, that means surgery to remove the cancer completely, if that can be done.

Types of Treatment

Surgery and Colostomies Surgery with complete removal of the cancer offers the best chance of curing the disease completely.

The exact nature of the operation depends on where the tumor is and whether it is stuck to any nearby crucial organs. Ideally the tumor should be removed and the bowel joined up again safely. It is possible, however, that the bowel will be so damaged after the removal of the tumor that it will not work properly. That can be very dangerous, because any leakage of bowel contents into the abdomen can

WHY A COLOSTOMY MAY BE NEEDED

Permanent Colostomy

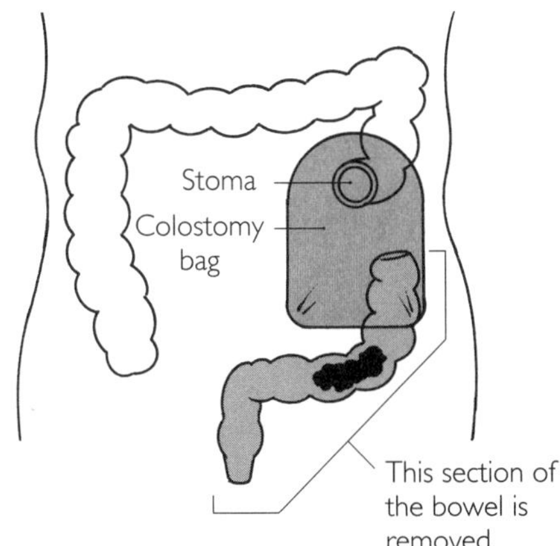

If, after removal of the tumor, it is not possible to reconnect the bowel, the surgeon will make a permanent colostomy.

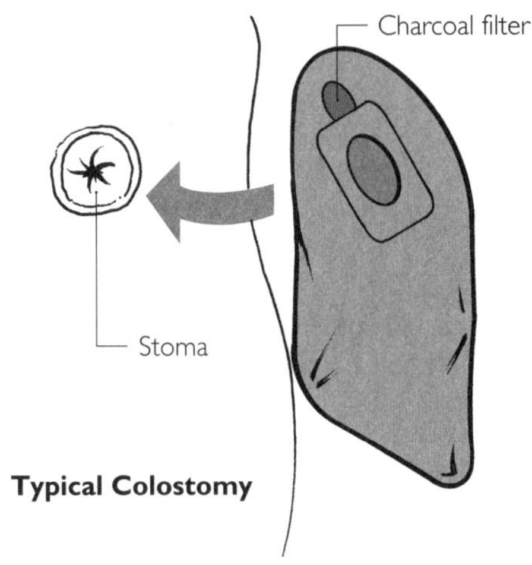

Typical Colostomy

Temporary Colostomy

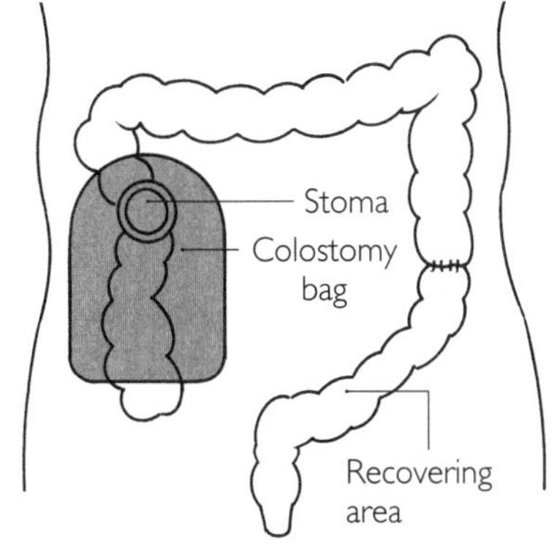

If, after removal of the tumor, the bowel is joined up but needs time to heal safely, the surgeon may create a temporary colostomy so that the stool leaves the bowel before it can reach the recovering area.

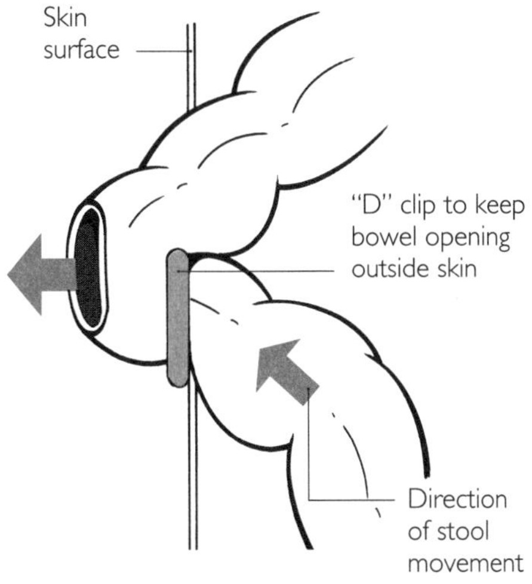

cause a major or even lethal infection. In that case, steps are taken to ensure that no bowel contents pass through the damaged area of bowel until it has fully recovered. A **colostomy** (see page 53) is done to divert the bowel contents (to the surface of the abdomen) before they reach the weak area or malfunctioning part of the bowel. A colostomy that is used to allow the joined parts of the bowel to recover may be temporary; if the damaged part of the bowel recovers, further surgery may be done to reconnect the bowel and close the colostomy.

If the tumor is very near the anus, surgical removal of the cancer may require the complete removal of the anus and the rectum as well (an abdomino-perineal resection). If this is necessary, it will not be technically possible to rejoin the bowel; in that case, a permanent colostomy will be required. In some cases, too, where the tumor cannot be removed entirely and the bowel cannot safely be reconnected, a permanent colostomy is necessary and will dramatically reduce pain and bowel problems by diverting the bowel contents away from the problem area through healthy functioning bowel.

More information on colostomies and how to live with them may be found in Chapter 10.

Radiotherapy Radiotherapy is often used before or after surgery, especially in cancer of the rectum, and is also used in some circumstances where surgery is not technically feasible, for instance, if the cancer happens to be very close to the anus or for some other reason is not surgically removable. By itself, radiotherapy has only a small effect on bowel cancer, but it is used as part of many treatment programs to reduce the chance of recurrence.

Chemotherapy Advanced or recurrent bowel cancer is very often resistant to treatment by chemotherapy. In certain other situations, however, chemotherapy has recently been found to help significantly. With various groups of patients in whom the cancer is moderately advanced and has spread all the way through the bowel wall or to the lymph nodes, it has been shown that giving certain types of drug therapy after surgery—in other words, as **adjuvant therapy**—increases the number of long-term cures. There are several different types of drugs used. Some, like the drug **levamisole**, seem to have a specific effect on the immune system, boosting certain aspects of its function, while others are chemotherapy agents often including **5-fluorouracil** (sometimes with **leucovorin**). You may therefore be recommended to receive one or several of these types of drugs after surgery. Because this area of cancer therapy is still being worked out, you may also be asked to enter a clinical trial (see page 233) comparing two or more different ways of using medications. As research into adjuvant therapy for bowel cancer is potentially very valuable, it is worth your giving serious consideration to any request to enter a trial.

The Possibility of Recurrences

Even though an operation may have removed all the visible tumor, recurrence can still, unfortunately, occur. Bowel cancer seems to recur when a few microscopic-sized fragments or cells of the cancer manage to establish themselves in normal tissues, often close to the site of the original operation. This is particularly likely to happen when the primary tumor has spread through the bowel wall or to the lymph nodes and is the main reason for considering therapy after surgery (adjuvant therapy). If there is no sign of recurrence after five years, the patient has a high chance of being cured, although there are occasionally recurrences after that time. In some circumstances, a recurrence in the pelvis can be removed surgically (though often this is not technically feasible), in which case the second operation may result in a cure. In some cases, even recurrence in the liver (if there are one or a few tumors and they are close to each other) can be treated surgically, and cure can sometimes be achieved. You will need to discuss the specifics with your surgeon.

TABLE 4.1: DECREASING THE RISK OF GETTING BOWEL CANCER
AVOID CONSTIPATION
Have **enough fiber** in your diet so that you pass a soft bowel movement once (or twice) a day without needing to strain or hold your breath. **Train** your bowel. Have a daily routine (perhaps after breakfast), and educate your bowel into acting at the same time every day! Try to get regular **exercise** (for example, work out, jog, walk).
DECREASE THE AMOUNT OF FAT IN YOUR DIET
A diet in which fat contributes 25 percent or less of your total energy (calorie) intake could reduce your risk of both bowel cancer and heart disease.
HAVE REGULAR CHECKUPS
Over the age of forty make sure you have a complete examination, including a rectal examination, at least once a year. The benefit of a rectal exam is not proven, but one is generally recommended.
GET A MEDICAL ASSESSMENT OF ANY POTENTIALLY DANGEROUS SYMPTOMS
These include: bleeding from the rectum or blood on the toilet paper, significant changes in bowel habit (for example, alternately having diarrhoea and constipation). Such problems are more likely to have noncancerous causes such as hemorrhoids, but you must get them checked just in case.
CONSIDER OTHER DIETARY FACTORS
It is important not to be deficient in calcium and perhaps other substances such as vitamin C and selenium. At present, however, it appears that most people have sufficient amounts of these in their diet.

Screening and Early Diagnosis

Screening for bowel cancer—in other words, testing the general population in order to detect bowel cancer at an early stage—would be extremely valuable if it could be done effectively. Because bowel cancer is so common, because in the early stages there may be no symptoms, and because it is so often curable if detected early, a really effective screening test would make a very large difference to people's health in this country. Unfortunately, although many large-scale and serious efforts have been made over the last twenty years, we still do not have a screening test that reliably detects all (or even most) bowel cancer. There have been many candidates for screening. Blood tests, such as the CEA, would have been useful, but unfortunately the test is usually normal in the early stages of bowel cancers, and some people (mostly cigarette smokers) have a slightly raised CEA anyway. Testing for occult blood has also been evaluated on a wide scale, but many of us have blood in the stool from other causes (such as hemorrhoids, anal fissures, blood from the mouth caused by dental problems or even by eating red meat). Thus occult blood tests were found to be positive in many people who did not have cancer, and were also negative in quite a few who did. Despite these limitations, the American Cancer Society currently recommends fecal occult blood testing and sigmoidoscopy.

Prevention: Tips to Reduce the Risk of Bowel Cancer

Table 4.1 summarizes the facts as far as we know them about ways of reducing the risk of getting bowel cancer in the long run.

BRAIN AND SPINAL CORD

Number of new cases diagnosed per year in the United States: 17,900

SUMMARY OF THE KEY FACTS IN THIS SECTION

- Cancers originating in the brain and spinal cord (in other words, **primary** cancers) are not very common.
- There are two peaks of incidence: one peak in childhood (when some of the cancers are rather primitive in their form and somewhat easier to treat and cure) and another peak in late adulthood when the cancers are in general more difficult to treat.
- The brain is also a place where **secondary** cancers may develop, having spread from a primary cancer elsewhere in the body.
- Primary cancers of the brain do not usually spread outside the brain and spinal cord, and therefore do not later involve other organs.
- Treatment consists of surgery, if technically feasible, or radiotherapy, or both, depending on the position and the type of the cancer, sometimes followed by chemotherapy in certain circumstances. The prognosis varies widely depending on whether the patient is a child or an adult, the type of the cancer, and also on what kind of treatment can be used.

The Most Important Features of the Tumor

Tumors originating within the brain or spinal cord are not very common, and there are many different types. The most important point, however, is that brain tumors that occur in childhood behave very differently from those that happen in adulthood.

In general, the brain tumors of childhood are easier to treat and are often curable. Unfortunately, in adults the prognosis is worse.

Treatment usually consists of surgery followed by radiotherapy. In some circumstances chemotherapy may play an important part.

What You Really Need to Know about the Brain and Spinal Cord (the Central Nervous System)

The Layout of the Brain and Spinal Cord The brain and the spinal cord together make up what we call the **central nervous system** or **CNS**. (The nerves, which carry information to and from the limbs, are called the peripheral nervous system.) The brain and spinal cord are wrapped in three layers of delicate and important membranes called the **meninges**. Within these membranes, the CNS is bathed in a fluid that is similar to serum (the fluid component of blood). The fluid in the CNS is called **cerebrospinal fluid** or **CSF**, and the meninges control the flow of it and also regulate some of the constituents and nutrients in it. Because the CNS is partly isolated by the meninges from the rest of the body, cancer cells that start within the CNS can circulate easily through the CNS but cannot get out into the rest of the body. For that reason, many primary tumors of the CNS can make secondary tumors only in other parts of the CNS and not elsewhere in the body.

Anatomy of the Brain There are four main parts to the brain. The back part of the brain is called the **cerebellum** and regulates most balance and coordination. The cerebellum is perched over an area of exceptional importance that could be called the **automatic brain**—the anatomical term is the **brainstem**. The brainstem controls all the vital functions that are essential to life, such as the breathing reflexes, control of the heartbeat, and so on. These functions are so essential to life that if the brainstem dies, we die. The third and fourth parts of the brain are two large structures on top of and

THE CENTRAL NERVOUS SYSTEM (THE BRAIN AND THE SPINAL CORD)

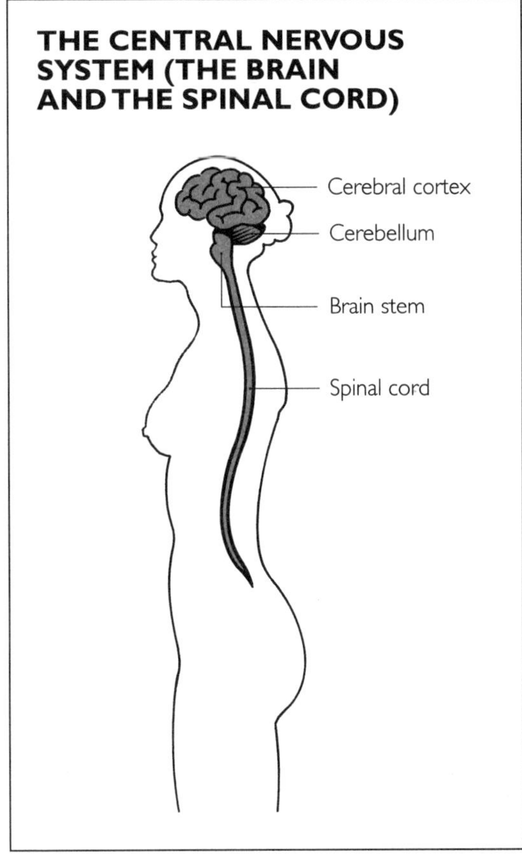

around the brainstem, the left and right **cerebral hemispheres** (half-globes). Together they make up the **cerebrum**, which is responsible for all the higher functions such as thinking, seeing, talking, and so on. The **left cerebral hemisphere** controls **the right half of the body**. The left hemisphere also controls **language**, our ability to speak. Because language is so important to us, we call the left half of the thinking brain the dominant hemisphere.

The **right cerebral hemisphere**, or nondominant hemisphere, controls the **left side of the body**, so that when you move your left hand, it is being controlled by the right side of the brain. The right hemisphere also controls the ability to interpret and make sense of the space around us. If something goes wrong in this area, you cannot make sense of the whole left side of your world, cannot find your way from place to place, and cannot do any activity—such as getting dressed—that requires understanding of how things are arranged around you.

Cells of the CNS The nerve cells that create and pass on information in the CNS are called **neurons**. They pass information to each other and to the rest of the body by means of long fibers. The neurons are physically supported by a type of specialized connective tissue in the brain made up of cells called **glial cells**. Shortly after birth, the neurons almost completely stop dividing, so that tumors of the neurons themselves are very rare after childhood. The glial cells go on dividing throughout life, however, so that cancers of the glial cells can occur in adulthood.

Age and Incidence

Brain tumors have two peaks of incidence, that is, they occur most frequently in two age groups. The first age group is children, with a peak between three and twelve years of age. The second group is older adults, with a peak between sixty and seventy years of age. The brain tumors that occur in children are quite different in type, position, and curability from those that occur in older adults. Most brain tumors affect males more than females. The male-female ratio varies from 2:1 up to 9:1 with the type of the brain cancer. Two types of brain tumor (including benign brain tumors, the meningiomas) affect females more than males.

Causes

We know almost nothing about the causes of tumors of the brain. We assume that some types of brain tumors in childhood originate from some defect in the cell-control system that was present as the fetus was developing. This does not mean that these tumors are inherited or passed on in the genetic material, but rather that the fault occurred in the system as the brain or spinal cord was forming. Many of the tumors that occur in children have cells that look like cells of the embryo and are called **embryonal tumors**. We have hardly any idea of what causes almost every other kind of brain tumor (apart from secondary tumors when the primary is elsewhere in the body).

How the Cancer Tends to Spread

Primary tumors of the brain may spread around the CNS using the CSF as a vehicle, but rarely spread outside the meninges. Moreover, not all brain tumors do spread around the CNS; and the most common type of primary brain tumors in adults—the gliomas—usually do *not* spread to other areas of the brain or spinal cord but are most likely to remain in one place. The cancer may recur in that place but is unlikely to crop up elsewhere.

Symptoms or Problems That You May Notice

There are many symptoms that can be caused by brain tumors, but the most common ones are **headaches** and **seizures**.

Headaches If a brain tumor is large, or causes swelling of the normal brain tissue around it, or if it happens to be in a position to block the flow of CSF, it may cause a rise in the pressure of the CSF inside the head. This is felt as a headache. Although one cannot distinguish with absolute certainty between an ordinary headache and a headache caused by rising pressure (for example, a brain tumor), some features are highly suggestive of the latter. If a headache is caused by a brain tumor, it will be quite severe and will occur every day. The pain is often made worse by coughing and may be accompanied by vomiting and sometimes blurring of vision. Any newly developing headache that has those features should be assessed by a physician.

Seizures A tendency to repeated seizures—epilepsy—is very common in the general population, and in the great majority of cases is, of course, not caused by a brain tumor. If epilepsy starts for the first time in adulthood, however, it *may* be a sign of an underlying brain problem (including the possibility of a tumor). Hence all epilepsy that begins in adulthood should be assessed by a physician. Any epilepsy that starts in childhood should also be assessed by a specialist in every case: there may be features in certain cases that lead the specialist to recommend a CT scan for the child, or some other test, to exclude the possibility of a tumor. To repeat: **seizures in childhood are common**, the **great majority of them are not caused by brain tumors**, but anyone (adult or child) with repeated seizures must be assessed by a specialist.

Other Symptoms Depending on the position of the tumor, a variety of symptoms may occur. These include difficulties in seeing (particularly double vision), difficulties in speaking (slurred speech or sudden and consistent inability to name things), unusual drowsiness, paralysis of one limb or of the arm and leg on one side of the body, difficulties in balance, excessive thirst and urination, or a marked change in the personality. Any of these can sometimes be caused by brain tumors. If any of these problems develop in a sudden and pronounced manner, they should be assessed by your doctor.

Diagnosis and Tests

After taking the history and performing a clinical examination, the doctor or specialist may want to recommend one or several of the following tests.

CT Scan CT scans of the brain are extremely useful in showing up tumors. A CT scan will often show the position of a tumor, whether it is causing swelling of the brain around it, and whether it is blocking the flow of CSF. A scan may also sometimes give clues about the type of tumor. If the CT scan reveals the problem, the newer type of scan, the MRI scan, will probably not be needed. However, there are some situations in which an MRI scan may be recommended as well.

MRI Scan Because the pictures in an MRI scan are obtained in a different way from those in a CT scan, an MRI scan is usually done and gives valuable information about a brain tumor and sometimes about spread. It may be useful if surgery is planned, or if certain types of radiotherapy are to be used.

EEG An EEG is an electrical recording of the brain activity (neatly referred to by most patients as "the brainwave test"). Recording electrodes are pressed onto the scalp, and the recording is made with the patient's eyes open, closed, and sometimes looking at flashing lights. If there have been seizures, the EEG may show whether the seizure activity is a problem caused by the whole brain or one part of it (the latter would suggest the possibility of a tumor).

Other Tests Often X rays or scans of other parts of the body and blood tests will be recommended, particularly if the patient is an adult rather than a child.

Biopsy A biopsy will almost certainly be recommended if the brain tumor is in a position where the biopsy can be done without a major risk to the patient. With a few parts of the brain, a biopsy is simply too hazardous, and the risk of leaving the patient with a major deficit (such as paralysis down one side of the body or inability to speak) is too high. If that is the case, your specialist may well recommend that treatment be started without biopsy. Also, if there is a known primary tumor elsewhere in the body—in the lung or in the breast, for example—a biopsy on a secondary tumor in the brain is usually unnecessary. In most other situations, a biopsy will be recommended in order to find out exactly what type of tumor is there and how aggressive it is likely to be.

A biopsy is usually done under a general anesthetic as part of an operation in which a piece of the skull is temporarily removed in order to allow the surgeon access to the tumor. This procedure is referred to as a **craniotomy**. In some centers and in certain circumstances, a biopsy may be done without removing a piece of the skull, using a thin needle which is guided to the tumor by the surgeon using CT or MRI imaging. This is called a **stereotactic biopsy**. In either case, the full details will be explained to you by the neurosurgeon. The procedure varies depending on the size and position of the tumor.

The Main Types of Brain and Spinal Cord Cancers

Primary Brain Tumors in Childhood

Medulloblastoma In children, some brain tumors are probably derived from cells that somehow remain from when the fetus was growing *in utero*. One of these is called the medulloblastoma. It is also sometimes called a **primitive neuroectodermal tumor** or **PNET**. It usually arises in the cerebellum, the back part of the brain, and may spread via the CSF to other parts of the CNS.

Gliomas There are several different types of gliomas (cancers of the supporting glial cells) of childhood. Because they vary a great deal, only a few general comments can be made about them. For reasons that we do not understand, gliomas occurring in children are likely to be situated in the cerebellum, and if so are easier to treat and even cure than they are in adults. They may also occur in the brainstem (where biopsy may be difficult). The prognosis depends on the grade of the tumor. If the tumor occurs higher up in the brain—in other words, in the cerebrum—and if it is of the kind called an **astrocytoma**, the grade of the tumor makes a considerable difference. **Low-grade astrocytomas** can often be removed in their entirety, and the prognosis is good. **High-grade astrocytomas** have a worse prognosis. Another type of tumor that occurs in childhood is called an **ependymoma**. With these tumors, the position in the brain and the grade are also important. Some are very slow growing and are often considered benign (not invasive). Others are clearly malignant and faster growing. Usually they occur in the back part of the brain. Of the more favorable types, more than half may be cured. (See also the section on meningiomas below, and the section "Rarer Cancers in Childhood.")

Primary Brain Tumors in Adults

In adults the most common type of primary brain tumor is a **glioma** (cancer of the supporting glial cells of the brain). There are several different subtypes of glial cells, which are named for their shape or appearance (astrocytes, oligodendrocytes, and so on). One particular type—the oligodendrogliomas—generally behave less aggressively than the other types. Oligodendrogliomas are also more responsive to chemotherapy than the other types. For the other types (that is, other than the oligodendrogliomas), the type of the tumor does not affect the prognosis, whereas the **grade** (high grade or low grade) does.

Lymphomas of the Brain or Spinal Cord

Lymphomas are cancers of the lymphocytes (see page 142) and can originate within the CNS; in other words, there can be a primary lymphoma of the CNS. Several other kinds of lymphoma may result from secondary spread from another part of the body—the bone marrow or the lymph nodes, for example—to the brain or the spinal cord. The behavior and treatment of lymphomas are dealt with in the section on lymphomas (see pages 142–148).

Secondary Cancers in the Brain or Spinal Cord

Secondary tumors in the brain or spinal cord may develop from primary cancers elsewhere in the body—the breast, lung, bowel, melanoma, kidney, and so on. With secondary tumors in the CNS, the behavior of the secondary tumor is usually similar to that of the primary tumor. For example, a secondary tumor from a primary such as a small-cell lung cancer (see page 140) is likely to be fast growing, sensitive to radiotherapy and chemotherapy, and with a tendency to recur. The prognosis for a patient with, say, a melanoma that has spread to the CNS is, unfortunately, less good than that for a patient without CNS secondaries.

Spinal Cord Tumors

Primary tumors of the spinal cord are uncommon. In general, they are likely to be benign tumors such as meningiomas, or ependymomas, which vary widely in their aggression and behavior.

Benign Tumors of the Brain: Meningiomas

I have included meningiomas in this section only for the sake of completeness. Meningiomas are benign brain tumors. They are by definition not cancers, in that they do not invade normal brain tissue. Because of *where* they are, however, they may cause severe symptoms and problems by compressing and putting pressure on adjacent parts of the brain. Furthermore, the treatment (surgery, if feasible) often causes worry and concern (not unreasonably). If they can be removed completely, however, they are usually cured, although recurrence may happen in some cases. Even if they do recur, they are benign tumors and do not carry the same prognosis as cancers.

Tumors of the Pituitary Gland

These tumors are almost always benign and are rare.

Factors That Influence the Treatment and Prognosis

A number of features of brain tumors have a major effect on the treatment and the outcome.

Age Age is important because the brain cancers that occur in childhood are of a completely different type from those that occur in adulthood. The age of the patient is an indicator of what type of cancer is present, and it is that which largely determines the chance of cure.

The Type of Tumor Childhood tumors are often curable. Adult tumors such as gliomas are curable much less often. Secondary tumors are incurable in the great majority of cases. Certain adult tumors, such as lymphomas, are easier to treat and even cure, although the relapse rate is very high. Among the gliomas, the oligodendrogliomas behave less aggressively than others and are more sensitive to chemotherapy.

Position The place in the brain where the tumor occurs may affect what can be done in terms of diagnosis and treatment. Tumors very close to or inside the brainstem are very difficult to deal with, because surgical intervention—whether biopsy or removal—may have very serious consequences. In such cases, it is often decided to treat the tumor without biopsy. It is more common for a tumor in childhood to be situated deep in the brain near the brainstem, whereas in the older adult tumors are usually situated in the cerebral hemispheres.

Grade (in Adult Gliomas) For most of the rarer types of brain tumors, the grade of the tumor is not as important as the type. In the gliomas, however—the most common type of adult brain tumor—the grade is very important. The lower-grade gliomas are often slow growing and may never recur after surgical removal, or if they do, only after many years. The higher-grade gliomas behave more aggressively and may recur earlier and enlarge more rapidly. The highest-grade gliomas—those most likely to be aggressive—are called **glioblastoma multiforme**. The subtype of the glioma, apart from the type known as oligodendrogliomas (see above), makes little difference to the treatment or the prognosis, once the grade has been taken into account.

The Main Objectives of Treatment

The objectives of treatment depend on what the tumor is. For those types that are curable, the objective, of course, is to cure the patient if possible.

Types of Treatment

The exact treatment recommended varies according to the individual circumstances. In what follows I discuss first some types of treatment and then some general treatment considerations related to the different types of tumor.

Surgery Surgery usually means a craniotomy (see page 60) in which a flap of bone is temporarily removed. In a few circumstances, newer surgical techniques such as lasers may be used. These offer an improvement in only a few special situations. In the majority of cases, standard neurosurgical techniques are considered to be as effective as lasers.

Dexamethasone Dexamethasone is a steroid that has been found to be highly effective in reducing swelling around brain tumors. It is often used if the CT scan shows that the tumor is surrounded by swelling of the brain tissue. The doses of dexamethasone used in treatment of brain tumors are likely to cause swelling of the face and abdomen, so do not be alarmed if this happens. Also, because it is customary to give dexamethasone for several weeks at a time, the dose has to be reduced very slowly. Stopping the drug suddenly may cause serious problems.

Radiotherapy For brain tumors, radiotherapy nowadays is commonly given just to the area involved, which reduces the side effects. Usually dexamethasone (see above) will be given at the same time to reduce any swelling that may result from the radiotherapy. The radiotherapy almost always makes the patient feel tired and lethargic, and the fatigue may continue for a few weeks after the treatment has finished. The treatment will almost certainly cause loss of hair. In most cases, this is temporary, though sometimes the hair does not grow back or grows back only thinly. Radiotherapy in childhood (and occasionally in adulthood) may affect the intelligence (IQ) and some other mental functions. However, because the treatment may often lead to a cure, it is important not to give too low a dose. The radiation oncologist will always try to select a dose that is large enough to give a good chance of curing the cancer, but small enough to minimize any negative effect on the child's intellect. These are matters for detailed discussion between you and the radiation oncologist, as the individual circumstances play a major part in determining the best type of treatment.

Treatment of Primary Brain Tumors in Childhood

Medulloblastoma These tumors occur at the back part of the brain, and if possible all or most of the tumor should be removed surgically. If that is feasible, then usually radiotherapy and in certain cases chemotherapy may be recommended afterward. If the tumor is large or has already spread, or if there is thought to be a high risk of spread, chemotherapy is recommended. There is a very good chance of a cure if all of the tumor can be removed and if therapy is given afterward. More than half of the children with this tumor will be cured.

Treatment of Primary Brain Tumors in Adults

Treatment of primary brain tumors in adults usually consists of surgical removal if that is feasible. The neurosurgeon will always try to remove the cancer completely if it can be done without major damage to the surrounding normal areas of the brain. In many circumstances, radiotherapy is given after surgery. Additional chemotherapy is not often curative but may prolong survival. Drugs such as **procarbazine**, **vincristine**, and the **nitrosoureas** may be recommended following radiotherapy. New drugs and new methods of giving established drugs are being investigated and may warrant consideration.

Lymphomas of the Brain or Spinal Cord

In general, surgery is not a major part of the treatment of lymphoma of the CNS, although it may be needed to make the diagnosis in the first place.

Usually the treatment consists of radiotherapy and chemotherapy. The exact type of treatment depends on the type of lymphoma and whether or not there is also lymphoma elsewhere in the body. Chemotherapy is usually essential if there is lymphoma elsewhere, and nowadays it may be recommended in many cases of primary lymphomas of the CNS as well. The intensity and duration of the chemotherapy vary depending on the individual circumstances, so the exact schedule and length of treatment will need to be determined in consultation with your doctor.

Secondary Cancers in the Brain or Spinal Cord

Even with cancers in which the primary is not very sensitive to radiotherapy, the CNS secondaries may respond to some extent, and symptoms (particularly headache) may often be relieved with radiotherapy and, in certain cases, surgery, or both.

Spinal Cord Tumors

The treatment of spinal cord tumors is usually surgery, radiotherapy, or both.

Benign Tumors of the Brain: Meningiomas

The treatment of meningiomas is usually surgical, with the aim of removing the tumor as completely as possible. The chance of a recurrence depends on the completeness of the removal, so that the chance of recurrence is slightly higher with a tumor in a very inaccessible area. Radiotherapy may be recommended in a very few instances.

BREAST

Number of new cases diagnosed per year in the United States: 185,700

SUMMARY OF THE KEY FACTS IN THIS SECTION

- Breast cancer is quite common, and about 185,700 new cases are diagnosed each year.
- The main danger of breast cancer is that it may have a high tendency to spread elsewhere in the body.
- The chance of distant spread can be partly predicted from whether it has involved the lymph nodes or not, from the size of the tumor, and from tests done on it called **hormone receptors**.
- Treatment given after surgery and radiotherapy may reduce the chance of distant spread; this is called **adjuvant therapy**.
- The type of adjuvant therapy is determined by whether you have had your menopause or not and by hormone receptors on the cancer.
- Treatment of the primary tumor is by surgery, radiotherapy, or both. The exact type and combination of these treatments depends on the size of the tumor, the size of the breast, and your own preferences when there are options that are equivalent to each other.

The Most Important Features of the Tumor

Breast cancer is a common tumor. The most serious problem with it is that it may spread to distant parts of the body.

Cancer of the breast—unlike many other cancers, such as cancer of the lung—varies a lot from patient to patient in the way it behaves. In some patients it may behave very aggressively and can spread to distant parts of the body very quickly. In other patients it may not spread at all, even after many years. Although at present we cannot predict precisely which women have cancers that are going to spread, we have some clues and can give each patient at least an estimate of the chance of her cancer spreading.

If the cancer in the breast does not spread elsewhere, it is quite often cured by surgery (which in certain circumstances may be limited in extent and leave much of the breast undisturbed). If the breast cancer has spread to the lymph nodes in the armpit at the time of diagnosis, however, it does have a higher tendency to spread later to other parts of the body, and that is serious. The good news is that in cases where the chance of spread is higher, some systemic treatment after surgery (with either hormone therapy or chemotherapy) can decrease that chance of spread. Hence what we know and can predict about breast cancer allows doctors to some extent to match the treatment to the individual patient and her cancer.

Age and Incidence

The chance of developing breast cancer increases with age. It is very rare before the thirties, begins to increase in incidence in the forties, and becomes more common in the fifties and beyond.

Is There an Epidemic of Breast Cancer?

You will often hear that *"one woman in nine will develop breast cancer"* (this figure actually refers to the risk that a female baby has at birth of developing breast cancer by the age of approximately ninety). Many people are worried that a few years ago that figure seemed to be one in twelve. There is, therefore, a widespread fear that breast cancer is becoming much more common. The brief answer is that breast cancer is becoming a little bit, but not much, more common. Once the incidence has been adjusted for age, it has increased by about 1 percent per year. Some of this increase, however, may be accounted for by the diagnosis of early lesions in successful screening programs, which means that the cancer seems to be more common but is actually being detected earlier. If that is true, we may see the incidence decrease or level off in the next few years, and there is some early evidence that that is beginning to happen already.

Causes

No one knows what causes breast cancer. We do know that, by and large, breast cancer is much more common in countries that have a Western lifestyle than in the developing countries. However, we do not know precisely what it is about the lifestyle in these countries that causes women to develop breast cancer. There is some evidence to suggest that it is partly due to our diet, particularly to the higher proportion of fat in what we eat. But that will remain an educated guess until more research has been completed. Even though we don't know exactly how breast cancer is caused, we do know some of the things that make an individual woman more liable than the average woman in her country to develop breast cancer. Several of these risk factors for breast cancer are listed in Table 4.2.

Close Relatives with Breast Cancer Among the proven risk factors for breast cancer, the most important is a history of breast cancer or ovarian cancer in the family. I stress that it is **only breast cancer and (probably) ovarian cancer in the family that matters**. If your mother or father had cancer of the lung or larynx or of some other site, that will not increase your chances of getting breast cancer. That may sound obvious, but cancer of any type in the family does cause considerable worry about the chance of inheriting it (see Chapter 3). Furthermore, it is only if *close* relatives had or have breast cancer that usually matters, and that means your mother, sister, or daughter. Aunts, cousins, and other distant relatives do not for the most part affect your chance of getting breast cancer. In a *very few* families, it may be relevant if a male relative has had prostate cancer, but such cases are rare.

TABLE 4.2: FACTORS THAT INCREASE THE CHANCE OF GETTING BREAST CANCER	
RISK FACTOR	**AMOUNT OF INCREASED RISK**
Breast or ovary cancer in a close family member—sister, mother, or daughter—especially if the breast cancer was in both breasts or was diagnosed at a young age	May increase the chance quite markedly
Never been pregnant or first pregnancy after the age of eighteen or so	Slight increase
Early start to menstruation (early menarche) and late menopause	Slight increase
A previous biopsy of a breast lump if it showed certain features under the microscope (atypical hyperplasia)	Moderate increase, particularly if associated with breast cancer in the family
The presence of an abnormal form of the BRCA1 or BRCA2 gene (applies to 5–10 percent of all breast cancer)	See text

Age at First Pregnancy The second risk factor is the age at which you had your first pregnancy. Women who have their first child early—and that means (in this context) before the age of eighteen or so—have a lower chance of developing breast cancer. We don't know why that is, but there is some evidence to suggest that the hormonal changes that accompany a full-term pregnancy in some way offer a degree of protection against breast cancer. Of course, having a child before the age of eighteen has very serious consequences of its own, for example, on the mother's education, her need for social support, and so on. Furthermore, the protection against breast cancer from an early pregnancy is only partial. In other words, an early pregnancy doesn't decrease the chance of breast cancer by very much—it's a "weak protector," not a "total preventer." Hence no woman should have her first child in her teens unless that is what she wants to do anyway.

Breast Feeding Breast feeding a baby also offers a small amount of protection against breast cancer. Again, this has a weak protective effect, and some research suggests that even this is not noticeable unless breast feeding has continued for several years. Nevertheless, women who have breast-fed an infant for a long time, possibly several years, do decrease their chances of breast cancer by a small amount.

A Previous Breast Lump That Had Atypical Changes Lumps in the breast are very common indeed. Most benign (that is, noncancerous) lumps in the younger age group are caused by benign tumors called **fibroadenomas**, which are common and pose no risk to health at all. In the older age group, noncancerous breast lumps are more likely to be caused by benign **cysts**—little, hollow, bead-like spaces in the breast filled with fluid. These are also of no risk to health.

The question *"Do ordinary benign breast lumps turn cancerous eventually?"* is, however, one of the most important in breast cancer research. It now seems that the answer to that question is *"Most ordinary breast lumps do not increase the chance of getting cancer later."* However, if under the microscope the benign breast lump showed certain changes that are called **atypical hyperplasia**, there seems to be a slight increase in the chance that the woman will later develop breast cancer. Although that particular lump will have been removed, we believe that atypical hyperplasia is a sign of instability in the breast generally; thus there is a greater than average chance that later on another part of the breast (or a part of the other breast) will develop a cancer. Again, this increase in risk does *not* mean that if you have had a biopsy that showed atypical hyperplasia, you *will* get a breast cancer later. It merely means that you should make sure that your breasts are checked regularly by your doctor (with mammography if recommended).

Recently Identified Genes Called BRCA1 and BRCA2 The two recently discovered genes BRCA1 and BRCA2 are present in probably fewer than one in ten women with breast cancer. When they are present, however, they indicate that the woman has a very high risk of later developing breast cancer. This research is still very new, but it suggests that (in the future), in families with a high incidence of breast or ovarian cancer, there may be value in testing unaffected individuals to see if they have either of these genes, which may indicate a high risk.

Can Breast Cancer Be Caused by Contraceptive Pills?

Many people ask whether breast cancer can be caused by the birth control pill (or BCP) and are confused by a large number of articles in newspapers and magazines on this subject. The answer is: contraceptive pills probably do not contribute to the development of breast cancer, and certainly do not if you take the pills for fewer than ten years. Furthermore, it is the dose of estrogen in the tablet that counts, and manufacturers have been putting less and less estrogen in BCPs over the last ten or so years. If you have been taking, or have taken, a BCP for fewer than ten years, there is no evidence that your chance of breast cancer is increased. In fact, there is some evidence that your chance of ovarian cancer may be decreased (that is, taking the BCP for fewer than ten years may reduce your risk of developing cancer of the ovary by up to one half). There is less clear evidence about taking the BCP for more than ten years, although there is a slight indication that taking the BCP for ten or more years increases the chance of breast cancer by a small amount. At present, we can say that any risk from contraceptive pills is very small, may be nonexistent, and comes into the picture only if you take the pills for more than ten years.

There is some recent evidence that suggests that the prolonged use of any estrogen therapy (including hormone replacement therapy) may increase the risk of breast cancer after many years. As with BCPs, use of estrogen for five years does not seem to increase risk, but there may be an increase after that. This situation is still unclear as the evidence is conflicting, and more research is needed before clear recommendations can be made.

This discussion of risk factors notwithstanding, **the majority of patients — nearly two-thirds — with breast cancer have no identifiable risk factors.** In other words, at present, at least two out of three cases of breast cancer seem (as far as we can tell) to be purely random or chance events.

How the Cancer Tends to Spread

In slightly less than two-thirds of cases, the breast cancer will not spread and therefore will be cured by surgery (with or without radiotherapy). If the cancer does spread, it is probably spread by the bloodstream, although we are not yet certain exactly how. We do know that the lymph nodes in the armpit are signals, or markers, of whether the ability of a particular breast cancer to spread is high or low. If the lymph nodes are not involved, the chance of spread is relatively low. If the lymph nodes are involved, the chance of spread is higher (although the cancer almost certainly does not spread from the lymph nodes themselves). If it does spread, it may spread to bone, the liver, or a lung, or sometimes other places such as the spinal cord or the brain.

Symptoms or Problems That You May Notice

Probably the most common way in which a woman (or her partner) finds a cancer in the breast is through feeling a lump in the breast, for example, while washing in the bath or shower. In a lot of cases, the lump has not caused any particular symptoms or problems but seems to appear quite suddenly (*"It wasn't there last week"*). To avoid causing any undue alarm, let me repeat that lumps in the breast are very common indeed, and **most lumps in the breast are not cancer!** But, of course, because of the risk of cancer, any woman finding a lump in her breast should see her doctor promptly. ("Promptly" means within a few days. It's not a middle-of-the-night medical emergency, but it should not be left for a month or more.)

Can a Woman Identify a Lump in Her Breast as Cancer?

Obviously it would save a great deal of worry and concern if a woman could reliably distinguish between ordinary (benign, noncancerous) breast lumps and cancer. Unfortunately, it is not easy to do so. There's not much that reliably distinguishes between benign lumps and cancer (see Table 4.3). Most cancers of the breast do not cause any specific symptoms or problems. Sometimes a cancer of the breast may cause a slight ache or tingling within it, but benign cysts in the breast are actually more likely to cause discomfort or pain than a cancer is. One important feature, however, is an inward-pointing nipple. If a cancer happens to arise near the nipple, it may cause the nipple to be drawn inward (the medical term is inverted), and that almost never happens with benign lumps. If one or both of your nipples have been inverted since puberty and you can evert them (pull them outward) easily, then don't worry at all. Nipples that have been inverted since puberty and can be everted easily are normal. It is only if one nipple becomes inverted later in your life and cannot be everted easily that there is a suspicion of a cancer near it. Very occasionally, too, a cancer may cause bleeding from the nipple or a discharge that contains blood or rust-colored material; but, as with pain, although cancers cause this occasionally, most cases of bleeding from the nipple are caused by benign problems rather than cancer. Sometimes you may also notice that the skin over the lump is dimpled or seems to be tethered to the lump when you move your arm. Again, that is not very common, but it may be indicative of cancer, so any

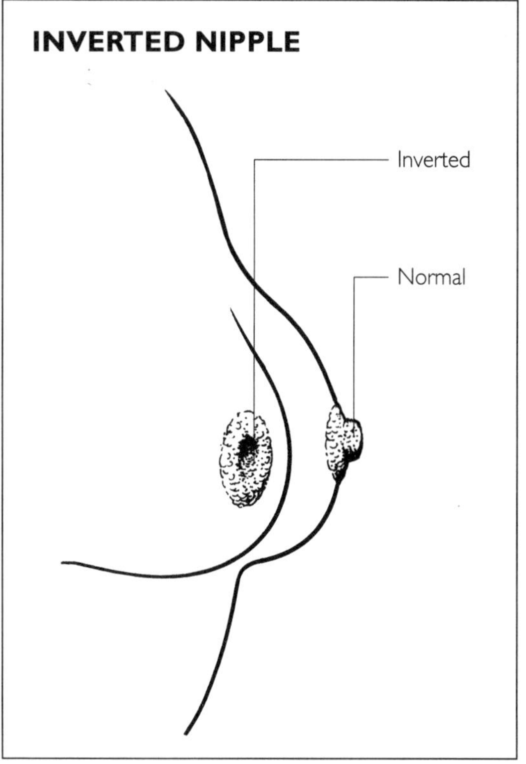

TABLE 4.3: SYMPTOMS THAT MAY HAPPEN WITH BREAST CANCER
A lump in the breast, often without any symptoms related to it, but sometimes with: • indrawing ("inversion") of the nipple • ache or pain around the lump • bleeding or blood-stained discharge from the nipple • dimpling of the skin over the lump or the skin looking somewhat like the peel of an orange
The whole breast may suddenly go red and feel hot (very rare)
A mammogram showing a lump when there is nothing detectable in the breast

dimpling or tethering of the skin (even if you don't see or feel a lump underneath it) should be checked by your doctor.

In very rare cases, the **whole breast may suddenly go red** and feel hot and swollen. This looks like an infection (such as can occur after breast feeding), but may be a rare form of breast cancer called **inflammatory breast cancer** for which the treatment is somewhat different from the usual approach.

To reiterate an important rule: **any breast lump (with or without any of the symptoms that I've mentioned) should be assessed by your doctor promptly**.

Finally, nowadays quite a number of cancers of the breast are first detected by routine screening using X rays of the breast (**mammography**). Women who have regular screening (as I discuss later) may have a mammogram that shows a cancer or something that might be a cancer, even when there is no lump detectable in the breast and there are no symptoms. Obviously it is very distressing to be told that there is (or may be) a cancer in your breast when you thought you were symptom-free; but you can take some comfort from the fact that tumors detected by mammography are usually very small and have an excellent outcome. And, of course, most abnormalities shown on a mammogram will turn out to be benign and noncancerous.

Diagnosis and Tests

Whether a lump in the breast is first detected by the woman herself, by a mammogram, or by a doctor at a routine checkup, the standard advice is that every breast lump should be assessed and then, depending on the age of the woman, either removed or observed closely. In many cases, any abnormality in the mammogram will be further investigated by an **ultrasound**, which can show whether the area is a solid lump or is a cyst.

In the younger age group, the chance that a lump will be malignant is very low. The great majority of lumps are fibroadenomas (see above) in the breast, which are quite normal and of no concern. In the somewhat older age group, lumps are more likely to be benign cysts. In both cases, the lump is likely to fluctuate in size with the menstrual cycle and may disappear. If a cyst is particularly prominent, it may be drained by your doctor using a fine needle (a procedure that is almost painless), and the fluid can be sent for analysis to ensure that there are no cancer cells in it. If the cyst doesn't recur and the fluid has no cancer cells in it, no further action is needed.

In the older age group, or if your doctor thinks the lump feels or appears suspicious in some way, then almost certainly a biopsy will be recommended. That can be done with a special needle on an outpatient basis or as a minor surgical operation using a local anesthetic or a brief general anesthetic, depending on your doctor's usual practice or your preferences. Sometimes (particularly if the abnormality on the mammogram is small) the biopsy is done in the X-ray department using a special needle under X-ray guidance to make sure the exact area of abnormality is sampled.

If the biopsy does show cancer of the breast, in most cases your surgeon will recommend two things to you: surgery on the breast to remove the tumor and removal of some of the lymph nodes in the armpit to see whether or not the cancer has spread there. There are several exceptions to this general rule, which I discuss in the next section.

If the biopsy of the breast lump does show cancer, a set of routine tests may be recommended in certain cases to make sure that the cancer has not spread anywhere else (for example, to the liver or the bones). Most women find the thought of these tests very alarming and are worried that their doctor has detected something sinister and isn't telling them. However, they are truly routine, and if it is recommended that you have them, please don't interpret that as a sign of doom.

In addition to the scans and X rays, there are blood tests (markers) used at some cancer centers that may be of value not only at the time of diagnosis but afterward during treatment (if it is needed) and follow-up.

The Main Types of the Cancer: Invasive and Noninvasive

Cancer of the breast can be classified in many different ways, based on what the pathologist sees under the microscope. Not all of the identifiable differences affect the way the cancer behaves, and therefore many of these features aren't very important to the patient's treatment and to the future. However, there is one basic feature that does make a difference: whether the cancer is invasive or not. Cancer of the breast begins either inside one of the tubes or ducts of the breast or within the balloon-like structures (lobules) at the ends of those ducts.

STRUCTURE OF THE NORMAL BREAST

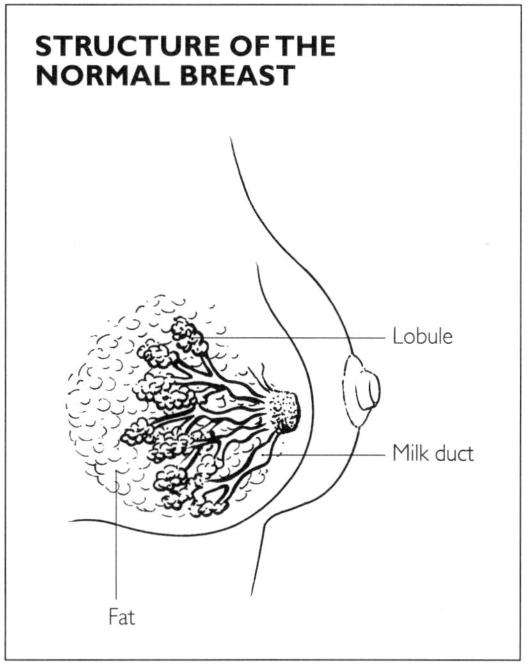

With cancer of the invasive type, the pathologist can see the cancer going through the wall of the duct or through the lobule out into the surrounding breast tissue. So "invasive breast cancer" means cancer that is spreading out of the duct or out of the lobule. In fact, most breast cancers are of the invasive type. However, some cancers stay within the duct or within the lobule, and they are called **carcinomas *in situ*,** meaning that they do not seem to be invasive. In the classification of breast cancer, there are two main types of noninvasive *in situ* cancer: **intraductal carcinoma** and **lobular carcinoma *in situ*.** They behave differently from the more common, invasive cancers and may not cause any trouble once they have been removed. They are also treated differently from the usual, invasive types of cancer and will be dealt with in a separate section.

If the cancer is invasive, the exact type and the microscopic classification of the cancer does not usually make a great deal of difference.

Factors That Influence the Treatment and Prognosis

There are two crucial questions in deciding what treatment is best in each case of breast cancer. First, is the chance of distant spread high or low? And second, what can be done to reduce that chance? The chance of distant spread will influence not only your doctor's recommendations but also your own choices about treatment options. If a particular cancer has a high chance of spreading to distant parts of the body, and if treatment can reduce that chance, your doctor will recommend that treatment more strongly, and you may be more likely to accept that treatment. If the chance of spread is low (and therefore the chance that you have already been cured by your operation is very high), you may be less motivated to accept more treatment. Although we cannot at present tell every woman with breast cancer whether her particular cancer will or will not spread, we can at least give some estimate of whether the chance of spread is high or low. At present, three features of breast cancer are routinely used to help in that prediction (see Table 4.4). Those three features are: whether or not the cancer has spread to the **lymph nodes** in the armpit (and if so, to how many of them), the **size** of the primary tumor, and whether the tumor is sensitive to hormones (these are the **hormone receptor** tests—the estrogen receptor test and the progesterone receptor test). There are additional tests that may help predict whether the cancer will spread or not (including certain appearances seen under the microscope such as invasion into lymph vessels, tests that show how many cells are actually multiplying at the time, and some others). At present these additional tests are still being evaluated and are not in routine use in every cancer center or clinic.

The Main Objectives of Treatment

Once a breast lump has been shown by biopsy to be a cancer, there are three main objectives to treatment. The first is to **remove the primary tumor** from the

TABLE 4.4: FACTORS THAT HELP PREDICT THE CHANCE THAT BREAST CANCER WILL SPREAD

FACTOR	NOTES
Whether the tumor has spread to the lymph nodes in the armpit	The number of lymph nodes involved is important here.
The size of the original breast tumor	This refers to the size as measured once it has been removed—the apparent size before the operation may be misleading.
Laboratory tests on the tumor for hormone receptors	These tests may not always be done, particularly if the original tumor was very small.
If the original cancer was inflammatory in type	See the "Symptoms or Problems" part of this section.
Other tests (S-phase, cathepsin D, invasion of lymph vessels, grade)	These are some of the different tests that can be done on the original tumor, but they are not yet universally accepted as predictive of spread.

breast, leaving the breast as undisturbed as possible. The second objective is to reduce the chance that the cancer will return in the breast or the armpit (known as **local recurrence**) using radiotherapy to the breast and, in certain cases, the armpit. The third objective is to reduce the chances that the cancer will establish secondaries elsewhere in the body (known as **distant spread**). Research studies over the last two decades have shown conclusively that when the chance of distant spread is high, treatment given after surgery may decrease that chance. Treatment, and selecting the right type of treatment, are therefore very, important.

Types of Treatment

The first three sections that follow all refer to the invasive types of breast cancer (by far the most common types). Because the noninvasive in situ cancers behave so differently from the invasive types, they are dealt with in a separate (fourth) section.

Surgery

Synopsis

The first objective of surgery for breast cancer is to remove the primary tumor from the breast. For the smaller tumors, we now know that it is as effective to do a less extensive operation that removes the tumor and some of the surrounding breast tissue, but leaves most of the remaining breast tissue undisturbed.

Lumpectomy with Radiation Therapy or Mastectomy

An operation in which the whole breast is removed (including the nipple) is called a **mastectomy**. Most commonly, at the time of this operation some of the lymph nodes from the armpit will be removed as well, so that they can be examined to see if the cancer has spread to them or not. Usually a mastectomy plus sampling of the lymph nodes is referred to as a **modified radical mastectomy** (because it was devised as a less mutilating and less extensive modification of an operation originally invented in 1894). There are other names for this operation, and there are variations on it depending which (if any) areas of muscle are removed as well. When a surgeon refers to a modified radical mastectomy, however, he or she means a single operation, with a single incision in which the breast and some of the armpit nodes are removed. Because of the removal of the breast, in the majority of cases radiotherapy is not needed after the operation. In many centers nowadays, after the mastectomy a second operation can be done to reconstruct the breast, and I discuss that under "Reconstructive Surgery" below.

In certain circumstances, an operation less extensive than the modified radical mastectomy may be used. In many cases, but not all, it is possible to remove the cancer and some surrounding breast tissue while leaving most or some of the rest of the breast undisturbed, and it has been shown that this type of surgery does not reduce the chance of long-term survival. This operation is usually called a **partial mastectomy** (or sometimes a **segmental mastectomy** or a **lumpectomy**, depending on exactly what is done). This operation normally leaves the nipple undisturbed (unless the cancer is very close to it). In most circumstances, however, the lymph nodes in the armpit have to be sampled through a separate incision. Thus, if you have a partial mastectomy, you will usually require two incisions, one for the breast cancer and another for the nodes. Furthermore, many research studies have now proven that after a partial mastectomy you should receive radiotherapy to the breast (and sometimes nodal areas as well) to reduce the chance of local recurrence. This means that in considering a partial mastectomy, you should be aware that you will be recommended to have radiotherapy after it.

Which Is the Right Operation for You?

There are four basic situations with regard to surgery for breast cancer. First, with tumors that are small enough and situated in an accessible part of the breast, the less extensive partial mastectomy operation can be done (accompanied by lymph

TYPES OF MASTECTOMY

Lumpectomy

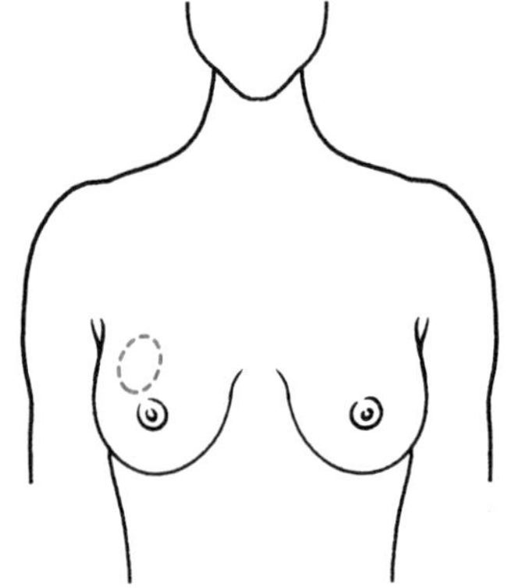

Partial Mastectomy

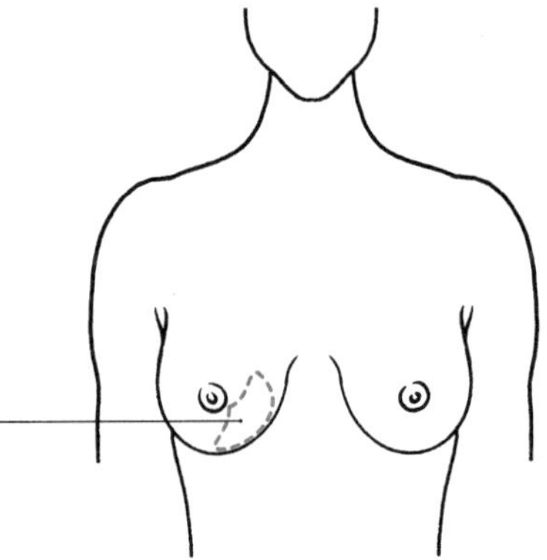

Partial or segmental mastectomy (depending on how much breast tissue is removed). In most cases, removal of the lymph nodes in the armpit will be done at the same time through a separate incision.

Modified Radical Mastectomy

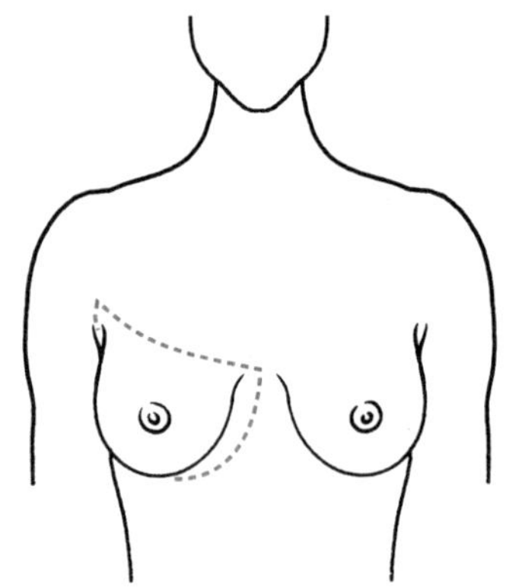

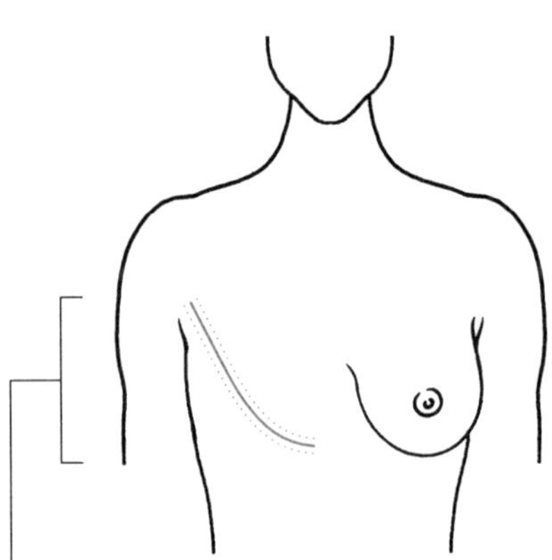

All of the breast tissue is removed (simple or total mastectomy), as well as many of the lymph nodes in the armpit.

node sampling and followed by radiotherapy). Second, with some tumors that are too large relative to the size of the breast or that are situated in a difficult position, a partial mastectomy cannot be done and the only operation that is technically possible is a mastectomy. Third, in many situations either of these operations could be done, and the choice will be made after discussions between you and your doctor. While many women prefer the less extensive partial mastectomy, many others prefer the mastectomy, either because they do not have to have radiotherapy afterward (thus avoiding many trips to the hospital) or for psychological reasons. Fourth, in a few cases the primary cancer cannot be removed for technical reasons. For example, it may be stuck to the chest wall underneath, or there may be other medical reasons that make the operation hazardous.

In your discussions with your doctor, make sure you understand which of these situations most closely resembles yours; and if you are in the third group, try to make sure that your doctor understands your preferences.

Reconstructive Surgery

After a mastectomy, it is often possible to reconstruct the breast area so that to some extent the contour and the cosmetic appearance of the previous breast are partly restored. This is quite a specialized procedure, and at present not every patient who has a mastectomy will have a surgeon nearby who can do this. There are several different methods of reconstruction, and your surgeon will explain the particular method that he or she uses. The reconstruction can be done using a flap of muscles from the abdomen, side, or back. Another method uses implants that are put in under the skin. These are breast-shaped bags made of synthetic material that can be filled with liquid; some of them can be filled progressively over a period of weeks or months so that the contour can be adjusted to match the other breast and the skin and other tissues have time to adapt. The nipple can be reconstructed, often using skin grafted from the other nipple, or sometimes using a tattoo. It may often be best to have reconstructive surgery several months after the original surgery, when the tissues in the area have settled down. You and your surgeon can then plan the operation effectively and with a clear idea of the likely result. In some centers, reconstruction is often done soon after the primary surgery or at the same time.

Radiotherapy

Radiotherapy is an important part of treatment in many cases. It is a local treatment; it can treat only the area where the radiation goes. This means that it may be effective and useful in breast cancer where local recurrence may be a problem. If there is a moderate (or greater) chance that local recurrence will occur, radiotherapy is used to decrease that chance. Radiotherapy will usually be recommended for all patients who have had a partial mastectomy and for certain patients who have had a mastectomy if there are features of the particular tumor that made local recurrence more likely than average.

Radiotherapy can be given to the breast and chest wall or (in certain cases) to the armpit and other areas that have lymph nodes in them, or to all these areas. The exact details of the radiotherapy needed in your case will be discussed with you by your radiation oncologist, but usually it involves having a daily treatment, five days a week, for about five weeks. Sometimes brachytherapy (see Chapter 5) may be used as well.

Adjuvant Therapy after the Surgery

The real problem with breast cancer is that it can spread to other parts of the body, and a great deal of research has shown that where the chance of distant spread is high, it can be reduced by giving systemic therapy after surgery. Treatment given to reduce the chance of such distant spread is called **adjuvant** treatment. The exact type of adjuvant therapy recommended will depend on three things: first, whether you have had your menopause or are still having menstrual periods; second, whether the cancer had hormone receptors on it when it was tested; and third (when there are several options to be considered), your own feelings and preferences. This is a very complex subject to summarize (and a lot of research is still going on). In brief, the important points are the following.

If the Lymph Nodes Were Involved

If the lymph nodes in the armpit did have cancer in some of them, there is a clear benefit (in terms of preventing recurrence and increasing survival) from having therapy. If you have had your menopause (are **postmenopausal**) and the cancer did have hormone receptors on it when tested, that therapy is usually a hormone therapy (sometimes with chemotherapy as well). If you are postmenopausal and the cancer did not have receptors on it, usually chemotherapy will be recommended. If you have not had your menopause (are **premenopausal**), chemotherapy will probably be recommended.

Hormone Therapy The most usual form of hormone therapy is a tablet called **tamoxifen**, which is taken once a day for five years (usually). Side effects from this tablet are relatively rare and mild; the commonest problem is hot flashes, very similar to those experienced during menopause. Some patients also experience mild nausea, and some have an increase in body weight. Others have generalized symptoms such as feeling tired. In most cases, if these symptoms are present, they decrease after a few months. Long-term treatment (over several years) with tamoxifen has been shown to carry a slightly increased risk of abnormalities in the lining of the uterus, including some cancerous changes.

Chemotherapy In premenopausal patients where the lymph nodes were involved, chemotherapy is usually recommended using combinations such as **cyclophosphamide**, **methotrexate**, and **5-fluorouracil** (**CMF**) or **cyclophosphamide**, **Adriamycin**, and **5-fluorouracil** (**FAC**). Usually six months of treatment are given, but the duration can vary a bit depending on your individual circumstances.

If you are postmenopausal and your cancer did not have hormone receptors on it (or in quite a few other circumstances), chemotherapy may be recommended.

CMF and FAC are not the only treatments there are. Depending on your individual circumstances, your doctor may discuss other types of treatment with you. If your particular cancer is unusual in any way (for instance, involving a large number of lymph nodes), your doctor may discuss using newer investigational types of treatment (again, see Chapter 5).

If the Lymph Nodes Were Not Involved

If the lymph nodes were not involved and you have had your menopause, and if the tumor had hormone receptors, you will probably be recommended to take tamoxifen for several years.

If you are premenopausal, the best type of treatment is still being defined. There is no doubt that chemotherapy used for premenopausal lymph-node-negative breast cancer does have some benefit. However, some people in this situation do not require chemotherapy. The difficulty at the moment is in deciding who among the people with node-negative breast cancer is at the highest risk for recurrence. In other words, current research is trying to identify those people among the "low-risk" group who have the highest risk. While we are waiting for the answers on this issue, some centers recommend chemotherapy to all node-negative people; other centers recommend chemotherapy only if the cancer appears to have been particularly aggressive (if it was very large, or if it was seen to be invading into lymph vessels when examined under the microscope). This is an area in which current practice is changing rapidly, and you will need to have a detailed discussion with your doctor about what he or she is recommending for you. You are also likely to be asked if you would be willing to participate in a clinical trial or new types of treatment (see page 233).

Treatment of the Noninvasive in Situ Types

Noninvasive cancers rarely (if ever) spread, which is very good. Curiously enough, however, that makes deciding on the best type of treatment more difficult. The problem is that noninvasive cancer increases your chance of getting invasive cancer later in life, so the purpose of treatment is primarily to prevent problems with a future invasive cancer. There are three basic approaches: to do a simple mastectomy and remove the breast; to give radiotherapy to the breast; or to monitor the breast with regular mammograms. At the moment, there is a small amount of evidence that radiotherapy is beneficial in some types of noninvasive cancer, but certainly a mastectomy is one option that you and your doctor should discuss, as is the use of regular mammograms. In particular, when you discuss the situation, your doctor may be able to give you some idea of the chance of your getting an invasive cancer later on.

Therapy If the Cancer Comes Back

In about two-thirds of cases, the cancer will not come back, and the surgery (with or without radiotherapy, if needed) will have been curative. In some cases, though, despite good surgery and adjuvant treatment, the breast cancer will recur. It may recur near the original operation (in the breast, in the scar, on the chest wall, or in the armpit), and that is called a **local** recurrence. It may also spread to other areas such as the bones, lungs, or liver, a situation that is more serious. There are two very important things you should be aware of. First, local recurrence does *not* mean you are definitely going to get distant spread. Although this doesn't sound possible (and many patients have great difficulty believing it), nevertheless it is true. If you get a recurrence in the breast or armpit, it does not necessarily mean that spread to other parts of your body is inevitable. In fact, if the initial operation was a partial mastectomy, and there is recurrence in the breast, further surgery (a second partial mastectomy or a simple mastectomy depending on the circumstances), sometimes with radiotherapy, may be curative. Second, even if it happens that cure is not possible, local recurrence and distant spread are treatable in the majority of cases. In other words, the chance of controlling the cancer is quite high. This is a situation that will need quite a lot of discussion between you and your doctor, but depending on the exact circumstances, radiotherapy, hormone therapy, chemotherapy (including drugs such as **Taxol** and **Taxotere**), and surgery may all have something to contribute, depending on where the problem is and what your symptoms are. The important point is to be aware that, with distant spread of breast cancer (unlike many other cancers), there is a great deal that can be done, even though, unfortunately, cure is rarely possible.

Cancer of the Male Breast

Cancer of the male breast is quite rare. In fact, it makes up less than 1 percent of all breast cancer. It tends to occur in later adulthood (in older age groups than female breast cancer) and is very rare below the age of forty or so. It is treated by removal of the breast tissue (also called, as in the female, a mastectomy), usually with lymph node sampling. By and large it usually behaves and is treated in the same ways as cancer of the female breast, although it is more often positive for hormone receptors, and so hormone therapy is used frequently. If there is recurrence, then tamoxifen can be used, as can other methods of altering the hormonal balance.

Screening and Early Diagnosis

In an ideal world, it would be possible to detect any form of trouble, particularly a common and potentially serious problem such as breast cancer, at a stage at which it could be dealt with and cured easily. Unfortunately, we are still a long way from that goal. In terms of screening, perhaps the most important point is that all women should be examined by a doctor at least annually. If you have never had breast cancer, then that doctor does not have to be a breast specialist (your gynecologist may be the right person, for example), but nowadays breast cancer screening centers are becoming much more common and are very useful in planning routine tests and giving advice.

The three most important elements in screening are assessment by your doctor, mammography (X ray of the breast), and breast self-examination (BSE).

Mammograms Although there has been some controversy over exactly which tests should be done and when, research now proves conclusively that mammograms are useful as part of the evaluation after the age of fifty and not before (unless the breasts are difficult to examine because of their large size or unusual lumpiness). We also know that, below the age of thirty, mammograms are of little value because the breast tissue appears so dense on the X ray that any suspicious areas cannot be seen. In addition, if one of your first-degree relatives has had breast cancer (mother, sister, or daughter), then you should have your first mammogram when you are ten years younger than your relative was when she had the breast cancer diagnosed. For women in the forty-to-fifty age group, at present it is not easy to make firm recommendations. Over the next few years we will have more information and may be able to state in which cases routine mammography is useful. One final point: ultrasound is useful as a test only after a mammogram has shown a suspicious area; it is of no value as a screening test. If you are in doubt about anything in this section, consult your family doctor, your local screening center, or the nearest branch of your Cancer Society.

Breast Self-Examination (BSE) There is no doubt that BSE is in general a good thing to do, although there is still some controversy about whether you should think of it as essential. Although it definitely can help in the detection of some cancers, it can be a cause of some alarm and concern. Of course, if you find a lump in a breast, you should see your doctor. Many women find doing BSE very difficult and then feel guilty that they are not doing it. Most specialists now say that if you can do it properly, go ahead, but if you can't bring yourself to do it don't feel guilty, as it is very far from being an infallible screening test. If you want to do it, get a brochure from your local Cancer Society or screening center and do the BSE properly and regularly. BSE is most beneficial when a woman does it regularly and gets to know what her breasts are like so that she can recognize any changes early on.

CANCER WITH NO KNOWN PRIMARY SITE

Number of new cases diagnosed per year in the United States: 45,230

SUMMARY OF THE KEY FACTS IN THIS SECTION

- Quite often a secondary cancer will appear (in a lymph node, for example, or on a chest X ray) with no sign of where the primary cancer is. This is called a cancer of unknown primary site, or CUP for short.
- In many cases, the primary source of the CUP will be found by special tests on the secondary and/or by X rays, scans, or endoscopy.
- In some of these cases the cancer can be cured or a remission can be produced.
- If the primary cancer cannot be identified, the situation is unlikely to be curable, and treatment should be directed at relieving symptoms or preventing them. A decision to undertake therapy such as chemotherapy should be made only after detailed discussions with your specialist.

The Most Important Features of the Tumor

A secondary cancer can appear in a lymph node or some other organ when there is no clue, even after several tests, as to where the primary cancer is. In some cases the primary source can be detected with one or more tests (see below), and in some of those cases, even though the cancer has spread, the patient can be cured. In some others there is a good chance of obtaining a remission.

In many cases, however, after the treatable types of cancer have been ruled out as possible primary sites, the actual primary cancer will not be found. Such tumors are often referred to as **carcinomas of unknown primary** (usually abbreviated **CUP**). Over years of studying thousands of such cases, we have gained some idea which tests are worthwhile and which are not in the search for a treatable (or even curable) primary cancer. In general, if a curable or treatable primary cannot be found (see below), the secondary is most likely to have been caused by a small primary cancer in the lung (non–small-cell) or the digestive tract. This has implications for the objectives of treatment, as discussed below.

Because a CUP might be caused by one of several different types of cancer, this section of the book is organized in a slightly different way from the others. I first discuss the ways in which your medical team may look for the primary site, then the ways in which a CUP might first be detected (by you or by your doctors). Finally, I discuss some of the treatment options.

Looking for the Unknown Primary

We know that certain types of cancer have certain "preferred" locations when they spread to other parts of the body. That association (of a secondary in a particular area with a certain kind of primary) may incline your medical team to look for certain kinds of primary cancers rather than others. The following lists the main areas of the body in which a CUP is likely to be found and some of the possible primary cancers that may be the origin of the problem.

Lymph Nodes in the Neck If the first sign of a problem is found in a lymph node in the neck and a biopsy shows that it is a cancer, the primary site might be in the mouth, throat, larynx, or upper parts of the airways. It may also be in the thyroid.

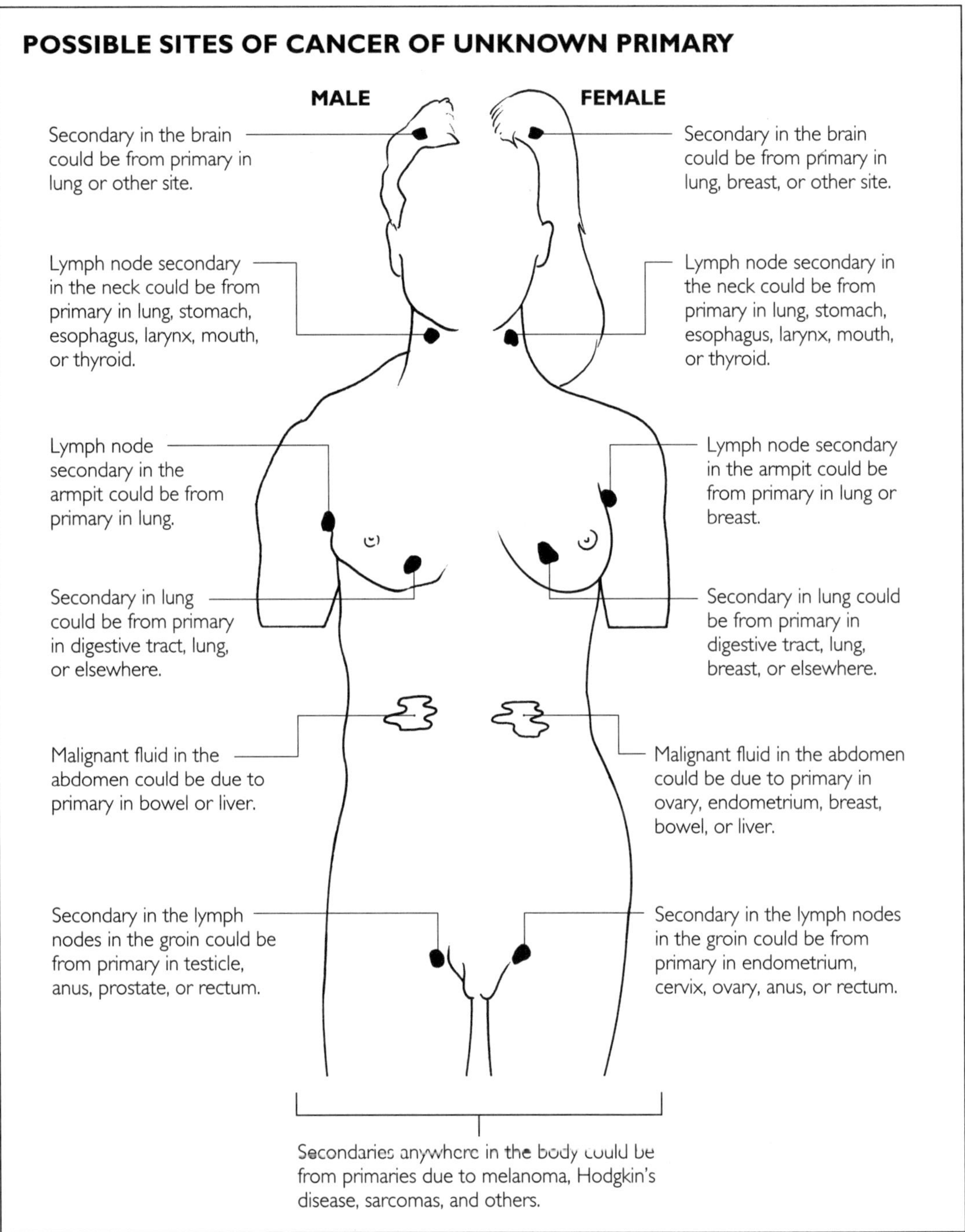
POSSIBLE SITES OF CANCER OF UNKNOWN PRIMARY
MALE
FEMALE
Secondary in the brain could be from primary in lung or other site.
Secondary in the brain could be from primary in lung, breast, or other site.
Lymph node secondary in the neck could be from primary in lung, stomach, esophagus, larynx, mouth, or thyroid.
Lymph node secondary in the neck could be from primary in lung, stomach, esophagus, larynx, mouth, or thyroid.
Lymph node secondary in the armpit could be from primary in lung.
Lymph node secondary in the armpit could be from primary in lung or breast.
Secondary in lung could be from primary in digestive tract, lung, or elsewhere.
Secondary in lung could be from primary in digestive tract, lung, breast, or elsewhere.
Malignant fluid in the abdomen could be due to primary in bowel or liver.
Malignant fluid in the abdomen could be due to primary in ovary, endometrium, breast, bowel, or liver.
Secondary in the lymph nodes in the groin could be from primary in testicle, anus, prostate, or rectum.
Secondary in the lymph nodes in the groin could be from primary in endometrium, cervix, ovary, anus, or rectum.
Secondaries anywhere in the body could be from primaries due to melanoma, Hodgkin's disease, sarcomas, and others.

Lymph Nodes in the Armpit In women, it is not rare for a cancer of the breast to spread to a lymph node in the armpit while the primary in the breast is undetectable. Studies show that in about half of women with cancerous lymph nodes in the armpit and no evidence of a primary, a primary cancer in the breast will be found in the next year or so. Most specialists would therefore recommend treatment as if there were a proven breast cancer. In men, an armpit node is most likely to be caused by a lung cancer, usually of the non–small-cell type.

A Shadow on a Chest X Ray A shadow on a chest X ray that on biopsy turns out to be a secondary is likely due to a primary in the lung (in an area where it is not visible) or in the bowel. Secondaries in the lung could be caused by many other types of cancer, however.

Fluid in the Abdomen (Ascites) If there are no signs of a primary cancer anywhere, ascites can be caused by cancer of the ovary, the cervix, or the endometrium in a woman or cancer of the bowel, liver, or pancreas in a man or woman.

Lymph Nodes in the Groin In women, cancer of the cervix, endometrium, vulva, ovary, or pelvis are possibilities; and in men and women, lymphomas, sarcomas, and cancer of the bowel are possible.

An Abnormality of a Liver Scan Secondary tumors in the liver are often caused by a primary cancer in the bowel, breast, or lung, although many other cancers can cause this as well.

"Generalized" Cancers Some cancers, such as lymphomas, sarcomas, and melanomas, can cause tumors almost anywhere. Tumors in the lymph nodes—in the neck, armpit, or elsewhere—could be due to one of these.

Tests That Might Help Decide Where the Primary Cancer Is

It is very important to find out whether there is or is not a curable or treatable cancer causing the secondary cancer. Germ-cell cancers, lymphomas, testicular cancers, choriocarcinomas, and thyroid, ovarian, prostate, lung (small-cell), laryngeal, oral, and other cancers can be treated and may in some cases be cured. Tests to determine the original source of the cancer are therefore an essential first step toward finding the appropriate treatment.

Pathology The appearance under the microscope of a secondary cancer (in a lymph node or the lung or liver, for example) often gives a clear indication of where the primary is. By definition, in the case of a CUP, that is not the case, and the tumor cells under the microscope usually look featureless and do not resemble, say, breast cells, lung cells, or whatever. In addition to a microscopic examination, the pathologist can do a variety of tests on the tumor. For instance, special stains can make visible certain proteins (antigens) on the surface of the tumor cells. In some cases, the presence of one of these proteins may provide strong evidence of where the tumor started. This procedure, called **immunohistochemistry**, can be very useful. For example, it can identify proteins in a group called the mammary mucins that are found mainly on breast cancer cells and more rarely on other cells. Other proteins that are found only on the surface of white cells strongly suggest that the tumor is a lymphoma. Similarly, other stains can show up the markers βHCG (beta human chorionic gonadotrophin) and AFP (alpha-fetoprotein), which suggest that the cancer is a germ-cell tumor. There are many other markers that can help diagnose a sarcoma, a brain tumor, prostate cancer, and so on. In addition to using immunohistochemistry, the pathologist can examine the tissue under an electron microscope. Often these tests are quite complicated and take several days, so, as I constantly say to my patients, a delay is not a sign of incompetence by your hospital.

Blood Tests In some cases the special tests done in the pathology department will reveal what the primary cancer is most likely to be. In cases where they do not, blood tests may help. The main blood tests are what are called markers. A marker that indicates an abnormal level of a protein in the blood called PSA (prostate-specific antigen) suggests prostate cancer; a high CEA (carcinoembryonic antigen) suggests bowel or breast cancer; a high AFP suggests liver cancer; a βHCG, a high AFP, or both suggests a germ-cell cancer, and so on.

Scans and X Rays In some cases, X rays and scans may also provide important information. For example, if the clinical picture suggests a lung cancer, a chest X ray is important; if there is involvement in a lymph node in the armpit in a female, mammograms are important; a lump in the neck may warrant scans of the thyroid, and so on.

Laryngoscopy and Endoscopy If the cancer is first detected in lymph nodes in the neck, your specialist will probably recommend a careful search for a possible cancer in the mouth, throat, larynx, pharynx, or esophagus. Usually this will require an examination of the throat and esophagus with a flexible endoscope (see the sections on cancer of the esophagus, mouth, and larynx).

What If the Primary Is Still "Unknown"?

If there is no evidence of one of the treatable or potentially curable tumors, locating the exact source of the primary cancer is not likely to be helpful to the patient. In other words, it is not helpful to do X rays of the bowel or a CT scan of the lungs if the patient has no symptoms, because if the primary is in the lung (non–small-cell) or bowel and has spread to, say, lymph nodes or the liver, proving that fact will not change the treatment. This may at first seem rather peculiar, but nevertheless it is true: if curable and treatable causes have been ruled out, then further exhaustive (and exhausting) tests will not help the patient.

If there is no evidence of a primary tumor, the treatment usually focuses on two things: the place in which the CUP first appeared and any symptoms that it may be causing. The likely treatment approaches, based on the way in which the tumor first appeared, are discussed below.

The Main Objectives of Treatment

The first objective is to find out if the primary cancer is curable or treatable, and if it is, to cure or treat as appropriate. If the situation is not curable or if the chance of a good remission is low, the objective of treatment must be the relief of symptoms or the prevention of symptoms or problems that are likely to develop. You and your doctors will have to discuss the potential risks and benefits of therapy in considerable detail to balance the potential advantages against the potential disadvantages.

Types of Treatment

Treatment of the Primary If the tests discussed above reveal the primary, then treatment will be recommended on the basis of the standard treatment for that particular primary. If the primary is undiscovered, the following treatments should be considered.

Radiotherapy This can be used effectively if the secondary cancer is causing discomfort or is likely to cause problems in the near future. Treatment of a secondary tumor for relief of symptoms is generally simpler than treatment of a primary and requires radiation to a smaller area of the body. Your radiation oncologist will discuss the details with you.

Chemotherapy Depending on your particular situation, your specialist may want to discuss with you the possibility of using a combination of drugs for the primary cancer that is most likely to be the cause. Or he or she may suggest a combination of drugs that are used in the treatment of CUPs. In general, only a fraction of true CUPs respond well to chemotherapy, so the decision to try chemotherapy is one you should make only after a thorough discussion of the pros and cons.

Surgery In a few circumstances (particularly if the tumor appears in lymph nodes in the neck), treatment with surgery and radiotherapy may be successful.

CERVIX

Number of new cases diagnosed per year in the United States: 15,700

SUMMARY OF THE KEY FACTS IN THIS SECTION

- Cancer of the cervix, and the precancerous changes that happen before it, can be reliably detected and monitored with the Pap test.
- Precancerous changes in the cervix, as well as the early stages of cancer of the cervix, can almost always be cured completely.
- Many of the factors that increase the risk of precancerous changes and cancer of the cervix are known (some of these factors are transmitted sexually), so prevention is a real possibility.

How This Section Is Organized

Because cancer of the cervix is, fortunately, so often detected before it has developed into a truly invasive cancer (in other words, because it is so commonly detected at the *pre*cancerous stage), I deal with the precancerous changes separately from the true, invasive cancer of the cervix. In this section, therefore, I begin by describing what the cervix is and what it does. I then explain how precancerous changes and cancer are caused, discuss the precancerous changes (detection and treatment), and, finally, deal with invasive cancer of the cervix.

The Most Important Features of the Tumor

Cancer of the cervix is an important disease for everyone to be aware of because it is relatively easy to detect and treat at an early stage before it has developed into a true, invasive cancer. When it is treated at an early stage, particularly in the precancerous stage, it is completely curable in a very large number of cases. Because we also know something about the factors that contribute to the development of cervical cancer, it is also possible to recommend precautions that will reduce a woman's chance of developing the cancer in the first place.

What You Really Need to Know about the Cervix

The cervix is the lower portion of the uterus or womb, the part of the uterus that is connected to the vagina. The cervix is like the neck of a balloon, except that it is, comparatively speaking, longer and has thick walls. It leads from the vagina into the cavity of the uterus. The lining of the vagina is quite thick and elastic and is actually well adapted to coping with the physical and biological challenges of intercourse and childbirth. However, because the lining of the uterus has to be capable of supporting a fertilized egg or ovum while it grows, it has to be extremely sensitive and receptive, an entirely different mandate from that of the vaginal lining. Between the vagina and the cavity of the uterus, the cervix acts as a true transitional area, where the relatively invulnerable lining of the vagina changes to the type of glandular lining needed in the uterus for hosting a developing fetus. In the cervix, the vaginal type of lining (called **squamous** epithelium) changes to the uterine type (called **columnar** epithelium), and that transitional area—the **squamocolumnar junction**—for some reason is particularly vulnerable to damage by the sort of agents that cause cancer to develop. Precisely what those agents are and how we think they cause the damage will be discussed in a moment. Encouraging features about cancer of the cervix are that it usually develops in a very methodical and predictable way and that the early changes can be detected easily. This is because the cervix, and particularly the part of it that contains the squamocolumnar junction, is accessible and can be assessed by a clinical examination and Pap test.

Age and Incidence

Cancer of the cervix occurs almost exclusively in women who have been sexually active at any time. The average age is in the mid-fifties, although the incidence is rising in younger women. For precancerous changes, the average age is younger, in the mid-thirties.

Causes of Precancerous Changes and Cancer

Precancerous changes and true invasive cancer of the cervix are caused by a combination of factors that are somehow present in seminal fluid. Epidemiological research (see page 24) has demonstrated that connection, as cancer of the cervix does not occur in nuns, and the chance of developing it is greater the more sexual partners a woman has and the younger she is when she starts sexual activity. In some respects, therefore, precancerous changes and cervical cancer are partially sexually transmitted diseases, as they develop only when a woman has had intercourse, and the factors causing the conditions are somehow transmitted by the male. Knowledge and acceptance of that fact means that sensible precautions can be taken and that the condition can be partly prevented and almost always cured if it is detected early.

Viruses The most likely causes of precancer and cancer of the cervix are certain viruses, particularly some particular substrains of a virus called the **human papilloma virus** (or **HPV**). Many males have these viruses, which are very common and do not cause any noticeable symptoms or problems. However, transmission of the virus to females may contribute to changes in the cells of the cervix. Another virus known as genital **herpes** (another sexually transmitted disease) may play a part in some cases, though precisely how this interacts with the HPV is not understood.

Because of the important role of viruses that are carried in seminal fluid, the chance of getting

THE FEMALE REPRODUCTIVE SYSTEM

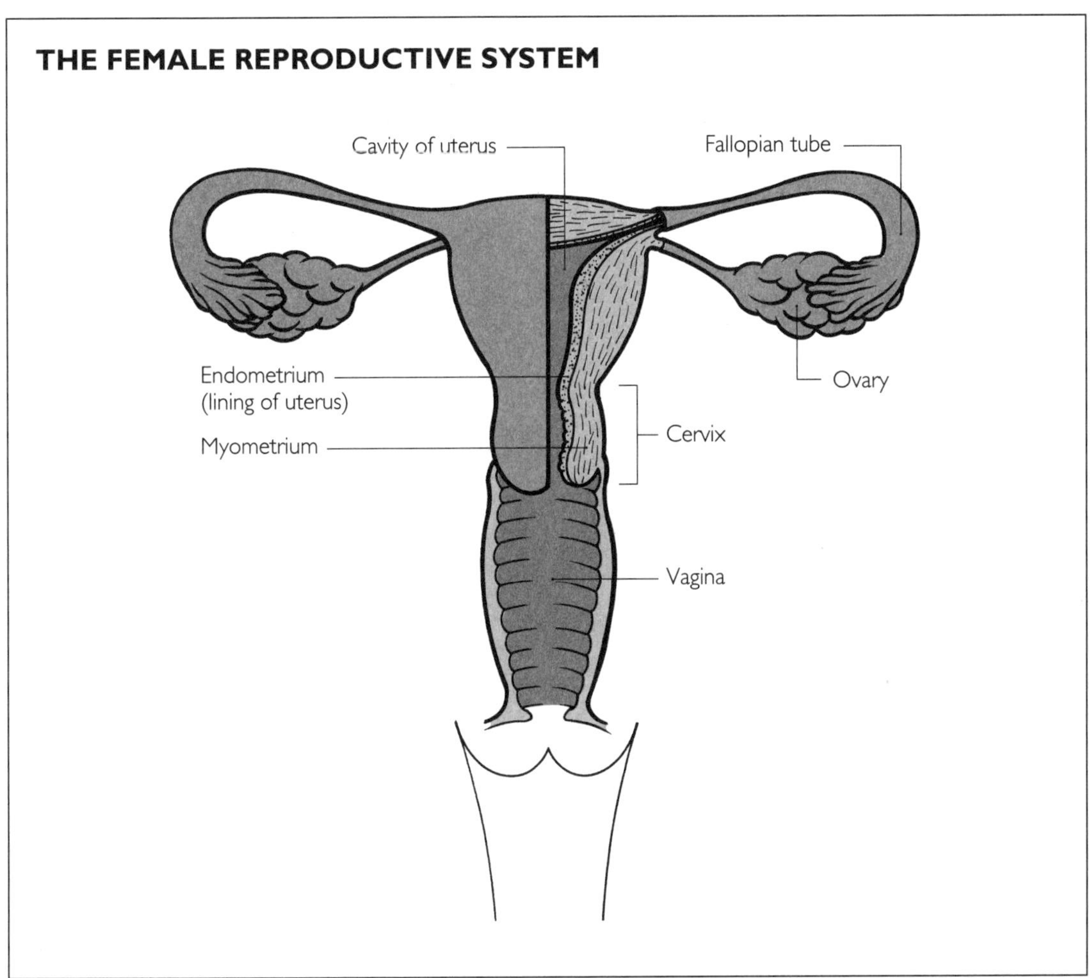

cervical cancer does increase the more sexual partners a woman has. That is simply a matter of statistics, although it can also happen that a woman who has had only one sexual partner in her life may develop a cancer of the cervix, while another woman who has had many partners may not. In addition to the number of sexual partners, the age when sexual intercourse begins also seems to be relevant. Starting intercourse early in the teens seems to be associated with a higher risk of cervical cancer. Whether this is because the cervix of a teenager is immature and in some way particularly vulnerable to damage by viruses is unknown.

Socioeconomic Factors Other factors may also increase the risk of cervical cancer. For example, the chance of developing cervical cancer is somewhat increased in the poorer socioeconomic groups of society and in smokers. Poor nutrition may play a part as well, but it is not known precisely how.

Although these risk factors are well established, it is important to note that **many women** with precancerous changes or with cancer of the cervix **have no known risk factors at all**, apart from having been sexually active.

Precancerous (Noninvasive) Changes in the Cervix and Screening

The Most Important Features of Precancerous Changes

Precancerous changes in the cervix are not the same as cancer itself. If left untreated, though, they may eventually turn into true, invasive cancer in the majority of cases. Unlike precancerous changes in most other parts of the body, however, these changes in the cervix can be detected easily with a screening test known as the Pap test (also called the cervical smear test) and if treated at the precancerous stage can be totally cured.

Symptoms or Problems That You May Notice

There are no symptoms associated with precancerous changes in the cervix. That is why it is so important to have a regular Pap test once you have started sexual activity, because having no symptoms is not a guarantee that there are no precancerous changes.

Diagnosis and Tests

Precancerous changes in the cervix can be readily detected with the Pap test. If necessary, further tests may be needed later on. These may include colposcopy and biopsy. Before any tests are done, however, your doctor will ask you some standard questions (including several about aspects of your sex life) and will perform a pelvic examination. During that examination the cervix is **palpated**

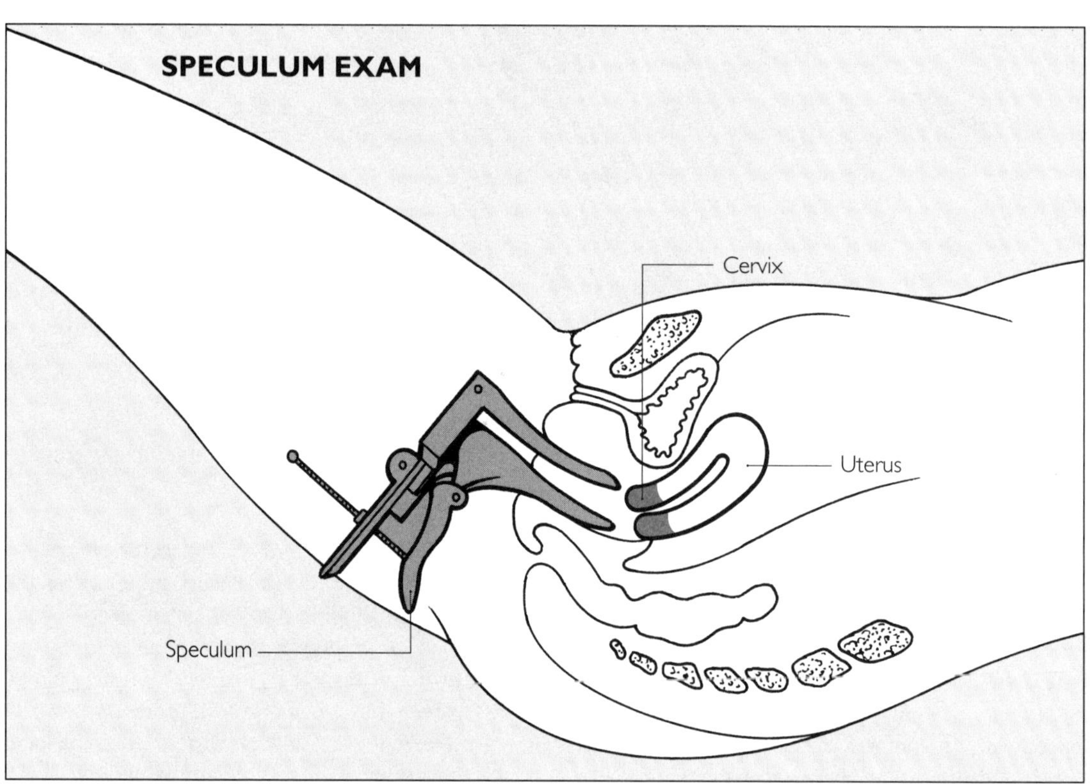

(that is, the physician assesses it by touch). The physician then introduces a small instrument called a **speculum** that allows the entire cervix to be seen, after which the Pap test is done.

The Pap Test or Cervical Smear Test The Pap test (named after its inventor, the pathologist Dr. George Papanicolaou) is a routine way of checking the health of the cervix by examining some of the cells from it to see if they show any signs of cancerous changes. The objective of the test is to obtain a sample of cells from the cervix, and in particular from the squamocolumnar junction, by gently wiping a specially shaped wooden spatula over the area and then using a cotton swab or a small brush to collect cells from the canal of the cervix. When the test is done correctly, the sample will contain cells from the squamous lining and from the columnar lining of the cervix. If there are precancerous changes in the cervix, or if there is a cancer developing, that will be visible in the cells collected by the Pap test. The cells are then put onto a glass slide (or rather smeared onto the slide; hence the term "cervical smear") and sent for examination under the microscope (this procedure is called **cytology**). The cytologist assesses several features of the cells and their nuclei and then, according to a set of stringent criteria, decides which category the cells belong in: normal, precancerous changes (which may be mild, moderate, or severe), cancer, or irritation of the cervix (including virus infections).

CELLS SEEN IN THE PAP SMEAR TEST

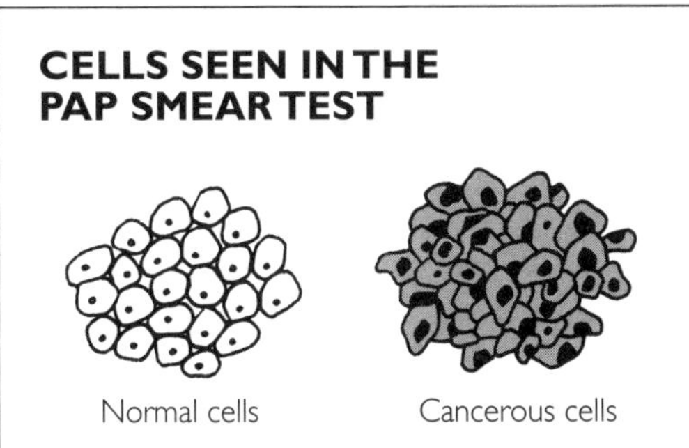

Factors That Influence the Treatment and Prognosis

The results of the Pap test largely determine what happens next. If the cells are normal, nothing need be done until the next screening Pap test. If there is evidence of virus infection, your doctor will discuss with you when the next test should be or if any further tests are needed. If the cells in the Pap test show some precancerous changes, what happens next depends on the degree of those changes and whether there were any other problems seen or felt in the cervix during the examination. If the precancerous changes are moderate or severe, your doctor will recommend a **colposcopy**.

Colposcopy A colposcopy is a technique that allows examination of the cervix in much greater detail than with a speculum. It also allows the doctor to use a substance that shows up abnormal areas and then to take biopsies of any areas that look abnormal. It does not require any form of anesthetic.

The colposcope is really a speculum with some very sophisticated equipment built into it that allows the doctor to look at the surface of the cervix through a microscope, to apply certain solutions to the surface that show up any abnormal areas, and then to take samples of the abnormal areas. Like a speculum examination, a colposcopy is somewhat uncomfortable and awkward, but neither it nor the biopsies cause severe pain.

Treatment of Mild Precancerous Changes

If the changes in the Pap test are mild, your doctor may suggest a repeat Pap test in a few months or a colposcopy. If there is no problem seen at the colposcopy, it may only be necessary to repeat the Pap test regularly, as in some or many cases the mild precancerous changes revert to normal.

Treatment of Moderate or Severe Precancerous Changes

If the changes in the cells seen in the Pap test or at a subsequent colposcopy show more severe changes,

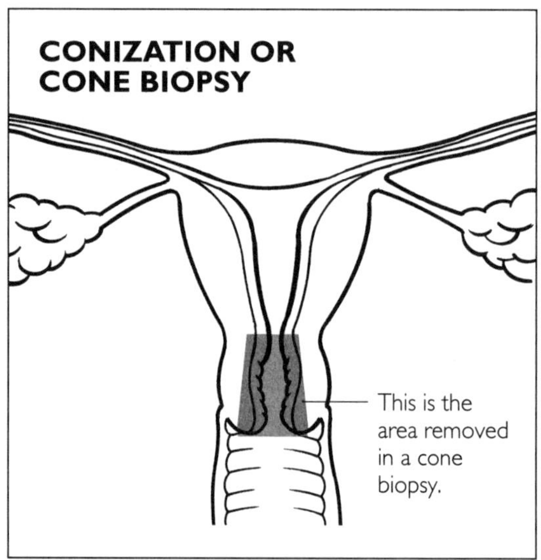

your doctor may decide to kill the cells in the problem area or remove the area itself, either of which will almost certainly cure the problem permanently. There are several ways of doing this. If the problem area is quite small, it is quite simple to kill all the precancerous cells in the area by applying a small instrument that freezes the area. This is called **cryosurgery**, and because the freezing temperature affects only a very small part of the cervix, it is extremely safe and effective. Exactly the same thing can be achieved by using high temperatures, and that is called **cautery**. If the area involved is not suited to cryosurgery or cautery, it can be removed using a **laser**, which in this procedure acts as a very sophisticated and accurate knife and vaporizes the cells in its path. Another method employs a fine wire in the shape of a loop, which is heated (as in cautery) but is used to remove the area rather than simply destroying the cells where they are.

In some circumstances you may be advised to have a larger area of the cervix removed in the form of a cone. This is called a **cone biopsy** or sometimes **conization**. It may be recommended to assist in diagnosis and may often be the only treatment needed. Usually this procedure requires a general anesthetic. A part of the cervix that includes the squamocolumnar junction is removed, and examination of the tissue under the microscope can show how widespread any changes were and if there was any true, invasive cancer. If there was very early cancer, it is quite common to find that all of the cancer was completely removed by the conization and that in certain circumstances no further treatment may be required.

How Often Should the Pap Test Be Done?

Every woman who is sexually active should have a Pap test done within a few years of starting sexual activity and then **annually** or **as recommended by your doctor**, if the Pap test has been negative three times. After the age of seventy, the Pap test should probably be repeated every five years or so.

(Invasive) Cancer of the Cervix

The Most Important Features of the Tumor

Cancer of the cervix that is truly cancerous, in other words, that invades the tissue of the cervix, will, if left untreated, grow and spread. If it is treated at an early stage, particularly before it has spread beyond the cervix itself, it is curable in the majority of cases. If it has spread beyond the cervix, the chance of cure is lower.

How Cancer of the Cervix Tends to Spread

If it spreads, cancer of the cervix first tends to invade more deeply into the cervix (sometimes causing enlargement) and then to adjacent tissues, including the top of the vagina and other parts of the uterus. It may also spread to other tissues in the pelvis, to lymph nodes in the pelvis and abdomen, and eventually to distant parts of the body such as the lungs.

Symptoms or Problems That You May Notice

The earliest stages of cervical cancer cause no symptoms at all; hence the importance of regular examinations and Pap tests for all women who are sexually active. If the cancer does cause symptoms, the most likely problems are vaginal **bleeding after intercourse** (postcoital bleeding), after the menopause, or at any time other than during the menstrual period, **pain** during intercourse, and sometimes blood-stained vaginal **discharge**.

Diagnosis and Tests

Very often the cancer will be suspected as a result of the doctor's examination of the cervix and confirmed with a biopsy. Depending on circumstances, this may be done during a speculum examination, a colposcopy, a conization, or, if the pelvis is particularly uncomfortable, as a separate procedure under an anesthetic.

If true cancer of the cervix is found, then it is important for your doctor to establish whether there is any spread or not. A variety of tests may be recommended to you, and these may include a CT scan of the pelvis and a lymphogram to see if any of the lymph nodes in the pelvis are involved. In a few cases, some other tests (further assessment of the kidneys or bowel, for example) may be required.

The Main Types of the Cancer

There are two main subtypes of cervical cancer. When seen under the microscope, the most common kind resembles the squamous part of the cervix and is therefore called **squamous carcinoma**. Some tumors show a different appearance; the most common of these resembles a glandular lining and is called **adenocarcinoma**. In most cases, the type of the cancer is not as important as the extent of the cancer and other features of its appearance under the microscope (such as invasion into blood or lymph vessels), although adenocarcinoma generally tends to behave somewhat more aggressively than squamous.

Factors That Influence the Treatment and Prognosis

The most important factor in determining the treatment and outcome is the extent of the cancer. If it has not spread beyond the cervix, it is curable in almost all cases, usually by surgery. If it has spread beyond the cervix but has not spread to the sides of the pelvis, it is still curable, in many cases, with radiotherapy. If it has spread to the lymph nodes or to the sides of the pelvis or beyond, the chance of cure becomes somewhat lower.

The Main Objectives of Treatment

For cancer of the cervix that has not advanced very far, the objective is cure, which may require surgery or radiotherapy. About two-thirds of patients with curable cancer of the cervix will be treated with radiotherapy alone. For the more advanced cancers, radiotherapy may be accompanied by chemotherapy. In some cases, surgery is not technically possible, and then chemotherapy or a combination of radiotherapy and chemotherapy may be used.

Types of Treatment

Radiotherapy Radiotherapy is often used with the objective of curing cancer of the cervix. If the cancer is small, radiotherapy is very often curative. If the cancer is large, the radiation may control the local disease within the pelvis. If the cancer happens to be very large and is causing bad symptoms, radiation can sometimes be used to control some or all of the local symptoms.

Depending on the exact circumstances, radiotherapy may be given by radiation beams from standard radiotherapy machines (**external beam irradiation**) or by small quantities of radioactive substances mounted in special tubes that are approximately the thickness of a pencil and are inserted into the uterus or vagina. In most cases, both are used for the same patient. The latter type of radiotherapy is called **brachytherapy** (which means therapy given from a short distance away). It involves your being admitted to the hospital for a few days, and the tubes are usually put in place under a general anesthetic. The potential advantage of using brachytherapy is that the dose of radiation is thereby concentrated on the area of the cancer, thus sparing more of the surrounding normal tissue. Brachytherapy is not always technically possible, however, and it requires a greater effort on the part of the patient. Your radiation oncologist will discuss with you the options that are applicable in your case.

Radiotherapy often causes mild diarrhea, which is temporary and easily controlled. It also makes you feel quite tired and occasionally a bit nauseated. Other complications, such as damage to the bowel or bladder, are rare. Many months after radiotherapy there may be some scarring in the irradiated area, and in a few cases this may cause some difficulty with sexual intercourse or with bowel function.

Surgery Involving the Cervix or Part of It If the cancer is very small, it may already have been removed by a biopsy procedure such as conization. If it has not been removed and is small, then any of the methods mentioned above may be used (cryosurgery, cautery, loop, laser, or cone biopsy). If the cancer is larger, or if the patient would prefer it and is past childbearing age, the uterus can be removed (**hysterectomy**).

Hysterectomy

Hysterectomy means removal of the uterus. In some cases of cancer of the cervix, it is recommended to remove the uterus together with a part of the tissues that surround it and some of the lymph nodes in the pelvis. This operation is called, rather off-puttingly, a **modified radical hysterectomy**; the operation in which only the uterus is removed without any of the surrounding tissue is called a **simple hysterectomy**.

Your surgeon will discuss with you the exact details of the operation recommended in your case.

A hysterectomy is not minor surgery; neither is it among the most major operations. Usually you will need to be in the hospital for a week to two weeks and may often require intravenous fluids and sometimes a catheter in the bladder immediately after the operation. Complications involving the bowel or the bladder are not common, but if they are more likely than average in your case, your surgeon will discuss them with you.

TABLE 4.5: DECREASING THE RISK OF GETTING CANCER OF THE CERVIX
1. The younger you are when you begin sexual activity and the more **sexual partners** you have, the greater your chances of developing cervical cancer.
2. If you are, or have been, sexually active, make sure you have a **Pap test once every year** to two years after the start of sexual activity.
3. Precancerous changes can be detected by the Pap test, and true cancer can be prevented if the **precancerous changes are treated**.
4. **Safe sex** (sex during which a condom is used) decreases the chance that you will acquire the human papilloma virus (HPV), which is one of the contributory causes of cancer of the cervix.
5. Get a **medical assessment** if you have any vaginal bleeding other than at the time of your menstrual period, or if you have pain during intercourse or pain inside the pelvic area.
6. Cigarette smoking also increases the risk of your getting cancer of the cervix.

Chemotherapy

At present there are no chemotherapy drugs that are effective against all or most cancers of the cervix. A few drugs, including platinum drugs and Taxol, have proved to be effective in some cases and may be recommended to you either by themselves (for example, if surgery and radiotherapy are not thought to be useful) or in conjunction with radiotherapy. Often, because there is not yet an established optimal combination of drugs, these treatments will be offered as part of a clinical trial (see page 233). With cancer of the cervix, it is certainly worth considering entering a clinical trial; you should therefore discuss with your doctor the potential benefits and side effects of the therapy being investigated.

Treatment and Sexual Function

Radiotherapy to the pelvis usually produces infertility and menopause, and it is customary to start hormone replacement therapy after the treatment. In addition, sexual function is often affected by the treatment, whether it is surgery or radiotherapy and may cause scarring or dryness of the vagina or other problems. You will need to discuss this with both your medical and nursing team and your partner (see also "Sexuality" in Chapter 10) and ensure that you know about the various options that may help including counseling, lubricants, and applicators.

Prevention

Because cancer of the cervix is a risk with any unprotected sexual intercourse, only those women who have never had and will not have sexual intercourse have a very low risk. You may decrease your chances of getting cancer of the cervix by taking the precautions listed in Table 4.5.

CHORIOCARCINOMA AND HYDATIDIFORM MOLE (TUMORS OF THE PLACENTA) AND RELATED TROPHOBLASTIC TUMORS

SUMMARY OF THE KEY FACTS IN THIS SECTION

- **Choriocarcinoma** is a cancer of the cells that form the beginnings of the placenta. It is usually the result of something going wrong during a pregnancy (by random chance rather than as a result of something the woman has taken or done).
- Sometimes choriocarcinoma develops after another type of growth problem during a pregnancy called a **hydatidiform mole** or **molar pregnancy**.
- These tumors may sometimes spread to distant parts of the body, particularly the lungs.
- Even when they spread, these are among the most curable cancers known and are cured in the great majority of cases.
- There are some similar cancers that develop when a women is not pregnant. These are called **nongestational trophoblastic tumors**, and they are also highly curable.
- A blood test—the βHCG—is a sensitive marker of all these tumors and can give the medical team an accurate picture of the state of the disease and how the treatment is working.

The Most Important Features of the Tumor

Choriocarcinoma and hydatidiform mole are tumors of tissue known as **trophoblastic tissue**, which is the part of the embryo that will eventually form, or has already formed, the placenta (the organ by which the fetus obtains oxygen and nutrients, also known as the afterbirth). For reasons that are not understood, but that are probably due to mischance and plain bad luck, a sperm fuses with an ovum that does not have a nucleus. Thus, instead of starting off a normal fetus and a normal placenta, the growth process goes wrong and may form a mass that resembles a bunch of grapes (within which there may or may not be parts of a fetus). This is called a **hydatidiform mole** or **molar pregnancy**, which in itself is a benign (noncancerous) condition. Sometimes a molar pregnancy may behave in a malignant way and invade deep into the wall of the uterus and occasionally metastasize. If it does that, or looks as if it will, it is called an **invasive mole** and is considered to be a malignant tumor, that is, a cancer. It can also develop into a choriocarcinoma, which is a true cancer. About half of the cases of choriocarcinoma are preceded by a molar pregnancy. In the other half, the choriocarcinoma seems to develop without a prior mole. A choriocarcinoma has a very high tendency to spread to other parts of the body, particularly the lungs, parts of the genital tract, and sometimes the brain. Fortunately, these tumors are all highly curable and are cured in the great majority of cases.

Sometimes tumors of trophoblastic tissue can develop when there is no pregnancy. These are called **nongestational trophoblastic tumors** and are unusual. They tend to be more aggressive but are in most respects similar to choriocarcinomas that develop during pregnancy.

Age and Incidence

Trophoblastic tumors occur only in women during the reproductive years, which means from the start of menstruation (usually in the early teens) until menopause (around the age of fifty). They occur at a rate of about one in every 4,000 pregnancies.

Causes

Although we do not know the cause (or causes) of molar pregnancies and choriocarcinomas, we do know that **they are not caused by anything the woman has done or taken**. It is important to stress this point, as everyone, particularly an expectant mother, feels very guilty when something goes wrong with a pregnancy. There is a great temptation to blame some medication that was taken, a lifestyle factor (such as drinking or smoking), an infection, or something similar. There is no evidence to support such a hypothesis. Trophoblastic problems appear to be a matter of pure bad luck, occurring by what is almost certainly random chance alone.

How the Cancer Tends to Spread

Molar pregnancies usually stay within the endometrium, the lining of the uterus (see page 93). Invasive moles tend to invade deeper into the muscular layer of the wall (the myometrium). Occasionally they spread to distant parts of the body. Choriocarcinomas have a high tendency to spread, commonly to the lungs, other parts of the genital tract (such as the cervix or the vagina), or sometimes the brain. Fortunately, this does not affect the outlook to a great extent, as the majority of these cancers are curable whether they have spread or not.

Symptoms or Problems That You May Notice

One of the most common signs of a molar pregnancy or a choriocarcinoma is bleeding during the first few months of a pregnancy. There are, of course, many other possible explanations for bleeding in the early stages of a pregnancy. Other symptoms include excessive nausea or vomiting or pelvic pain (for which there are also much more common causes).

In these circumstances the examination by your doctor may show that the fetus is not developing as it should, which may be another indication of a molar pregnancy. Occasionally, however, the first sign of trouble from a mole can be when the grape-like cysts of a mole are expelled from the uterus. Less frequently, an invasive mole can invade through the wall of the uterus and cause rupture with severe abdominal pain. This is an emergency, and you should have a prompt assessment done in the nearest emergency department.

Diagnosis and Tests

If a woman has a pregnancy with abnormal bleeding and pain or some of the other symptoms listed above, after a clinical examination the doctor will probably recommend an ultrasound. If there is a molar pregnancy or a choriocarcinoma, the ultrasound will show that there is something wrong with the fetus or there is no fetus visible and that the image of the contents of the uterus shows cysts suggestive of a molar pregnancy. Hence the diagnosis is often suspected after the ultrasound. The βHCG (beta human chorionic gonadotrophin) blood test will show very high levels of the hormone βHCG (which is produced in large amounts by trophoblastic tissue). Generally a chest X ray will be recommended. Whether any other tests are required before starting treatment depends on the particular circumstances.

Factors That Influence the Treatment and Prognosis

The most important feature of a molar pregnancy or a choriocarcinoma is whether or not it has spread or is likely to. With a molar pregnancy, that chance can be estimated, to a certain extent, after the condition has been treated and the mole removed. With a choriocarcinoma it is often important to give treatment with chemotherapy and to continue that treatment until the βHCG level falls to normal.

The Main Objectives of Treatment

These tumors are among the most curable cancers, and therefore the objective of therapy is to cure the patient.

Types of Treatment

Treatment of a Mole (Molar Pregnancy) A molar pregnancy is treated by removing the contents of the uterus by suction curettage, in other words, by a therapeutic termination of pregnancy. In about one-third of cases, the high quantities of hormones produced by the mole will have caused enlarged cysts in the ovaries. These disappear of their own accord. The mole that has been removed will then be examined extensively by the pathologists, and if there is any evidence of a choriocarcinoma within it, or if the βHCG blood test it still abnormal a few weeks later, a course of chemotherapy will probably be recommended to kill any remaining tumor cells. The exact schedule and duration of chemotherapy vary considerably depending on the particular case, so your specialist will explain in detail what he or she is recommending for you.

Treatment of an Invasive Mole or Choriocarcinoma Generally an invasive mole or a choriocarcinoma is treated in the same way as a molar pregnancy, but with the difference that chemotherapy is almost always recommended. A suction curettage is done. There may be additional tests, such as CT scans of the lungs, to see if there is any evidence of metastases. Then chemotherapy will be recommended. There are many drugs that are effective in this context, and usually a combination of several is used. These may include: **methotrexate**, **etoposide**, **Adriamycin**, **cyclophosphamide**, **platinum**, **vinblastine**, **bleomycin**, **actinomycin-D**, and others. The exact combination and schedule of drugs recommended, together with the duration of the planned therapy, will be explained by your specialist.

Pregnancies after Treatment for Trophoblastic Tumors Since these treatment methods have been used, many thousands of women have been cured, and many hundreds of those have gone on to have a successful pregnancy after treatment. These pregnancies show that there is no long-term ill effect of the treatment on subsequent pregnancies. If you wish to become pregnant when the treatment is finished—the standard recommendation is to wait twelve months—your chances of a normal pregnancy are the same as everyone else's.

Follow-up

The βHCG blood test is extremely useful for detecting early signs of any recurrence of the tumor and for alerting the medical team to the possibility that the cancer is resistant to the chemotherapy drugs. Hence **it is very important—more important than with almost any other tumor—for you to attend all your planned follow-up visits and blood tests.**

ENDOMETRIUM (WOMB)

Number of new cases diagnosed per year in the United States: 32,800

SUMMARY OF THE KEY FACTS IN THIS SECTION

- Cancer of the lining of the womb (endometrium) is relatively common and also highly curable.
- It usually causes vaginal bleeding after menopause as the first symptom.
- Treatment is by surgery (hysterectomy) and/or hormone tablets and is curative in most cases.

The Most Important Features of the Tumor

Cancer of the main part of the uterus (womb) is a fairly common type of cancer and in many cases is relatively easy to treat and cure. It begins in the lining of the uterus (the **endometrium**), which is particularly susceptible to hormonal changes such as those that occur in every menstrual cycle. Often the growth and repair of the lining may become abnormal after many decades, and in some cases may progress to precancerous changes. In some cases, precancerous changes may progress to cancer. Endometrial cancer generally occurs in late adulthood, and the most usual symptoms are bleeding after menopause or very irregular or heavy bleeding during menopause. If detected in the early stages, both endometrial cancer and these precancerous changes that carry the highest risk of progressing to cancer are curable in most cases, usually by surgery but sometimes by hormone treatment if surgery is not feasible. As regards early detection and prevention, although we do not yet know all the details of how endometrial cancer develops, there is sufficient information to make a few useful recommendations.

What You Really Need to Know about the Womb and the Endometrium

The womb or uterus is shaped a bit like a balloon. The neck of the balloon is called the cervix (see page 83), and the rest of the womb is called (rather inelegantly) the **corpus** or body of the uterus. The body of the womb consists of a thick wall made up of muscle (the **myometrium**) and an inner lining (the **endometrium**), which is where most cancers develop. Cancers of other components of the uterine wall, such as sarcomas, may develop from the myometrium, but they are much less common. The uterus is capable of expanding greatly to accommodate the fetus as it grows. In most women after menopause, the uterus usually contracts and shrinks until it is smaller than a fist.

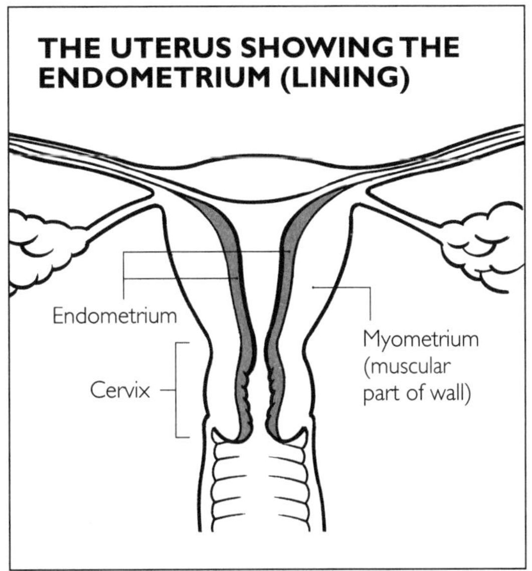

Age and Incidence

By and large, endometrial cancers occur in women of middle age and older. In fact, the peak incidence is in the late fifties and early sixties, and more than three-quarters of all cases occur in women after the age of fifty.

Causes

Although we do not yet know the precise way in which endometrial cancer develops, and therefore do not fully understand all its causes, we do know some of the contributory factors. Most of these are factors that increase the amount of the female hormone estrogen in the body or prolong the time that the uterus is exposed to it. In other words, anything that prolongs or increases the amount of estrogen to which the uterus is exposed increases the risk that the uterus will develop a cancer.

Current explanations suggest that an excess of estrogen may cause the endometrium to grow excessively. This condition, known as **hyperplasia**, is very common. In many cases the excessive growth does not progress to precancerous changes or to cancer, that is, it carries a **low risk** of progression. In some cases, however, the excessive growth is accompanied by abnormalities in the growth pattern of the cells of the lining, a condition that carries a **high risk** of progression. In some cases, then, the abnormal growth may progress to precancerous changes, and in some of those cases, progression to true, invasive cancer may follow. We do not know that this stepwise progression is the way in which every endometrial cancer develops, but there is some evidence to suggest that this is the most common way.

Too much estrogen, therefore, is very important in the development of endometrial cancer and the factors that are most likely to carry the highest risk are the following.

Age Over Forty Women under forty rarely get endometrial cancer unless there has been some other unusual risk factor. By and large, the tumor is more common after menopause, perhaps because it takes several decades of exposure to estrogen to contribute to the cancer.

Certain Types of Menstrual Problems Certain types of menstrual problems often accompany a relative excess of estrogen. These include: irregular bleeding during and after menopause, infertility due to failure of the ovaries, a late menopause (after the age of fifty-two or so), and periods that are particularly irregular. Because all these problems may involve an excess of estrogen, women experiencing them have a somewhat increased risk of later developing endometrial cancer.

Obesity Obesity can affect the hormonal environment. The body handles several hormones, particularly estrogen, in many different ways and in several different areas of the body. Moreover, fatty tissue contains some of the important enzymes used in the production of estrogen. The more fat there is in the body, the more estrogen it can make, and the greater the risk of endometrial cancer. Because excess body weight is also associated with high blood pressure and diabetes, people with diabetes and high blood pressure have an increased likelihood of developing endometrial cancer, not because of the diabetes or high blood pressure but because of the excess weight.

Birth Control Pills (BCPs) or Other Hormone Preparations Containing Only Estrogen Another possible source of estrogen is from medication. There is good evidence now that those pills that contain only estrogen (as opposed to estrogen combined with another hormone, progesterone) may increase a woman's chance of developing endometrial cancer. Nowadays most BCPs contain both estrogen and progesterone. In fact, since the association between estrogen and endometrial cancer is well known, you will not be given a prescription for an "estrogen only" medication unless your doctor has discussed the potential risks and benefits with you in some detail.

A reassuring fact about endometrial cancers associated with estrogen medications is that they are in general less aggressive than average, likely to be lower grade as seen under the microscope, and are curable by hysterectomy.

Tamoxifen Tamoxifen is a very important hormonal medication used in the treatment of breast cancer. It works in breast cancer partly because it blocks the action of estrogen on the cancer cells, thus cutting them off, as it were, from an ingredient that is important in their growth. In some respects, however, tamoxifen acts somewhat like an estrogen itself. Some research studies have shown that women who take tamoxifen for breast cancer have a slightly increased risk of developing endometrial cancer. This risk is very small compared to the risk to life and health posed by the breast cancer, and in many cases even if an endometrial cancer does develop, it can be cured. This risk does mean, though, that patients should be given tamoxifen only if there is good evidence that they really need it and that the risk posed by the breast cancer is much greater than the risk of developing endometrial cancer.

The existence of identifiable risk factors notwithstanding, in approximately **half of the cases of endometrial cancer, there are no identified risk factors** apart from the woman's age.

How the Cancer Tends to Spread

Endometrial cancer tends to spread in a fairly predictable manner. In the early stages, the cancer is found in the innermost layer of the endometrium, but as it progresses it may cause the size of the uterus to enlarge and may also be found deeper in the muscle layer (the myometrium). It then tends to spread into the cervix of the womb or through the full thickness of the wall of the womb or both. Thereafter, it may spread in three different ways. It may spread directly into adjacent parts of the pelvic organs, including the vagina, the ovaries, and the supporting tissues around the uterus and cervix. It may spread to lymph nodes in the pelvis, or it may spread around the cavity of the abdomen. After that it may spread to distant areas of the body, the most common sites being the lungs or sometimes the bones.

If the cancer has not spread deeply into the wall of the uterus or beyond, the chance that it will spread to any other part of the body is very much lower.

Symptoms or Problems That You May Notice

Occasionally an endometrial cancer may cause no symptoms at all and be discovered during tests done for some other reason. In most cases, however, it does cause symptoms, the most common one being vaginal bleeding. Bleeding may occur after menopause, that is, the menstrual periods stop for several months and then intermittent bleeding starts again. In some cases, particularly heavy bleeding may occur at the time of menopause. In addition to bleeding, occasionally the tumor may cause cramping pelvic or abdominal pain, and very occasionally it may cause distension or bloating of the abdomen. Because most symptoms are readily noticed by the patient, endometrial cancer is usually detected and diagnosed at an early stage.

Diagnosis and Tests

The history and examination are quite important in the diagnosis of endometrial cancer, and the pelvic examination is an important part of the initial assessment. Usually, though, it is not possible to be certain whether there is endometrial cancer inside the uterus until samples of the endometrial lining are taken.

There are several methods for taking samples of the endometrial lining (**endometrial biopsy**). Some do not require any anesthetic, while others usually require a brief general anesthetic.

One of the outpatient procedures involves gentle insertion of a long, thin, plastic tube through the cervix. Samples of the lining of the uterus are then sucked into the tube and sent for analysis. This is called **aspiration curettage**, and the amount of discomfort it causes is slight.

The most common inpatient procedure, which does require a brief general anesthetic, is called a **dilatation and curettage**, usually abbreviated **D and C**. Because the cervix of the womb is normally tightly closed, in the first part of the D and C, the specialist gently widens the opening using a series of smooth rounded rods of increasing thickness. That is called **dilatation**. The specialist then takes samples of the uterine lining (using an instrument called a **curette**, hence the name of the procedure) that are then examined under the microscope to see if they contain any cancer cells.

Other tests that may be recommended include **hysteroscopy**, in which a thin telescope is introduced into the uterus so that the specialist can examine the lining of the uterus directly, and **hysterography**, an X ray of the uterus using a dye to show up any tumor. Both tests may be helpful in determining how much tumor there is and where it is situated.

If the D and C does show some cancer, a chest X ray will be recommended, but often no other tests are necessary. In some cases an ultrasound of the abdomen and pelvis (or sometimes a CT scan or an MRI scan) may be recommended.

The Main Types of the Cancer

Precancerous Changes As mentioned above, excessive growth of the endometrial lining (hyperplasia) is very common. In many cases it carries a low risk of progressing to true precancerous changes or cancer, but in some cases there is a higher risk.

Endometrial Cancer Most cases of endometrial cancer are of one particular type when viewed under the microscope. There are other types as well, some of which may be somewhat more aggressive than the main type. In general the grade of the tumor (high or low, depending on how aggressive it appears under the microscope) makes a bigger difference to the outcome and the treatment than the type.

Factors That Influence the Treatment and Prognosis

The factors that affect the outcome and determine the treatment to the greatest extent are the **stage** of the condition (whether it has spread beyond the uterus), the **depth** of penetration (whether it has invaded into the myometrium, and if so, how far), and the **grade** of the tumor. If the tumor is at an early stage and of a low grade (that is, least aggressive in appearance), it will be cured in almost all cases.

The Main Objectives of Treatment

Endometrial cancer is curable in most cases in the early stages. The primary objective is therefore to cure if that is feasible. If that is not possible, the next objective of treatment is to keep symptoms and problems to a minimum, particularly in the pelvis where tumor (or recurrence of tumor) can be very troublesome.

Types of Treatment

Surgery The mainstay of treatment for the early stages of endometrial cancer is surgery. Because the cancer is predictable, if it has not invaded deeply into the tissues of the uterus, only the uterus and the ovaries need be removed, and other structures such as the lymph nodes may remain. In some cases, samples of lymph nodes may be taken. The ovaries are removed because the great majority of patients are postmenopausal (so the ovaries are not manufacturing estrogen), because the ovaries may otherwise be the site of future recurrence of endometrial cancer, and because the ovaries themselves may be potential sites of future primary ovarian cancer.

Radiotherapy In certain situations, radiotherapy may be given after the operation. Radiotherapy is particularly likely to be recommended if the tumor has invaded deeply into the muscle layer of the wall of the uterus, or if there is some reason for suspecting aggressive behavior from the tumor. Radiotherapy may also be recommended if the primary tumor cannot be removed, if the medical condition of the patient makes surgery hazardous, or if there is a recurrence in the pelvis.

In the treatment of endometrial cancer, **external beam radiotherapy**, the standard method of radiotherapy, is most often employed, using standard radiotherapy machines. However, in addition, some centers use **brachytherapy**, that is, radioactive substances held in place within the pelvis by means of little tubes about as thick as a pencil. If this is recommended in your case, it will involve a short admission to the hospital for a few days. The exact details of the treatment proposed in your case will be discussed by your radiation oncologist.

Hormone Therapy Both endometrial cancer and precancerous changes may respond to hormone therapy of various types (given by tablet or injection), and this treatment can be used in cases where surgery is either not feasible or unnecessary. Hormone therapy is quite commonly used as the first type of treatment for many cases of precancerous changes, and the right type of hormones will often cause the uterus to shed the endometrial lining and with it the precancerous changes.

Endometrial cancer itself may also shrink or even disappear completely if the patient takes hormones given by tablet or injection. This may be of a great advantage because the side effects of hormone therapy are relatively slight. Various hormones can be used (megestrol, medroxyprogesterone, and others). Most patients experience no side effects at all; if there are problems, they most commonly include flushing, sweating, weight gain, fluid retention, and sometimes nausea.

Chemotherapy In cases where the cancer has spread to distant areas of the body, or does not respond to hormone therapy, or in a few other rare cases, chemotherapy may be recommended. Several different chemotherapy drugs have been used for endometrial cancers, and several are being evaluated at present. While chemotherapy drugs may produce remissions, they are very unlikely to cure. Thus you should thoroughly discuss the potential benefits and expected side effects of any recommended chemotherapy with your specialist.

Screening and Early Diagnosis

At present there are no tests sufficiently sensitive to be used effectively to screen the general population, that is, women without any symptoms at all. Because endometrial cancer and precancerous changes are so curable in the early stages, **it is extremely important for any woman with symptoms that might be early signs of endometrial cancer to seek medical advice.** In particular, if you have bleeding that starts after menopause, or if you have particularly irregular or heavy bleeding around the time of menopause, make sure you are assessed by your doctor. In any case, every woman should have a full general examination, including a pelvic examination, annually.

Prevention

Awareness of the known risk factors is an important element in prevention. If you happen to be overweight, it may well be worth trying to keep your weight close to your so-called ideal body weight. If you have taken estrogens or if you are diabetic or have high blood pressure, you should be aware of the somewhat increased risk of endometrial cancer, ensure that you get regular checkups, and report any postmenopausal bleeding.

ESOPHAGUS

Number of new cases diagnosed per year in the United States: 12,300

SUMMARY OF THE KEY FACTS IN THIS SECTION

- Cancer of the esophagus is not very common and can be caused by a combination of smoking and drinking.
- It usually causes difficulty in swallowing or pain as food or drink goes down.
- In some cases, if the cancer is situated in the lower part of the esophagus, it may be cured by surgery, and in some others by radiotherapy. Unfortunately, in many cases it is not curable, and treatment is directed at reducing the symptoms and controlling the growth.

The Most Important Features of the Tumor

Cancer of the esophagus is not very common. It is partly caused by a combination of smoking and drinking alcohol. Unfortunately, it is often diagnosed when it has already spread to lymph nodes in the area. In some cases, particularly if the cancer is located in the lower part of the esophagus and has not spread, it may be cured by surgery. In some other cases, radiotherapy with chemotherapy (sometimes after surgery) can be used and may be curative in some circumstances. In most cases, treatment can control the cancer and the symptoms for a time.

What You Really Need to Know about the Esophagus

The esophagus is the gullet, the tube that leads food from the mouth to the stomach. It is about thirty centimeters (twelve inches) long and has powerful muscles in its wall that propel food downward to the stomach (and occasionally in the opposite direction during vomiting). The lining of the esophagus at the top is similar to the lining of the mouth: it is squamous lining and resembles skin when seen under the microscope. The bottom one-third or so of the esophagus, the part that leads into the stomach, has a glandular type of lining.

Where the esophagus joins the stomach, muscular reflexes normally prevent the contents of the stomach from flowing up into the esophagus. These reflex mechanisms often weaken with advancing age, however, and allow stomach contents, including stomach acid, to reach the bottom part of the esophagus. This is called esophageal **reflux**, and in some people it may cause **esophagitis**—irritation of the bottom part of the esophagus. In some cases the irritation may cause changes in the lining of the esophagus, and these may predispose to cancer.

Age and Incidence

In this country, cancer of the esophagus is predominantly a disease of people over the age of sixty, and particularly of people who drink alcohol and smoke. It occurs more frequently in men than in women and in black people than in white. In other parts of the world—China, other Asian countries, and Indonesia—it is more common than here

THE DIGESTIVE TRACT SHOWING THE ESOPHAGUS

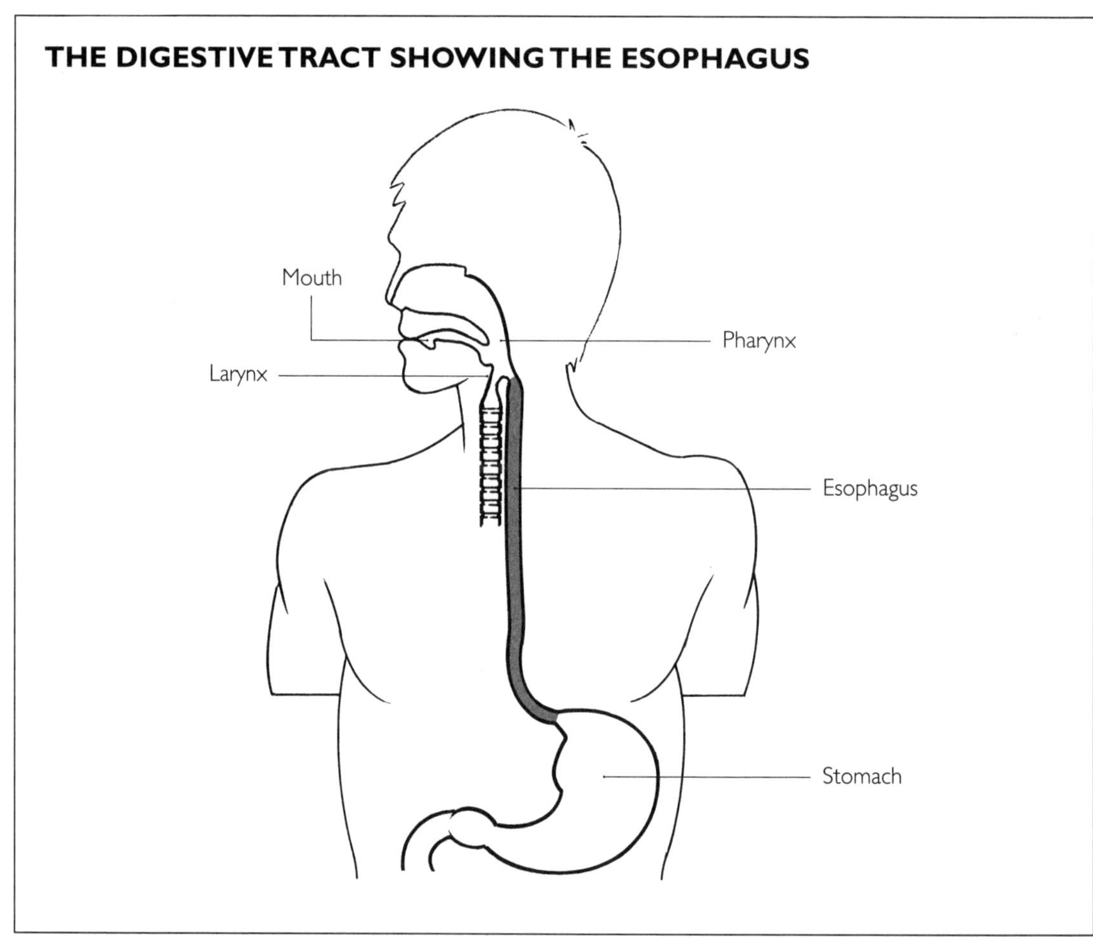

(probably as a result of carcinogenic substances in the diet) and occurs in younger people.

Causes

Tobacco and Alcohol In this country, long-term use of tobacco and alcohol are risk factors and increase the chance of getting cancer of the esophagus.

Medical Conditions Affecting the Esophagus

If there is long-standing esophagitis due to reflux, there may, in some cases, be changes in the lining of the esophagus, known as **Barrett's esophagus**. If Barrett's esophagus is diagnosed (by esophagoscopy), the risk of cancer is increased. Other conditions of the esophagus, such as a condition called **achalasia** in which the esophagus is unable to propel food and drink normally, may also increase the chance of cancer somewhat. People who often drink very hot fluids may sustain chronic damage to the esophagus, and this may also increase the risk of cancer.

Other Factors In other areas of the world, especially Asia and Indonesia, it seems that certain substances in the diet are common contributing causes of esophageal cancer. These substances include nitrosamines, and possibly some nitrites, probably assisted by certain dietary deficiencies that can be found in those areas (insufficient nicotinic acid, zinc, or riboflavin, for example).

How the Cancer Tends to Spread

Cancer of the esophagus starts in the lining of the esophagus and may later invade through the wall of the esophagus. It may also spread to lymph nodes in the area (around the bottom of the esophagus and the stomach or in the chest) and later to distant areas of the body, including lungs, liver, and bone.

Symptoms or Problems That You May Notice

The most common symptom caused by cancer of the esophagus is difficulty in swallowing or pain when food or liquid is swallowed. When you swallow food or liquid, it may feel as if the material will not go down properly and is stuck in the esophagus somewhere—a very important symptom. If there is pain, it may be dull or sharp and is often felt behind the breastbone (sternum) a few minutes after food leaves the mouth. Of course, this type of pain is also quite common with esophagitis caused by reflux, so not everybody who experiences it will have cancer. Nevertheless, pain on swallowing is an important symptom and should be reported to your doctor and assessed. If the tumor is in the upper part of the esophagus, the pain might be felt in the throat.

Unplanned weight loss is another symptom. Because they find eating and drinking uncomfortable, people with cancer of the esophagus often lose weight. In some cases the cancer can affect the nerves that go to the vocal cords and may cause hoarseness of the voice. In some cases the tumor may bleed, causing you to cough up blood.

Diagnosis and Tests

Your doctor will first discuss the details of the problem with you and examine you carefully. Because the esophagus cannot be examined without special tests, your doctor may recommend some or all of the following.

Endoscopy Endoscopy involves using a flexible scope to look down the esophagus and take biopsies of anything that appears suspicious.

CT Scans A CT scan may be used in determining the extent of a tumor, whether it involves any neighboring structures, and whether any lymph nodes are involved.

Barium X Rays In some situations, a barium X ray may be recommended. You will drink a dye that shows up white under X rays, allowing a tumor to be seen and also showing how the rest of the esophagus is moving.

The Main Types of the Cancer

Because the lining of the esophagus is of two types (squamous at the top and glandular at the bottom), two main types of cancer may develop. In the upper parts of the esophagus, the tumors are more usually squamous cancers and account for about 60 percent of the cancers. The cancers of the lower parts tend to be adenocarcinomas. Other types of tumors can occasionally occur in the esophagus (such as lymphomas or melanomas), but these are rare.

Factors That Influence the Treatment and Prognosis

The most important feature of any cancer of the esophagus is whether it has spread or can be completely removed. That, in turn, depends on the position of the tumor. In general, tumors that are situated lower in the esophagus are more removable, although the surgery is a considerable undertaking.

The Main Objectives of Treatment

If the cancer can be removed surgically, you and your surgeon will want to discuss the operation in some detail. The surgery is considered to be a major operation and requires considerable care afterward. In other cases, particularly with a cancer in the upper part of the esophagus, radiotherapy, often in combination with chemotherapy, may be recommended to try to cure the cancer. If surgery is not feasible, or not appropriate from your point of view, radiotherapy, chemotherapy, or both may be used with the objective of trying to control the disease and reduce your symptoms.

Types of Treatment

Surgery If the cancer is situated in the bottom part of the esophagus and has not spread, it may be possible to remove it, often along with the upper part of the stomach. In some cases, it may be possible to bring the remaining part of the stomach up into the chest and join it to the remaining part of the esophagus. If that is not possible, it may be possible to use another part of the digestive tract (usually a length of colon) to bridge the gap. This type of surgery is usually only done in centers that specialize in it (because of both the nature of the surgery and the supportive care needed afterward), so you and your surgeon should discuss the various aspects in some detail.

In cases where the cancer is blocking or threatening to block the esophagus, it may be possible to reduce the symptoms by doing a bypass operation or by putting a tube directly into the stomach (a gastrostomy). If either is being considered in your case, your surgeon will explain the reasons and the procedures to you.

Radiotherapy If the cancer is in the upper part of the esophagus, particularly if it is small, radiotherapy may be recommended with the intention of curing the cancer. The treatment may consist of external beam radiotherapy with or without additional chemotherapy and with or without further radiotherapy in the form of brachytherapy. In other circumstances, even if cure is not possible, radiotherapy may provide some measure of symptom relief by shrinking the tumor or controlling its growth. Again, the details of your own particular situation will need to be discussed with your radiation oncologist.

Chemotherapy In general, only a fraction of cancers of the esophagus respond to chemotherapy drugs, but chemotherapy, including drugs such as **5-fluorouracil** and **cis-platinum**, may have a role as additional treatment for esophageal cancer that has not advanced or spread. In addition, some centers are investigating the use of drugs with, for example, radiotherapy, and new drugs are being tested. It is important for you and your specialist to discuss the potential benefits, side effects, and risks of any drugs that are being recommended.

HODGKIN'S DISEASE

Number of new cases diagnosed per year in the United States: 7,500

SUMMARY OF THE KEY FACTS IN THIS SECTION

- Hodgkin's disease is the name given to one particular type of lymphoma (cancer of the lymphocytes).
- It generally occurs in young adults, usually starting off in the lymph nodes in the neck, armpits, or chest.
- Tumors of Hodgkin's disease have a characteristic appearance when seen under the microscope.
- Selecting the correct treatment depends partly on an accurate assessment of where the disease is located and how far it has spread (in other words, the *stage* of the disease).
- With modern treatment methods (radiotherapy, chemotherapy, or both), the disease is curable in the majority of cases, and in the early stages it is curable in almost all cases.

The Most Important Features of the Tumor

Hodgkin's disease is actually a particular type of lymphoma, a cancer of the lymphocytes. It was first studied in detail and described in 1832 by a physician (Thomas Hodgkin) who noted that there was a characteristic pattern to most of the cases (the areas in which the cancerous lymph nodes first appeared and so on). He linked that pattern with the characteristic appearance of the tumor he saw under the microscope. As a result of his work, this type of lymphoma was named after him, and it has always been thought of and treated differently from other tumors of lymphocytes studied in the years that followed. In practice, this has worked out rather well, because of all the lymphomas, Hodgkin's disease is the easiest to cure. In fact, curative therapy was discovered for Hodgkin's disease many years before it was discovered for any other lymphoma. Hence setting Hodgkin's disease apart from the other lymphomas turned out to be useful and practical.

Hodgkin's disease, although not common, is one of the types of cancer in which there has been dramatic improvement in treatment. Treatment depends, first, on accurately staging the disease, that is, determining exactly where the disease is and how far it has spread. Then, depending on the location of the disease, it is treated with radiotherapy, chemotherapy, or both. If the disease is in its early stages, it can be cured in almost all cases. Even in the later stages, it is curable in the majority of cases.

What You Really Need to Know about the Bone Marrow and Lymph Nodes

Please see the section about bone marrow and lymph nodes under "Leukemias" later in this chapter.

Age and Incidence

Hodgkin's disease is somewhat unusual in that it seems to have two peaks of incidence: one in young adulthood and one in older age. It is rare before the age of ten, but then the incidence rises with a peak in the late twenties. After that, the incidence declines but rises again after the age of forty-five, so that older people make up a considerable proportion of people with Hodgkin's disease. Overall, the condition is somewhat more common in males than in females, with a male-female ratio of approximately 1.5 to 1.

Causes

The cause of Hodgkin's disease is unknown. Many theories have been investigated, including some theories that it was an infectious, probably viral, disease. Although it is possible that a virus may be involved in some way in some cases, it is not yet clear how.

How the Cancer Tends to Spread

Hodgkin's disease tends to spread via the lymphatic system. It usually begins in lymph nodes in the neck, armpit, or chest. It then tends to spread to other lymph nodes nearby, then to lymph nodes elsewhere in the body, then to the bone marrow and the liver. It can sometimes spread to other areas of the body that are in contact with lymph-node-bearing areas, such as the lungs or the skin.

Symptoms or Problems That You May Notice

Enlarged lymph nodes, most commonly in the neck, are one indicator you may notice. Other, generalized symptoms (called B symptoms) are important in determining the type of treatment.

Symptoms Related to Enlarged Lymph Nodes

With Hodgkin's disease, enlarged lymph nodes are quite often the first problem a person may notice. (Please note that enlarged lymph nodes, usually resulting from an infection, are very common in the general population. **In the vast majority of cases, enlarged lymph nodes are not caused by Hodgkin's disease.**) Usually the nodes are **painless** and are **not tender** when touched. They may first be noticed when the person washes, showers, or shaves. If the lymph nodes are inside the chest, in the space between the lungs, they cannot be seen or felt. Sometimes lymph nodes in this area are first detected on a **routine chest X ray** or if they cause mild symptoms such as a long-standing **nonproductive cough** (a cough without any sputum) or, occasionally, **breathlessness**.

Generalized Symptoms Called B Symptoms

It has been known for many decades that certain people with Hodgkin's disease may have one or more of three particular types of generalized symptoms. If these symptoms are not present, the stage of the disease is given the letter "A" (stage IA or IIA, for example). If any of these symptoms *are* present, the stage is given the letter "B" (stage IIB, for example). The symptom type is relevant in determining the type of treatment. The **B symptoms** consist of:

- **weight loss.** If you lose more than 10 percent of your previous body weight at the onset of Hodgkin's disease, that is a B symptom.
- **unexplained fever.** Several episodes of fever (with a temperature higher than 100.5°F, or 38°C) without any explanation (such as a cold or flu) is a B symptom.
- **night sweats.** Profuse sweating at night that requires you to change your nightclothes or bedclothes is a B symptom.

Other generalized symptoms may include tiredness or, rarely, itching all over your body or an ache in the affected lymph nodes after you drink alcohol. Although these symptoms are associated with Hodgkin's disease, they do not influence the type of treatment and are not therefore called B symptoms.

Diagnosis and Tests

There are two important parts to the diagnosis of Hodgkin's disease. One is the diagnosis itself—establishing that the problem is Hodgkin's disease and not something else. The second is the accurate assessment of the stage of the disease.

Diagnosis Usually the diagnosis is established by taking a **biopsy** of a lymph node. If there are nodes that can be felt in the neck or the armpit, the procedure is usually very straightforward (although it may require a general anesthetic if the node is not easily accessible). If the node is in the chest, a **mediastinoscopy** (see page 331) may be required or (less commonly) a **thoracotomy**, involving an incision to open the chest cavity so that lymph nodes may be removed in their entirety. The tissue from the lymph node is then examined by the pathologist. In most cases the diagnosis of Hodgkin's

MAIN AREAS OF LYMPH NODES

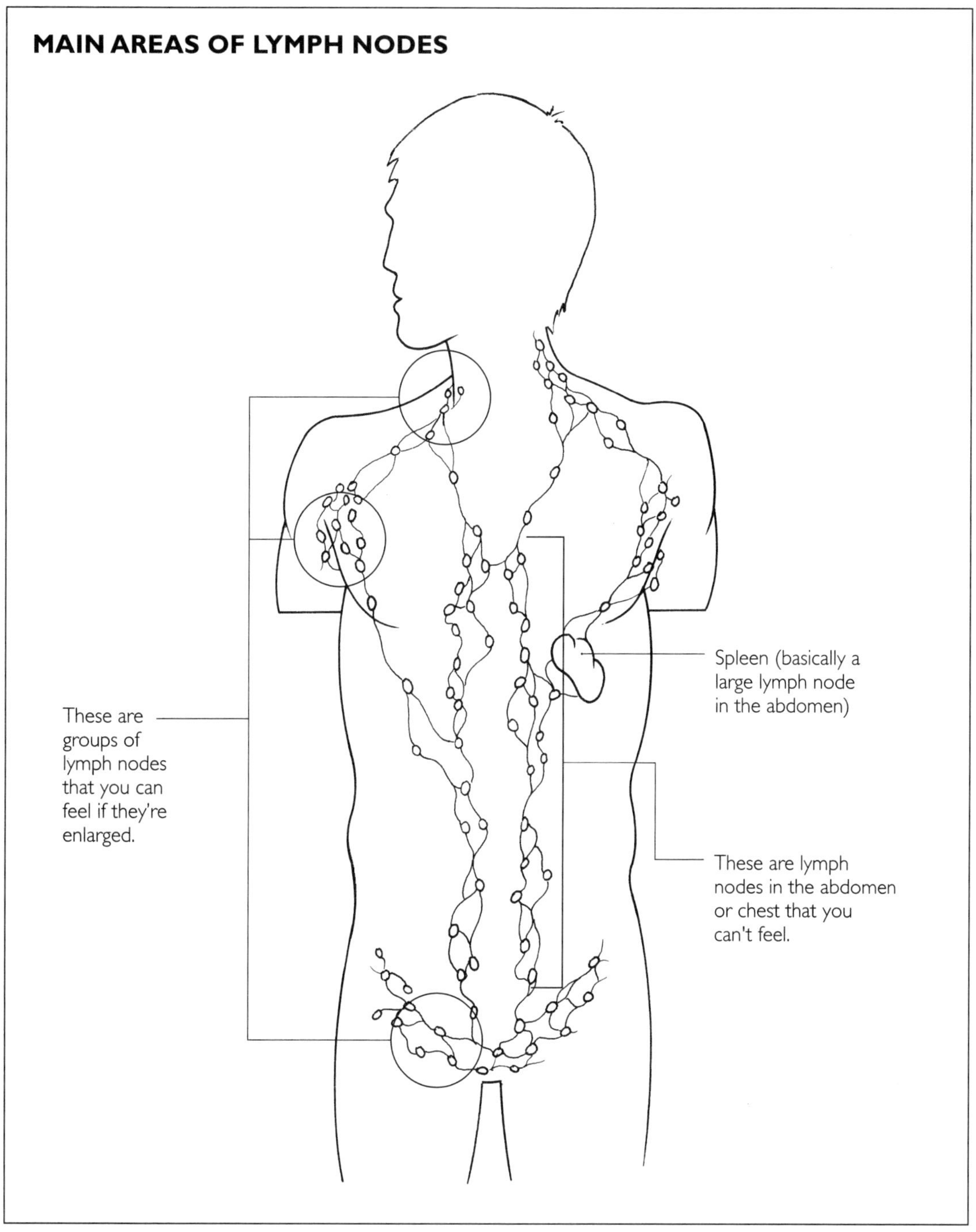

disease is fairly straightforward, but in a few cases the appearance under the microscope is quite difficult to distinguish from other types of lymphoma. Special staining techniques may then be required to assist in a firm diagnosis, so if it takes a few days, have patience: the delay is not due to incompetence in your medical team!

Staging Tests

If the diagnosis is Hodgkin's disease, it is very important to establish exactly where the disease is and how far it has spread. Depending on where the initial lymph nodes are, some (or all) of the following tests may be recommended to you.

Ultrasound and CT Scan of Abdomen and Liver An ultrasound, a CT scan, or both may be useful in certain cases in showing up groups of lymph nodes in the abdomen, an enlarged spleen, or abnormalities in the liver. CT scans of the chest may show lymph nodes in other areas (for example, in the mediastinum).

Lymphogram A lymphogram may be useful in certain circumstances in Hodgkin's disease. If it shows that certain nodes in the pelvis or abdomen are enlarged, ordinary X rays may be taken over the months that follow to show the nodes shrinking during treatment.

Bone Marrow Biopsy Because Hodgkin's disease can spread to the bone marrow, most people with the condition should have a sample of the bone marrow analyzed for any signs of the disease.

Laparotomy A laparotomy involves making an incision in the abdomen to allow the surgeon to assess all the organs within it. The procedure used to be a major part of the staging of Hodgkin's disease and is still used in some situations, though increasingly other forms of staging (such as scans) plus different criteria for treatment have made laparotomy less necessary. Customarily, at the time of laparotomy, the spleen is removed, partly because it is a focus (or potential focus) of Hodgkin's disease, partly because its absence makes subsequent radiotherapy easier. Practice varies from one cancer center to another.

Liver Biopsy In certain circumstances, a biopsy of the liver may be required, using a fine needle put in under local anesthetic.

Gallium Scans The cells of Hodgkin's disease are particularly active in taking up a metal called gallium. In a gallium scan, you will be given an injection of gallium, which shows up on a scan. This test is used to show nodes that are difficult to see otherwise. It may also give information about the status of any suspicious nodes.

Other Tests Several blood tests will be done as a matter of routine. Other tests being investigated in some cancer centers may provide useful information in certain circumstances.

The Main Types of the Cancer

There are several different classifications of the ways Hodgkin's disease appears under the microscope and four or five different subtypes or categories of the disease. Two features are particularly useful. One is whether fibrous scars (called **nodular sclerosis**) are present within the lymph node. Lymph nodes with nodular sclerosis may take longer to shrink back to normal, so your medical team will be aware that the nodes could take weeks or months to return to normal after treatment. By and large, nodular sclerosis is found more often among young adults with Hodgkin's disease and when the disease occurs in the neck or chest. The other important feature is whether there are many or few lymphocytes in the node. If there are many, it usually means that the Hodgkin's disease will behave less aggressively; if there are few, it may behave more aggressively. The more aggressive types of the tumor tend to be more common in the older age group.

Factors That Influence the Treatment and Prognosis

Stage The most important factor in deciding which type of treatment to use is the stage of the disease. By and large, if the Hodgkin's disease is limited to one site of the body (say the neck) and if there are no B symptoms, it is usually treated with radiotherapy. If it involves lymph nodes in the chest and in the abdomen or if there are B symptoms (or in a few other circumstances), it is customary to use chemotherapy or a combination of chemotherapy and radiotherapy. If it involves non–lymph node areas such as the marrow or liver, generally the treatment will be with chemotherapy.

B Symptoms If B symptoms are present, your medical team may recommend chemotherapy as part of the treatment.

Type of the Tumor To a lesser extent, if other factors are not decisive in pointing to radiotherapy or chemotherapy, the type of the tumor (for example, the number of lymphocytes present in the tumor) may influence treatment.

The Main Objectives of Treatment

Because Hodgkin's disease is curable in the majority of cases, the primary objective of treatment is to cure the patient.

Types of Treatment

Radiotherapy Radiotherapy is the treatment frequently used if the disease is limited to one area of the body (or a few areas that are close to each other). It is also used in other circumstances in combination with chemotherapy. Generally speaking, the radiotherapy is given not only to the areas in which there is (or was) a tumor, but to some of the adjacent areas as well. This "extended field" radiotherapy increases the chance of eradicating the disease completely. The exact details of the therapy in your particular case will need to be discussed between you and your radiation oncologist. Any side effects that you experience will depend on which areas of the body are included in the radiation.

It should be noted that if the Hodgkin's disease recurs after radiotherapy, there is still a high probability that it can be cured by chemotherapy. For that reason, chemotherapy is being used more frequently nowadays as the first treatment even if the disease is limited.

Chemotherapy If the disease is widespread (in both the chest and the abdomen or involving the bone marrow or liver) or if there are B symptoms, chemotherapy will be recommended, either by itself or in addition to radiotherapy. Many different drugs are effective in treating Hodgkin's disease, and they are usually given in combinations. The first combination to be used in this context comprised four drugs whose initials are MOPP. This combination proved to be very effective, and both MOPP and variations on it are still sometimes used. Another combination of four drugs, ABVD, has now become the standard, and some cancer centers use alternating courses of MOPP (or a variant) and ABVD, or a combination of some of the drugs in these regimens, as the first-line therapy. Again, your specialist will discuss with you the full details of the particular regimen being recommended in your case.

Treatment If There Is a Recurrence

High-Dose Therapy If the Hodgkin's disease recurs after chemotherapy, the situation is more difficult. In many cases, it may respond to other chemotherapy drugs (used as what is termed **salvage therapy**). The long-term prognosis may also be improved by using high-dose treatment with bone marrow rescue or peripheral stem-cell rescue (see page 228). These are intensive and arduous forms of therapy but may be very effective in some cases. If one of these treatments is recommended, you and your doctors will need to discuss the potential benefits and hazards in detail.

Long-Term Effects of Therapy

There are some long-term effects of therapy that, although not common, are significant. There is a chance that the radiotherapy and chemotherapy may affect the working of your thyroid gland (so that tests and hormone tablets may sometimes be required). Also the strength of the heart muscle may sometimes be reduced, leading to shortness of breath. In addition, there is an increased risk that patients may develop a second type of cancer, particularly a non-Hodgkin's type of lymphoma, several years after successful treatment for Hodgkin's disease.

KAPOSI'S SARCOMA AND AIDS-RELATED LYMPHOMA

SUMMARY OF THE KEY FACTS IN THIS SECTION

- Kaposi's sarcoma (KS) is a cancer that most commonly appears in the skin or in the linings of the digestive tract or lungs. It is one of the conditions that is used as a defining criterion for AIDS (when it is called epidemic KS). It occurs in other situations but much more rarely.
- Individual lesions of KS are often sensitive to radiotherapy and can be controlled.
- Chemotherapy and some biologic agents are also active against KS.
- The main problem with KS is that new lesions of KS are likely to occur in other areas, and therefore complete cure is rare.
- People with AIDS also have a higher-than-average tendency to get lymphomas, and the lymphomas that occur in AIDS often behave somewhat differently from those that are not AIDS related.

The Most Important Features of the Tumor

Before the 1980s, Kaposi's sarcoma (abbreviated KS) was an uncommon type of cancer. It was until then known as a rare purplish-colored sarcoma of the skin usually seen in elderly men of Italian or Eastern European background in whom it was generally slow growing. It was also seen in younger Africans, initially in North Africa, in whom the disease seemed to be faster growing. Then the syndrome (the group of symptoms or conditions) that we now call AIDS began to emerge. It was first recognized as a separate and new disease entity when physicians noted a group of young men who developed a rare form of pneumonia (caused by pneumocystis carinii, previously rare except in immune-suppressed individuals) associated with KS, a hitherto uncommon form of cancer. At the present time, KS is quite common in people with AIDS, and, in fact, most cases of KS occur in people with AIDS. This form of the disease is usually referred to as epidemic KS.

KS is a sarcoma that begins in connective tissue (see page 183) usually from the dermis layer of the skin (see page 149).

Age and Incidence

Most KS occurs in homosexual or bisexual males in the twenty- to sixty-year-old age group.

Causes

Although it is clear that epidemic KS is caused by infection with the HIV (human immunodeficiency virus), the exact mechanism is unknown, nor is it known why KS and lymphoma are the tumors whose development is most promoted by the HIV infection.

How the Cancer Tends to Spread

KS is basically a multicentric disease, appearing in several places almost at the same time. It is therefore not considered to have spread from one place to another.

Symptoms or Problems That You May Notice

Individual lesions of KS appear as purplish, painless skin lesions. KS often appears in several areas over the face, torso, and limbs in a short time. In addition, there may be lesions in the lining of the mouth. In more than half of people with KS, many lymph nodes are enlarged at the time of diagnosis, though this may be part of the AIDS picture and not caused by the spread of KS in at least some cases. KS can also occur in any part of the digestive tract and may be found in the lungs. There may be constitutional symptoms as well, such as lethargy, night sweats, and weight loss.

Diagnosis and Tests

The clinical history and examination may provide the diagnosis, particularly in an HIV-positive person. In most cases, a biopsy of one of the KS lesions will be recommended to confirm the diagnosis. Other tests (scans, X rays, or endoscopies) may be recommended as well, depending on the person's symptoms and the particular circumstances.

Factors That Influence the Treatment and Prognosis

In general, the outlook for people with KS depends to a considerable extent on the severity of the other aspects of the immune deficiency. If the immune deficiency is severe, with frequent and severe infections and with a marked decrease in the helper (CD4 or T4) lymphocytes, the outlook is poorer. If, on the other hand, the person is well, apart from KS lesions on the skin, the outlook is better.

The Main Objectives of Treatment

Because KS is considered a multifocal disease, the main objective of therapy is to control the condition and reduce the symptoms. It is particularly important to do so because, as a result of the immune suppression, many people with AIDS do not easily tolerate the usual doses of chemotherapy.

Types of Treatment

Radiotherapy Lesions of KS are quite sensitive to radiotherapy and may respond to extremely small doses, such as 20 Gy or 2,000 rads, compared with 45 to 60 Gy or 4,500 to 6,000 rads for other types of cancer ("Gy": abbreviation for "gray," meaning a unit of absorbed radiation dose equal to 100 rads; "rad": acronym for radiation absorbed dose).

Chemotherapy Several drugs may be of use in KS. They include: **vinblastine**, **vincristine**, **etoposide**,

Adriamycin, and **bleomycin**. It may be difficult to give adequate doses of these drugs, however, because the person may have severe immune suppression.

Biologic Therapy Of the biologic response modifiers (biologic agents), **alpha-interferon** has been most extensively investigated and used. It may produce good responses, particularly in those patients in whom the immune suppression is not too severe.

AIDS-Related Lymphoma

Lymphomas—cancers of the lymphocytes—are the only other tumors apart from KS that are definitely associated with AIDS. You will find a detailed discussion of the lymphomas on pages 142–148, but a few points about the types of lymphomas that occur in HIV-positive people are noted here.

Types of Lymphoma In general, the lymphomas that occur in AIDS patients are mostly of the high-grade type rather than the intermediate or low-grade types.

CNS Lymphomas In people with AIDS, lymphomas occur more commonly within the brain and spinal cord (the central nervous system, or CNS). In fact, lymphoma of the CNS is one of the criteria for the definition of AIDS. Generally it tends to occur late in the disease and to be severe. It responds to treatment with radiotherapy and steroids in some cases, but if there is no response, unfortunately the outlook is poor.

Treatment of Lymphomas in AIDS Patients

The biggest problem in treating lymphomas in AIDS patients is that there may be severe immune suppression, which may make chemotherapy more hazardous than usual. Furthermore, additional therapy to the central nervous system is sometimes required because spread to the CNS is relatively common. Many drug combinations can be used but often with some limitation on the amount that can be given safely. The drugs that are most commonly used include: **methotrexate**, **bleomycin**, **Adriamycin**, **cyclophosphamide**, **steroids**, **etoposide**, **cytosine arabinoside**, and others. The details of each case will vary considerably, and so you will need to discuss the specifics of what is being recommended with your doctor.

KIDNEY

Number of new cases diagnosed per year in the United States: 30,600

SUMMARY OF THE KEY FACTS IN THIS SECTION

- The most common type of kidney cancer is **adenocarcinoma** of the kidney, also called **renal-cell carcinoma** (and formerly called **hypernephroma**).
- Renal-cell carcinoma occurs in men twice as frequently as in women, and smoking is often a contributory cause.
- It has a marked tendency to spread to distant parts of the body, but if it is treated before it has done so, it is curable in many cases.
- A rarer kidney cancer that occurs in childhood is called **Wilms' tumor** and is curable in most cases with a combination of surgery and chemotherapy. (See "Rarer Cancers in Childhood" later in this chapter.)

The Most Important Features of the Tumor

Renal-cell carcinoma is one of the types of cancer that is often associated with smoking. This is probably because some of the most important carcinogens in tobacco smoke pass unchanged into the urine and, as they collect and become concentrated there, expose the linings of the kidney and the bladder to a high risk of cancer. Renal-cell carcinoma has a high tendency to spread to other parts of the body, particularly via the bloodstream, and may cause secondary tumors in the lungs. If treated (with surgery) before spread occurs, there is a relatively high probability of cure. Unfortunately, detection of kidney tumors at an early stage is difficult. Because the kidney (like the liver and other visceral organs) is not very well supplied with nerves, tumors can grow there without causing pain or discomfort. Renal-cell carcinoma is among the few types of cancer that have been shown to respond to substances that alter the response of the immune system. The most important of these for this particular cancer are the agents interleukin-2 and interferon.

What You Really Need to Know about the Kidneys

Most people have some idea of what the kidneys are and what they do. There are two of them, and they produce urine in a two-step process. First, the kidneys **filter** the blood through billions (literally) of tiny filters called **glomeruli**. These separate the cells of the blood (red cells, white cells, and platelets)

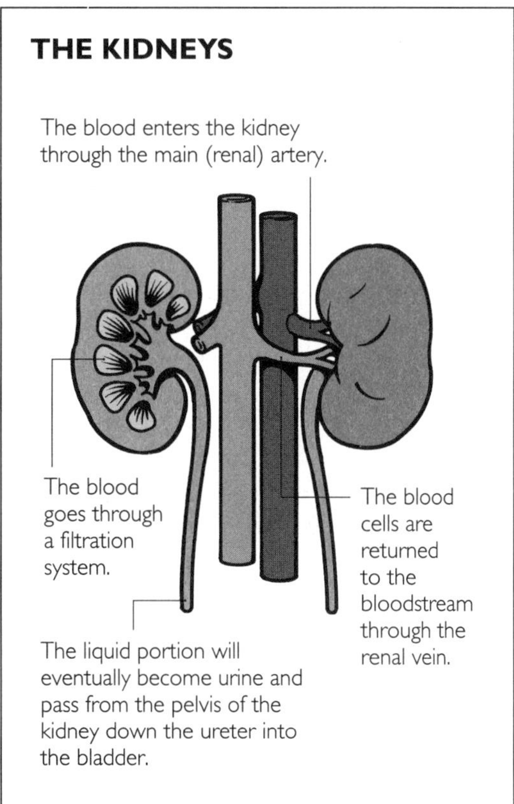

from the liquid (plasma) so that the liquid component passes out of the body's circulatory system into a set of tubules. As the liquid passes through those tubules, it is processed in a highly complex way so that necessary substances are absorbed back into the blood and unwanted waste products pass onward.

In the second part of the process, **collecting** the fluid, the processed fluid that will eventually be urine passes into tubules that lead into bigger and bigger tubules until they reach the collecting "port" of the kidney. On the way, some minor adjustments to the urine are made. The collecting port is called the **pelvis** of the kidney, and the urine flows out of the pelvis into the **ureter**, which is a thin tube leading down into the bladder.

Many people do not realize that the kidneys have a far greater power of filtering the blood than we actually need. In fact, we can easily exist with only one kidney (as, of course, thousands of living kidney donors prove), and we could probably exist with only a third or a quarter of one kidney. Hence anything that damages only one kidney, or necessitates its removal, does not create a medical problem.

The Main Types of the Cancer

Note: I depart from the usual order of topics in this section because I need to clarify that there are different types of kidney cancer. The most common kind, **renal-cell carcinoma**, will be the subject of this section. There is a rare type of kidney tumor that occurs in childhood, called **Wilms' tumor**. I deal with that in the section "Rarer Cancers in Childhood" (pages 203–204).

The most common type of kidney cancer is renal-cell carcinoma (which used to be called hypernephroma). This type accounts for about 85 percent of all kidney cancers. It appears to develop from the cells lining the tubules of the kidney.

In childhood there is a completely different type of cancer called Wilms' tumor that has a different way of behaving and is easier to cure, although the treatment is usually complicated and somewhat difficult.

As well as these two types, there are some other kidney cancers that are rarer. Cancers may develop in the pelvis of the kidney. These are not usually adenocarcinomas but are similar to cancers of the bladder (pages 36–41) and behave in a similar way. One or two other types of cancer, such as sarcomas, occur in the kidney but only rarely.

Age and Incidence

Renal-cell carcinoma has a peak incidence in the fifties and is quite rare in young adulthood (say, before age forty). It occurs twice as frequently in men as in women. We suspect that this is the result of smoking patterns, and therefore that this gender difference may change as smoking habits change.

Causes

About one-third of the cases of renal-cell carcinoma are associated with smoking. As with cancer of the bladder, many carcinogens in tobacco smoke are processed by the kidney and are then concentrated as they pass through the collecting systems of the kidneys and the bladder.

In previous eras, factors that used to cause kidney cancer included exposure to chemicals involved in working with coke ovens. Nowadays the operation of coke ovens is strictly regulated, and there is now no risk to such workers. In a very few cases, kidney cancers may be inherited in families, associated with problems in the cerebellum.

How the Cancer Tends to Spread

Renal-cell carcinoma is somewhat unusual in that it tends to spread first via the bloodstream (rather than the lymph nodes). It may spread to the lymph nodes as well, but it is not unusual to find that the bloodstream is the first means of spread. In such cases, any secondary tumors are most likely to be found in the lungs, though other organs of the body may also be involved.

Symptoms or Problems That You May Notice

It is often difficult to detect renal-cell carcinoma in the early stages because the kidneys are situated at the back of the abdomen and are not richly supplied with nerves. Hence it is comparatively easy for a tumor to grow there without causing any pain or discomfort. In fact, the most common symptom caused by kidney cancer is **blood in the urine** (**hematuria**). It must be stressed that **most cases of hematuria are not caused by kidney cancer**. In the vast majority of cases, hematuria is caused by some benign problem such as infection, enlargement of the prostate, or kidney stones. However, because a possible cause of hematuria is renal-cell carcinoma, it is essential for all cases of blood in the urine to be assessed by a physician.

In some cases the kidney cancer may cause mild **pain** or discomfort, which is usually felt in the **flank** region, that is, around the back and side of the abdomen. The pain is usually rather dull in nature and tends to be constant—a continuing ache for many hours at a time. By contrast, the pain of a kidney stone experienced in the same area is usually very sharp in nature and comes and goes in waves (a colicky pain rather than a constant ache).

LOCATION OF THE FLANK

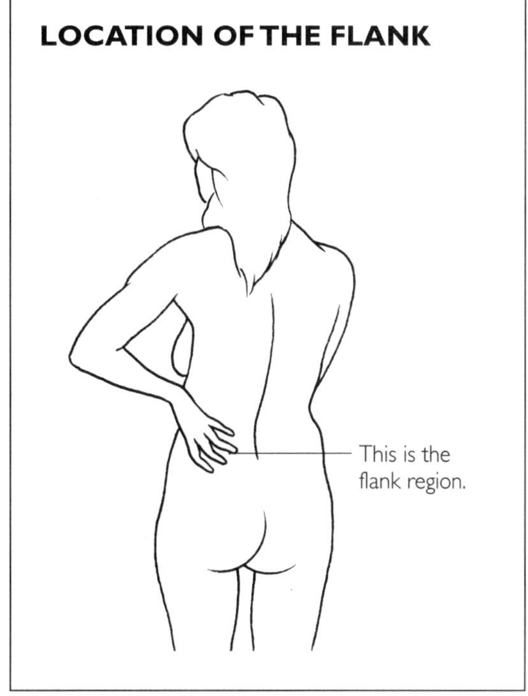

Diagnosis and Tests

The diagnosis of renal-cell carcinoma depends on some or all of the following tests.

Urine Tests Urine tests are usually done as a preliminary screen to confirm the presence of blood cells in the urine and also to look for other explanations (such as infections).

IVP (Intravenous Pyelogram) The IVP is an X ray in which a special dye is injected into a vein in your arm and X-ray pictures are taken as the dye passes through the kidney and ureters. The test can show up irregularities in the outline of the kidneys (as well as other problems such as stones).

Ultrasound and CT Scan Both ultrasounds and CT scans of the abdomen and pelvis can be very useful in suspected cases of renal-cell carcinoma. They may show other problems such as involvement of the lymph nodes. Usually an MRI scan is unnecessary if the CT scan shows the problem clearly.

Other Kidney Tests Several other tests may be done to assist in planning any surgery. For example, an **arteriogram** may be recommended. In this procedure, a dye is injected that enters the kidney through the arteries in the area, enabling the biggest arteries to be seen so that the surgeon knows where they are (in your particular case) before the surgery. Other tests may be recommended to make sure the other kidney is functioning normally.

Other Tests to Detect Any Spread Other tests may be recommended to check whether the cancer has spread. These may include a bone scan or special X rays or CT scans of the lungs in certain circumstances.

Factors That Influence the Treatment and Prognosis

In renal-cell carcinoma the most important factor is whether or not the tumor has spread. If it has not spread, complete removal of the kidney (and some surrounding tissue) may be curative in many cases.

The Main Objectives of Treatment

If the cancer has not spread, complete removal of the kidney (usually with some surrounding tissue) is performed with the intention of curing the patient completely. Even if the cancer has spread to other parts of the body, it is worthwhile considering surgery for two reasons. First, and most important, removal of the kidney will relieve any pain or discomfort and will also prevent future local problems (such as bleeding). Because the course of kidney cancer is somewhat unpredictable, this may give a high quality of life for up to several years. Second, in a very few cases, the secondaries may disappear after the primary has been removed. Such cases are very rare but happen occasionally with renal-cell carcinoma.

Types of Treatment

Surgery Surgery is the mainstay for treatment for cancer of the kidney. Even if tests show that an operation may not be curative, it is still recommended for the control or prevention of symptoms in many cases, unless the general medical condition of the patient makes it too hazardous. The usual operation consists of removal of the kidney plus the lymph nodes in the area and is called a **radical nephrectomy**. It is fairly major surgery, but often the incision is made in the flank region, which makes the healing process quicker and easier. As the operation removes the kidney and does not affect the bladder, you will not need a urostomy (surgical creation of a means of collecting the urine in a bag), though you may have a urinary catheter (drainage tube in the bladder) for a few days after surgery.

Hormone Therapy For reasons that we do not understand, some cases of kidney cancer respond to hormone medications of the progesterone type. This effect is rare, but as there are very few side effects from the hormone tablets, they are sometimes recommended. In fact, the major side effect of the hormone tablet is an increase in appetite and energy.

Biological Response Modifiers Again for reasons that are not well understood, renal-cell carcinoma is among the types of cancer sensitive to treatments that alter the response of the immune system to the cancer. The substances that have proved most successful in such treatments are **interferons** and **interleukin-2**, sometimes in combination with chemotherapy. The treatments may be quite intense, and the side effects can be debilitating and sometimes hazardous. These treatments are not available at all centers. The details should be discussed with your specialist.

Chemotherapy Chemotherapy drugs have an effect in some cases of renal-cell carcinoma. Your specialist may have investigational drugs available, and the treatment is worth considering.

Spontaneous Remissions Renal-cell carcinoma is one of the four types of cancer that account for more than half of all documented spontaneous remissions. (The other three types are melanoma, neuroblastoma, and choriocarcinoma.) It is well documented that shrinkage or even complete disappearance of renal-cell carcinoma (including secondary tumors in the lungs) does occur. This characteristic is thought to be connected in some way to the way in which kidney cancer responds to biological response modifiers and hormones. I must emphasize that spontaneous remission is very rare (the incidence is approximately one case in every 100,000 cases of cancer), but if it happens it is very welcome and may last for a considerable time.

Other Therapy In certain circumstances, it may be possible to inject material into the artery supplying the tumor, and part of the kidney, with blood. This is called **embolization** or **angioinfarction**. This treatment may kill some tumor cells and may produce shrinkage in some cases. If it is recommended in your case, you will need to discuss the details with your doctor.

Other Types of Kidney Cancer

Sometimes a cancer that is not an adenocarcinoma when seen under the microscope may arise in the pelvis of the kidney. Usually these cancers are of the transitional-cell type and resemble cancers of the bladder. You can find an outline of treatment in the section on bladder cancer (pages 36–41).

LARYNX (VOICE BOX) AND PHARYNX (THROAT)

Number of new cases diagnosed per year in the United States: larynx 11,600, pharynx 9,100

SUMMARY OF THE KEY FACTS IN THIS SECTION

- Cancer of the larynx occurs in men five times more frequently than in women and is mostly caused by a combination of cigarette smoking and alcohol.
- If detected and treated in its early stages, it is curable in the great majority of cases.
- Treatment is with surgery, radiotherapy, or both, or with a combination of chemotherapy and radiotherapy.
- Because the causes of these cancers are known, prevention is a real possibility.

The Most Important Features of Cancer of the Larynx

Cancer of the larynx develops in the voice box, the front part of the area at the back of the throat, in the region of the vocal cords. Because of its location near the vocal cords and its function, it is often detected at an early stage when there may be changes in the voice. If diagnosed and treated at an early stage—with surgery, and radiotherapy, or both, or with a combination of chemotherapy and radiotherapy—it may be cured in the majority of cases. In some cases the vocal cords may have to be removed to provide the maximum chance of permanent cure, and if that happens a new way of producing speech can be learned, using either electronic devices or a different method of producing sound. Laryngeal cancer is mostly associated with a combination of cigarette smoking and alcohol, so that prevention of this particular cancer is a real possibility.

What You Really Need to Know about the Larynx and Pharynx

The **pharynx** is the curved area that leads from the back of the mouth to the top of the esophagus (gullet) and the **trachea** (the airway that leads to the lungs). In other words, the pharynx is basically the throat plus the area at the back of the nose. At the front of the pharynx is the **larynx** (often called the voice box), which contains the apparatus that creates the voice. The larynx is shaped rather like a box and is situated on top of the trachea. The **epiglottis** is a little spur of cartilage that is attached to the top end of the larynx. Inside the larynx are the **vocal cords**, which create sound when they are vibrated by air coming out of the trachea as we talk.

For convenience, different medical terms are used for different areas in the region of the pharynx, so that the back of the nasal passages is often called the **nasopharynx**, the back of the mouth is called the **oropharynx**, the laryngeal area is sometimes called the **laryngopharynx**, and the area behind it is called the **hypopharynx**. You may hear your medical team using terms like these. They are useful for indicating specifically which area is involved.

Age and Incidence

Cancer of the larynx occurs predominantly in middle to late adulthood and is rare in the thirties or younger. It is currently five times as common in men as in women, and this almost certainly reflects smoking habits. As smoking has increased among women, the incidence of laryngeal cancer has followed it fifteen to twenty years later.

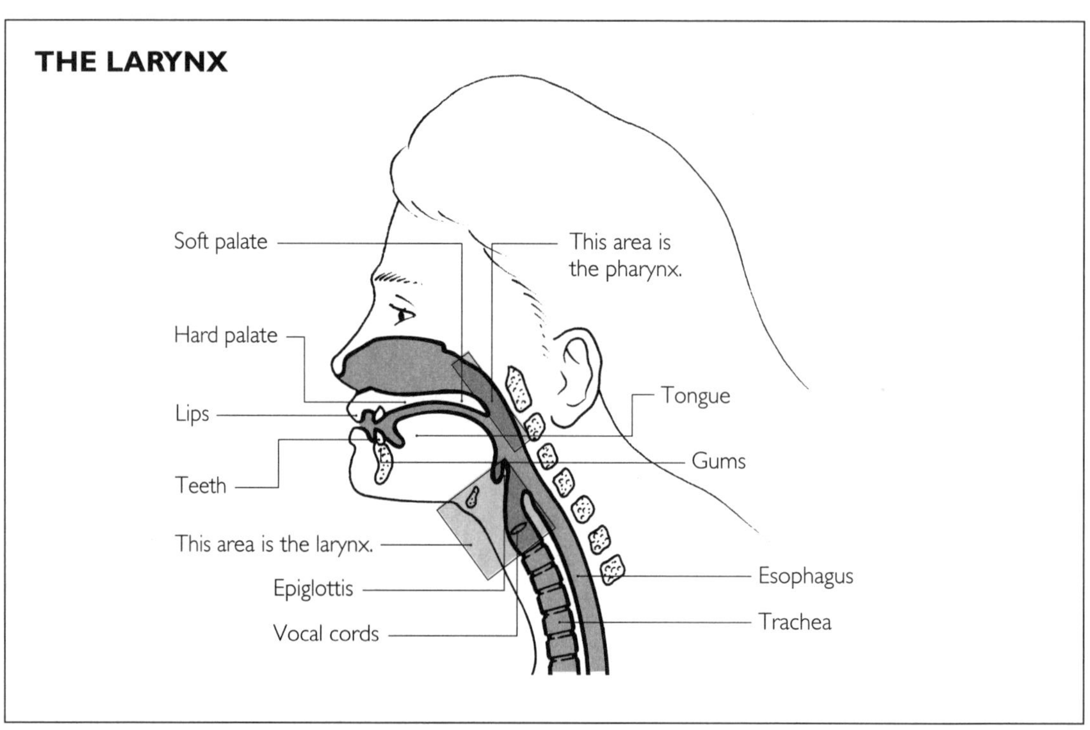

Causes

The main cause of laryngeal cancer is cigarette smoke, often combined with alcohol. Other factors may sometimes contribute, particularly with cancer in the nasopharynx, which has different causes and treatment and behaves in a different way.

How the Cancer Tends to Spread

If the cancer develops close to the vocal cords, it usually stays localized in that area for some time and does not spread to lymph nodes until later. We think this is because the vocal cords have fewer lymphatic vessels in them than other organs. If the cancer develops farther from the vocal cords, it may spread to lymph nodes at a somewhat earlier stage.

Symptoms or Problems That You May Notice

If the cancer develops near the vocal cords, there is a good chance that it will be detected at an early stage because it will affect the voice while the tumor is still small. In fact, the earliest symptom is usually **hoarseness** or, with cancer of the pharynx, **pain** and **difficulty with swallowing**. If the cancer remains undetected and grows within the larynx, it may cause some discomfort later on, sometimes involving the ear. It may also sometimes cause bleeding, which may result in **coughing up or spitting blood**.

Diagnosis and Tests

Usually the diagnosis of cancer of the larynx starts with the examination of the area by a specialist using a thin, flexible, fiberoptic instrument (a **laryngoscope**) or (less commonly) a light-and-mirror system that is used to see the back of the throat. The laryngoscope is introduced through the nose and is uncomfortable but not painful. Depending on exactly where the problem is, further assessments of the airways may be needed, often with an examination performed under a brief general anesthetic. This is usually called an **EUA** (examination under anesthetic) and is performed in the hospital without

LARYNX INSPECTION

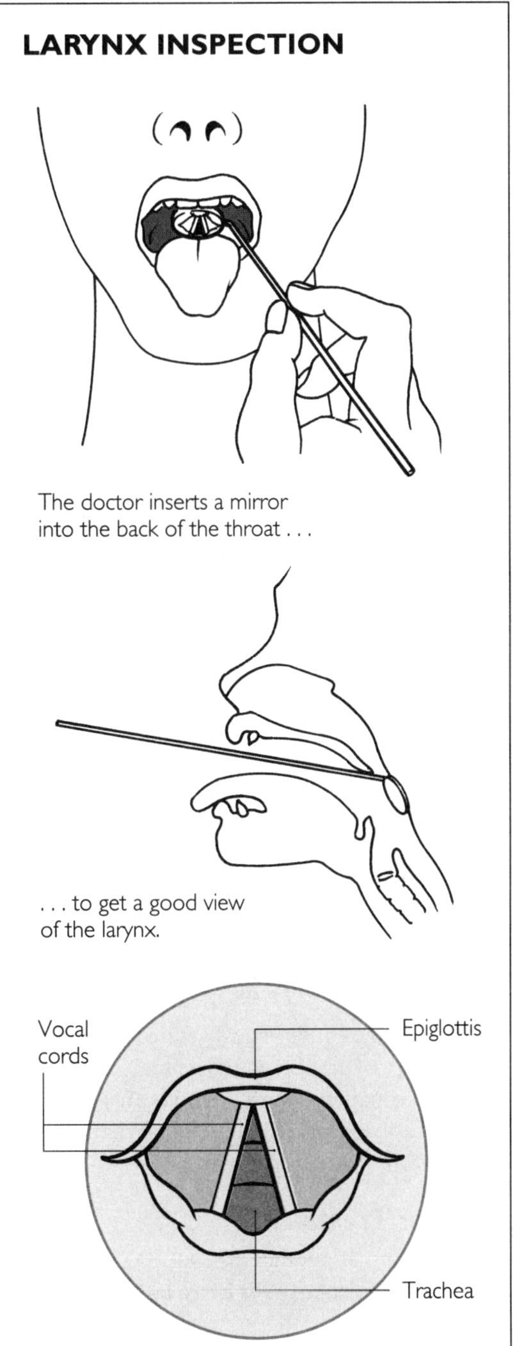

The doctor inserts a mirror into the back of the throat . . .

. . . to get a good view of the larynx.

having to say overnight. Biopsies may be taken during the EUA.

In some cases the area is examined using an instrument that allows the physician to see the vocal cords magnified with a microscope system. The procedure is called microlaryngoscopy and also requires a general anesthetic.

In many cases a CT scan will be recommended to assess the extent of the tumor and to see if there are any enlarged lymph nodes in the area.

Factors That Influence the Treatment and Prognosis

Site and Extent of the Tumor One of the most important factors determining the treatment and the future is the exact location of the tumor. As mentioned above, the site is important because a tumor close to the vocal cords will usually cause symptoms early in its progress and will therefore be detected before it has spread extensively. If the tumor develops farther from the vocal cords, the cancer may grow and spread within the area for some time before it is detected. Once the cancer is detected, what matters next is how far it has spread. Usually, if the tumor is removable and if the vocal cords can move relatively freely, the cure rate is very high. If the tumor has spread far enough so that one or both vocal cords are stuck fast to their surroundings, the condition has a lower cure rate. If it has spread to the lymph nodes, the cure rate is lower still.

The Main Objectives of Treatment

The early stages of laryngeal cancer are curable in the majority of cases, and the primary objective is to cure the patient using methods that minimize any aftereffects, particularly those that interfere with speech.

Types of Treatment

Radiotherapy Radiotherapy is often the treatment of choice, particularly for early laryngeal cancer, because it combines the best chance of cure with preserving the voice. In many cases, radiotherapy alone is curative. In cases where the cancer recurs, surgery is still possible, and a proportion of those patients will be cured. The full details of your radiotherapy treatment will be explained by your radiation oncologist.

Surgery In certain circumstances, surgery may be recommended. Surgery is likely if the cancer has recurred after radiotherapy, and in some other situations as well. The surgery planned will vary considerably from person to person. Your surgeon will discuss the details with you.

In a few cases, if the tumor is relatively small, it may be possible to remove it with a **partial laryngectomy** in which part of the larynx is removed, leaving the vocal cords unaffected (or affected only slightly) in most cases. The details depend on the individual case and require discussion with your surgeon about the exact type and extent of the operation. In some circumstances, and in some cancer centers, **laser surgery** may be used to remove small tumors. If this treatment is available and is thought to be advantageous in your case, your surgeon will discuss it with you.

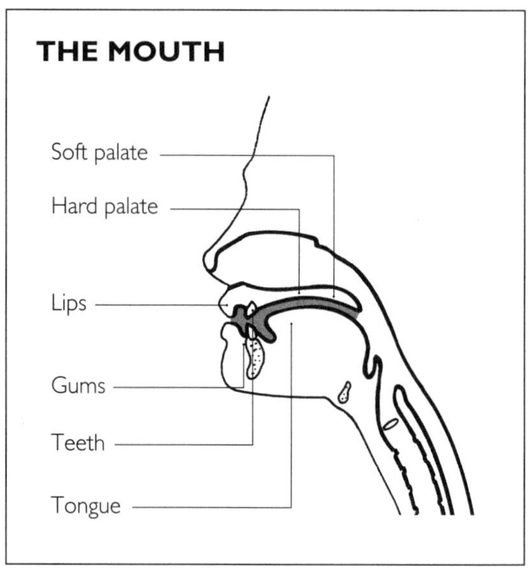

Chemotherapy Nowadays many centers recommend the use of chemotherapy and radiotherapy instead of surgery and radiotherapy. **5-Fluorouracil**, **cis-platinum**, and other drugs are used. This is an area of active research and investigation, so it is important to discuss all the options with your medical team.

Speech after Surgery

In some cases, surgery that involves removal of all of the larynx including the vocal cords may be recommended. This is called a **total laryngectomy**. After the operation you will need to learn to speak in a different way. During the operation, your surgeon will create an opening in your trachea through which air can get in and out of your lungs. The opening is called a **tracheostomy** and is, of course, essential to allow you to breathe. It will not by itself restore your speech, however. Generally, there are three different ways by which speech can be restored.

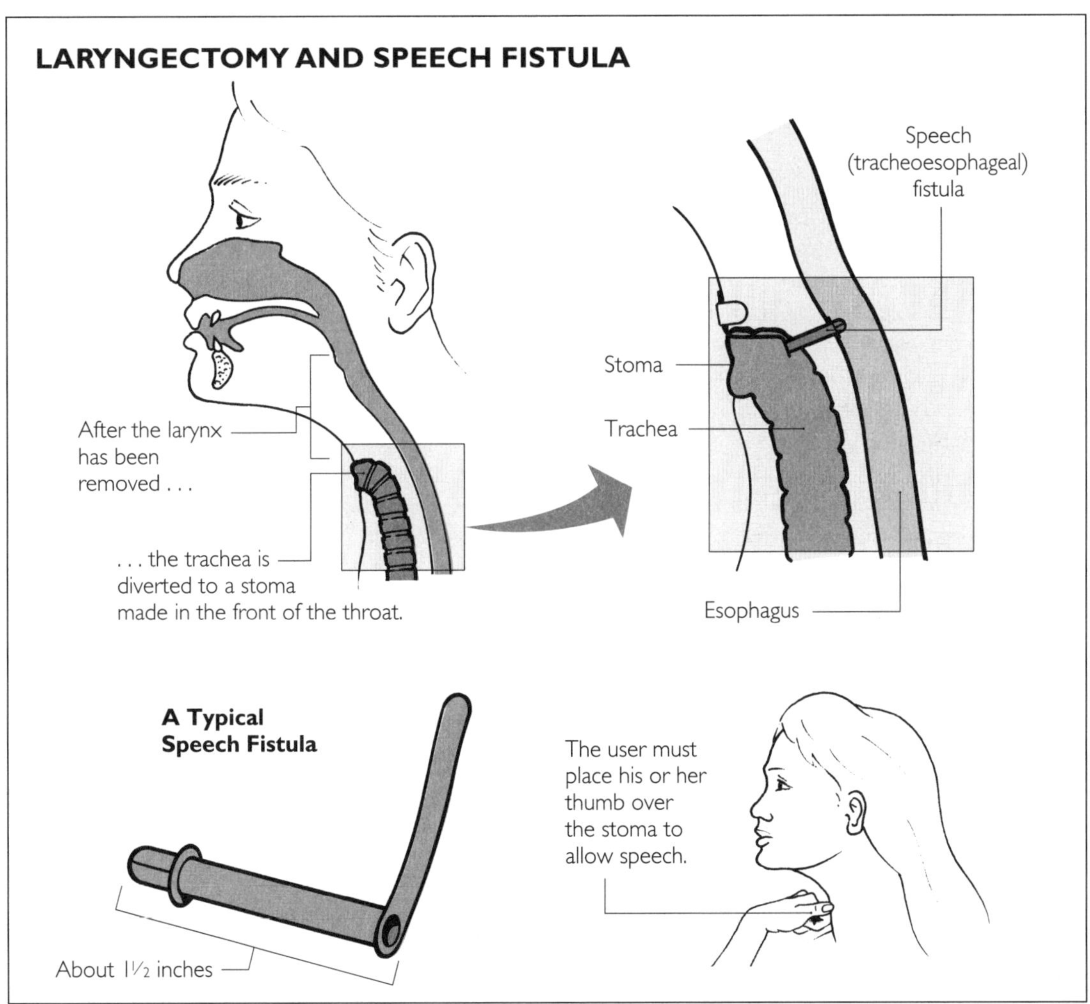

Tracheoesophageal Fistula After the larynx has been removed, you will breathe through the tracheostomy. In addition, your surgeon will create an opening from the upper end of your trachea into your esophagus. Air that you have breathed in can be forced up through this opening (called a tracheoesophageal fistula) into your mouth. You can use that air to talk by blocking the tracheostomy opening with your thumb or finger and using your mouth to make the sounds instead of your vocal cords. This technique, which requires some training, is the most common method of restoring speech in most cancer centers. The fistula requires a one-way valve system (which is built in) to prevent food from your mouth from going down into your lungs. The valve is usually changed and cleaned by the patient.

The Electrolarynx The electrolarynx is a small, hand-held device that creates vibrations. When you hold it to your throat, under your jaw, or even against your cheek, it creates vibrations that you can then change into clearly intelligible words by using your mouth. Each person needs to find the best place to hold the electrolarynx, and it requires some practice to get the best effect.

Esophageal Speech A third method requires the patient to learn to trap air in the esophagus and then expel it (almost like a controlled belch). This also requires some training and practice.

Relearning how to speak after the operation is a very important part of the planned surgery, and you will need to discuss the exact details with your surgeon. It may be helpful for you to see a speech therapist before the operation in order to become familiar with some of the techniques or devices. It may also be possible for you to meet a patient who has had a similar operation so that you can hear at firsthand what the voice sounds like and how he or she coped with the surgery and relearned to speak. Many people who are about to have surgery greatly appreciate this; others feel differently. Do make sure that your views are known.

Cancer of Adjacent Areas of the Pharynx

A cancer may begin in other parts of the pharynx. As I mentioned above, the larynx can be thought of as part of the whole area called the pharynx. If the cancer begins in another part of the pharynx (for example, at the back of the nasal passages or in the upper part of the throat behind the larynx), the basic principles of treatment are the same as those mentioned above. The details of the treatment, however—whether surgery, radiotherapy, or chemotherapy is the first option and what aftereffects may be expected—depend on the specific circumstances. Several factors will need to be considered: the nature of the tumor, its size and site, any other medical conditions that the patient might have, how he or she might cope with any disability after the treatment, and so on. Hence it is important to make sure you understand from your specialists where the problem is and the options they are considering for treating it.

LEUKEMIAS

Number of new cases diagnosed per year in the United States: 27,600

SUMMARY OF THE KEY FACTS IN THIS SECTION

- There are four main types of leukemia: two are called acute because they may progress rapidly, and two are called chronic because they often progress slowly and intermittently.
- Leukemias are also classified according to whether they arise from lymphocytes (lymphocytic and lymphoblastic leukemias) or from another type of white cell, granulocytes (granulocytic or myeloid leukemias).
- Each type of leukemia has a characteristic way of behaving and requires different treatment.
- The most common leukemia in childhood is acute lymphoblastic leukemia, which responds well to chemotherapy and is often curable.
- In early adulthood, acute myeloid leukemia is more common and can sometimes be cured with intensive therapy.
- Chronic lymphocytic and chronic myeloid leukemia can both be controlled with medication for periods of time.

Leukemias: A Summary

Even among the cancers, the word "leukemia" seems to be particularly feared and dreaded. In fact, the main types of leukemia are basically four different diseases, all of which are cancers of the white cells in the bone marrow or the lymph nodes (of which I explain more in a moment) or both. Two different types of white cells are particularly important: the **lymphocytes** and the **granulocytes**. Each of these types can become malignant, thus giving rise to the **lymphocytic leukemias** and the **granulocytic leukemias**. The granulocytic ones are also often called (for unimportant historical reasons) **myeloid leukemias**.

Another aspect of the leukemias is also very important: how immature the leukemia is (a question in some ways comparable to how aggressive it would be if left untreated). If the leukemia produces extremely immature white cells (called **blast** cells), they will appear in the bloodstream. Such a condition is called acute leukemia (so there is **acute lymphocytic leukemia** and **acute myeloid leukemia**). Several years ago, before the modern era of treatment, these acute leukemias would usually progress very rapidly and would often bring about the patient's death in a short time. Nowadays a good proportion of patients can actually be cured.

If the leukemia produces lesser degrees of immaturity in the white cells, there will not be any highly immature blast cells in the bloodstream, and the abnormal cells in the bloodstream will appear (under the microscope) to be more mature and will more closely resemble normal white cells. Leukemias in which that happens are termed **chronic** leukemias (and there is therefore **chronic lymphocytic leukemia** and **chronic myeloid, or granulocytic, leukemia**). The word "chronic" means *goes on for a long time.* Although many people think that "chronic" means *very bad,* it does not, and in the context of leukemias actually means that the situation is *less urgent* and *slower moving* than the acute leukemias.

In addition to these four main types of leukemia, there are one or two other, rarer types, but they usually behave in a way similar to one of the four main types. I deal briefly with one of those other types at the end of this section.

The white cells are made and spend most of their time in the bone marrow and lymph nodes. After discussing those tissues in more detail in order to see what they are and what they do, I deal with each of the types of leukemia in detail.

THE BONES THAT CONTAIN RED MARROW

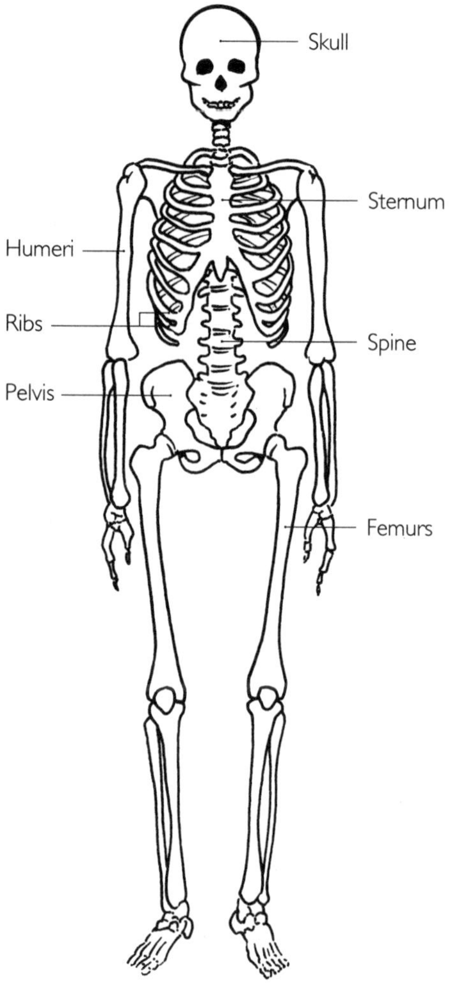

These are the bones that continue to contain blood-making marrow after childhood.

What You Really Need to Know about the Bone Marrow and Lymph Nodes

The bone marrow is the soft tissue inside the hollow center of the major bones of the body—the spine, pelvis, upper arms, legs, and so on. The bone marrow is responsible for making three main types of cells that are in the bloodstream. They are: (a) the **red cells**, which are red from the hemoglobin in them and which **carry oxygen**; (b) the **white cells**, which **are part of the body's defenses against infection** and include the **granulocytes** (also called **neutrophils**) and the **lymphocytes**; and (c) the **platelets**, which are important in helping the blood clot when it needs to, that is, they **control bleeding or bruising** after an injury. These are the three most important types of cells made in the marrow. If the marrow is not working properly, you might have insufficient numbers of any of those three, which could cause a variety of problems. If you have too few red cells or too little hemoglobin in your red cells (**anemia**), you feel tired and breathless because with too little hemoglobin your blood cannot carry enough oxygen to meet your body's needs. If you haven't got enough white cells (a condition called **neutropenia**), you can't fight infections very well. And if you haven't got enough platelets (a condition called **thrombocytopenia**), you might bruise easily or bleed from your gums or nose, or might notice small purple spots (called **petechiae**) in the skin over your arms or legs.

To assess how well the bone marrow is working, a **bone marrow sample** test might be recommended. The test is done under local anesthetic. A thin needle is introduced into the bone at the back of your pelvis (slightly above and to the side of the buttock). This procedure is somewhat uncomfortable (you will be aware of the pushing and prodding), but in many cases is not actually painful. (I have had one done, so I speak from experience!)

MAIN AREAS OF LYMPH NODES

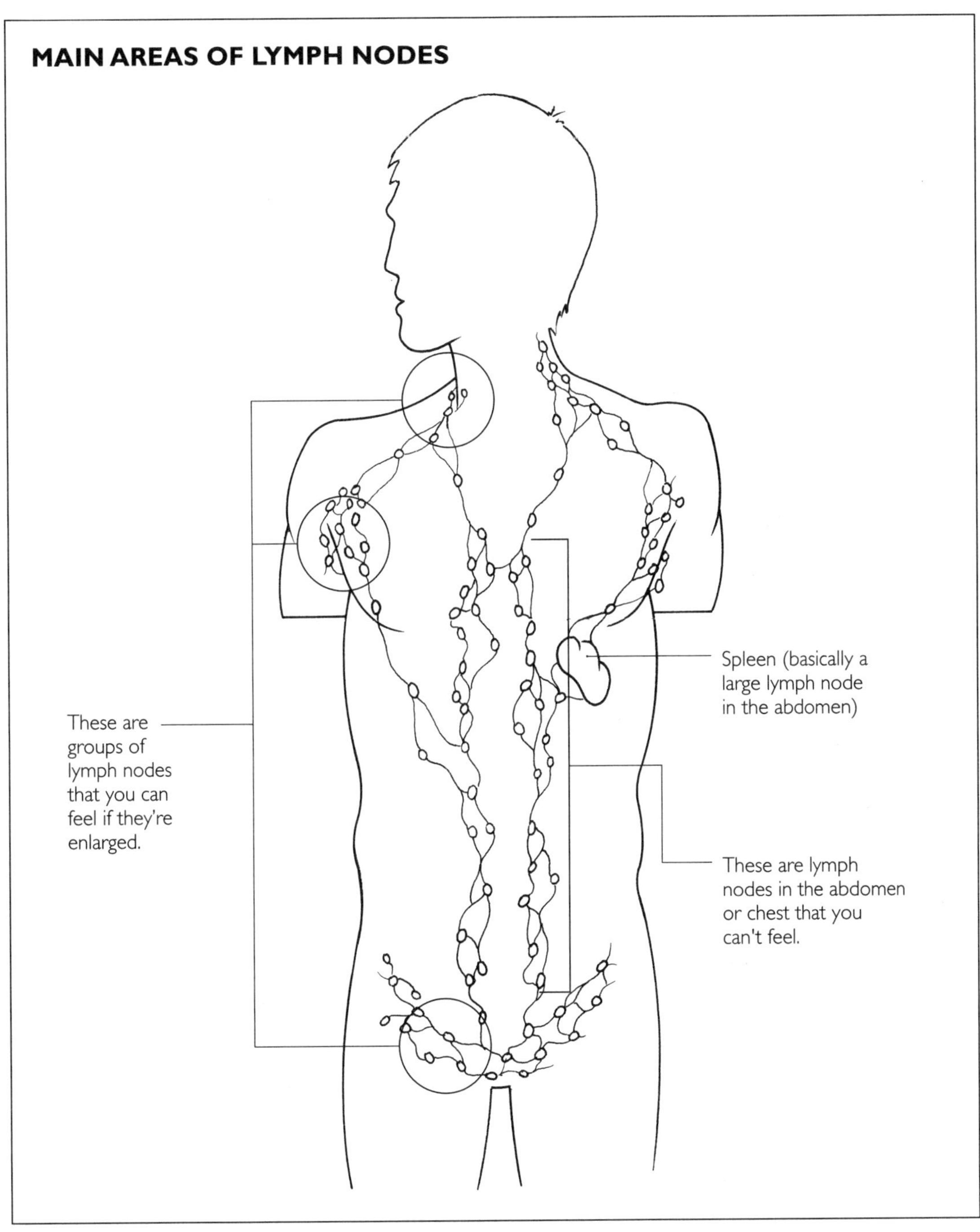

Lymphocytes are found not only in the bone marrow but also in the **lymph nodes**. These are tiny little soft pieces of tissue that are not normally palpable (in other words, you cannot feel them). They are scattered all over the body, with particularly large collections in the neck, the groin, and the armpit. Usually you aren't aware of them and can't feel them at all. Sometimes if you get an infection—say, a boil on your hand or a virus illness such as flu—some of the lymph nodes (in the armpit or neck, for example) might get bigger. They might also feel a little tender when you touch them. These changes occur because the nodes are engorged with lymphocytes produced in response to the infection. Any problem in an enlarged lymph node can be diagnosed by a **lymph node biopsy**. A lymph node biopsy is usually done with a local anesthetic, though if the node is in an awkward location, a general anesthetic might be needed. It is not a major procedure, and a part or the whole of a node is simply taken out.

In addition to the nodes in the neck, groin, and armpit, there are lymph nodes in many other areas, including the abdomen and chest. Also, inside the abdomen there is a large organ, the **spleen**, that is composed mostly of the same tissue that lymph nodes are made of. The spleen is approximately the size of a clenched fist and is situated on the left side of the abdomen. Normally it is not possible to feel it because of its position under the ribs. In the context of the leukemias, it is possible to think of the spleen as simply a very big and important lymph node. Thus the phrase "lymph nodes" used in regard to lymphocytic leukemia really means "the lymph nodes and the spleen."

A Special Note about "Spread"

Many leukemias are cancers that begin, or seem to begin, in several places at once. The medical term is multicentric. Thus we tend not to think of leukemias as spreading in the way that other cancers do. For that reason, there is no section about the possible spread of the tumors in this chapter.

CHRONIC LYMPHOCYTIC LEUKEMIA (CLL)

The Most Important Features of Chronic Lymphocytic Leukemia

Chronic lymphocytic leukemia (usually abbreviated **CLL**) is a cancer of the lymphocytes (one type of white cell). However, it is the word "chronic" that really matters in helping explain the disease. Because CLL is a chronic and therefore slow-moving type of condition, it is much less alarming than almost any other form of cancer or leukemia. Furthermore, cancers of the lymphocytes in general (and particularly CLL) are almost always responsive to chemotherapy, which may often consist of tablets only. Thus most people with CLL have a condition that is not only slow moving but that is also easily treatable and whose symptoms may usually be controlled.

Age and Incidence

CLL is predominantly a condition of the older age group, with approximately 90 percent of cases occurring after the age of fifty. It accounts for a quarter or more of all cases of leukemia.

Causes

As with most cancers, the true cause or causes of CLL are unknown. There seems to be no common link between cases of CLL. On the other hand, we do know that it is not caused by smoking, diet, stress, or pollution and is not caught from anyone else. Nor can it be passed on to anyone else; so if you have CLL, your children, friends, and others in your circle are not in danger of catching it from you.

Symptoms or Problems That You May Notice

In many cases, CLL causes no problems or symptoms at the time of diagnosis, a state that may continue for a long time. Often people with CLL have no specific symptoms related to CLL at all, and the diagnosis might be made when a routine blood test is done for some other reason. At some stage, however, there will be symptoms. The major symptoms of CLL are of two types: problems created when lymph nodes get too big and problems created in the blood system and the immune system when the normal cells begin to be crowded out by the malignant lymphocytes.

Problems Created by Enlarged Lymph Nodes Usually lymph nodes are small and cannot be felt unless there has been a recent infection such as a boil or a viral illness. In CLL the lymph nodes can grow to a few centimeters (an inch or two) in diameter, and, although they do not usually hurt, they can cause some local inconvenience—an **ache** or **discomfort** in the groin, neck, or armpit, for example. What is true of the lymph nodes is also true of the spleen. In CLL the spleen is quite often enlarged, which may cause some discomfort in the upper left part of the abdomen, particularly when you bend over or exercise, or may give you a feeling of fullness in the abdomen soon after eating a relatively small meal.

When there are a large number of lymph nodes involved in many different places, you may have some **constitutional symptoms**. For example, you may feel **generally unwell** or **tired and lacking in energy**. You might **lose** some **weight**, with or without a **loss of appetite**, and you might get occasional bouts of **mild fever** or experience marked **sweating, particularly at night** (so that, for instance, you have to change your nightclothes or bedclothes).

Problems Related to the Blood and Immune Systems Although CLL may interfere with the blood system and the immune system in several different ways, the easiest way of thinking about it is to imagine that the marrow is filled with too many malignant lymphocytes, and the normal marrow cells are crowded and unable to function normally. In CLL the most important effect of this overcrowding is that the marrow's ability to make white cells to combat infection is reduced. Hence in CLL the most common problem created by impaired function of the marrow is **lowered resistance to infection**. This means two things. First, when you get an infection such as a cold or flu, you cannot shrug off the infection in a few days as you used to. Infections are likely to take longer to deal with and may often require treatment (for example, with antibiotics). Second, you get infections more easily. In other words, you catch things from other people more easily. This has general implications for the way in which you should take care of yourself (see the information on treatment below).

Although some or all of these symptoms may occur, I want to emphasize that many people with CLL will have **no symptoms** at all from it, often for many years. So if your doctor has told you that you have CLL, that doesn't mean you will automatically have symptoms or problems!

Diagnosis and Tests

The diagnosis of CLL is usually suspected when there are too many lymphocytes in the bloodstream. Almost always the suspicion of CLL will need to be confirmed with further blood tests, a **sample of the bone marrow**, or both (see page 120).

In some cases, blood tests are the only tests needed. In other cases, further tests—such as X rays or scans—may be required, to see if the spleen is enlarged and so on. If other tests are needed, your doctor will discuss them with you.

How Is Chronic Lymphocytic Leukemia Treated?

Because CLL is a chronic, slow-moving condition, and because there are often no symptoms at all at the outset, it is quite usual for no treatment to be given until the patient develops symptoms. Although this policy of *"no treatment until problems arise"* usually causes some surprise, it is the best policy for someone who has no symptoms and is the usual approach to most patients with CLL.

At some stage, medications will be required. These are described in the following paragraphs.

However, because CLL is often accompanied by a weakening of your immune system, it is also very important for you to follow the guidelines for reducing infections, given here after the section on medications.

Medications Used for CLL

If you begin to suffer from tiredness, infections, or bruising (caused by, respectively, anemia, lack of white cells, or lack of platelets), your doctor might start you on some medication. The medications used most commonly in CLL are of two kinds: **steroids** and **chemotherapy** drugs. Either or both may be prescribed for you.

Steroids In CLL the steroids used most often are **prednisone** or sometimes **prednisolone**. They are useful because they suppress the immune system. They reduce the number of immune cells in your body and in your bloodstream. Because CLL is a malignancy of the immune system, steroids happen to work very well. They may reduce the number of lymphocytes, including the malignant lymphocytes, in your bloodstream; they may make any particularly large lymph nodes get smaller or even disappear; and they may cause a really useful improvement in any constitutional symptoms you may have (such as tiredness, weight loss, low appetite, and sweating). The steroids are almost always given by mouth as tablets. The schedules for taking them can vary. Sometimes they are given every day for two weeks followed by a two-week break. Sometimes they are given on alternate days or daily but in a lower dosage. Don't be worried if your doctor gives you a different schedule from someone else, but do **stick to the doses exactly as prescribed and don't miss a single dose**.

You may experience some side effects from the steroids. They can, and usually do, increase your appetite and make you hungry. Depending on the dose and on for how long they're needed, they can cause skin problems such as acne, and they can also make your face rather swollen and moon-shaped. All of these side effects stop when you stop the steroids. In a few people, steroids also have the potential to cause **bleeding from the stomach**, which may result in **jet-black bowel movements** or **vomiting up** material that contains **fresh blood** or that looks **like coffee grounds**. If any of these things happen, **get immediate medical advice**. Steroids can also **reduce your ability to fight off infections**, so if you get an **infection** (flu or bronchitis, for example) or a **fever**, you must **check with your doctor**.

Chemotherapy Drugs The other drugs used in CLL are chemotherapy drugs. In CLL, chemotherapy is usually given by tablets only. The drug most commonly used is **chlorambucil**, though others, such as **cyclophosphamide**, can be used. Because chemotherapy agents kill all growing cells, they may suppress your normal bone marrow cells at the same time as they control the malignant leukemic cells. The medications may therefore affect your blood and immune system as well as the leukemia. In monitoring your treatment, your doctor will be treading a relatively fine line trying to control the CLL while at the same time trying not to suppress your bone marrow, as that could make you more anemic or decrease your platelets or ability to fight infection. Hence the exact dose and how often you need your medication will be tailored by your doctor to your individual case. You, in turn, must make sure that you **let your doctor or nurse know within a few hours** if you develop a **fever** or **shivering**, if you have any major **bruising or bleeding** for which there's no obvious explanation (such as a cut), if you develop **little purple spots** on your skin, or if you develop an infection, say, around a finger, a toenail, or the anus. Let your doctor or nurse know at once if you get any of those while you're on chemotherapy. If you do, quite often the problem can be treated quite easily, although you may need to be in the hospital for a few days to get antibiotics intravenously or platelets or transfusions.

Other chemotherapy drugs can be used, and often are, at various stages or in various situations. If the CLL does not respond to chlorambucil, or if the disease is behaving in an aggressive manner, other drugs might be needed. Drugs that can be used include combinations of drugs given by injection, including **fludarabine**, **Adriamycin**, and also newer chemotherapy drugs, particularly a group of agents called **purine analogues**. In fact, these may nowadays be used as the first type of therapy. This is an area of active research, so do discuss the details with your medical team.

Guidelines for Reducing Infections

The most common type of problem you are likely to get with CLL is an infection. The following guidelines can help you decrease your chances of catching an infection and speed up your recovery from any infection you do catch.

Stay away from people who have an infection—a cold, flu, gastroenteritis, or anything similar. In particular, **do not shake hands** with them and make sure that you **do not touch your own mouth or face** after you've been in the room with them. Viruses are passed via household surfaces, so they can easily get onto your hands and then into your body if you touch your mouth or eyes. Also, **report any infection at once to your doctor or nurse**. Things to watch out for include: a **boil** on the skin, **pus** around a nail fold, **bronchitis**, or even just a **fever** without any visible sign of infection.

Next, make sure that every year you have a vaccination against flu (a "flu shot"). Flu can be particularly unpleasant if you have CLL, and a flu shot may prevent it altogether or may reduce its severity if you do get it. Any other vaccinations you may need should be discussed with your doctor. Some vaccines (not the flu vaccine) contain live viruses and may be dangerous for people with compromised immune systems. That means you should also **discuss foreign travel plans in advance**. You might ask your travel agent what diseases (if any) are common where you want to go and then ask your doctor what you should do.

One particular infection, **shingles**, is quite common in CLL patients and can be a great nuisance. Shingles is a rash with little blisters that look like chicken pox on the skin. It is caused by a reactivation—a reawakening—of the chicken pox virus. If you had chicken pox as a child, the virus will remain dormant in your body. Decades later it may be reactivated and cause shingles. Shingles may develop and may be quite unpleasant in patients with CLL. Furthermore, it may start on your back, where you cannot see it easily. If you feel any prickling or stinging or other peculiar feelings on your back or

SHINGLES

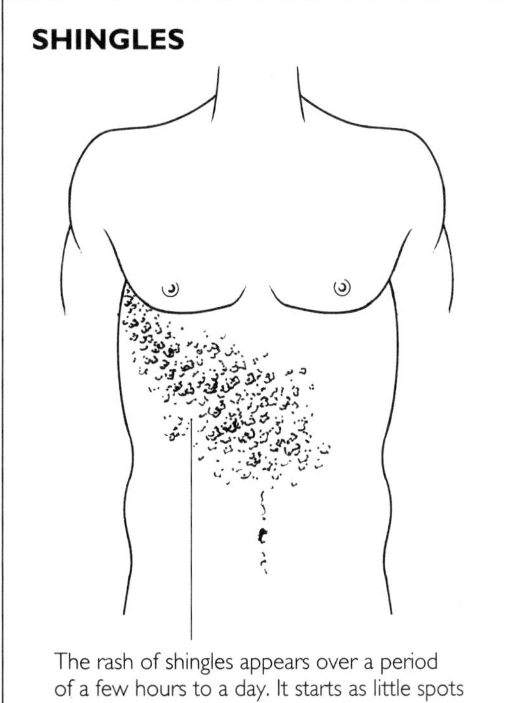

The rash of shingles appears over a period of a few hours to a day. It starts as little spots that get bigger and develop into blisters. It is often painful.

trunk, get someone to look at it. If you start getting shingles, let your doctor know at once because in CLL it can spread all over your body, and there are very good antiviral medications available that may reduce any trouble if they are started early.

CHRONIC MYELOCYTIC (OR GRANULOCYTIC) LEUKEMIA (CML OR CGL)

The Most Important Features of Chronic Myelocytic Leukemia

Chronic myelocytic leukemia (often abbreviated CML) is—like CLL, the other main type of chronic leukemia—a slow-moving condition that may not cause symptoms or problems for a long time. In general, however, it progresses more steadily (and more rapidly) than CLL, and so the treatment is somewhat different. In some cases it can be controlled with relatively simple chemotherapy for a time (often tablets to start with, with injections later on). In recent years, it has been shown that aggressive treatment early on may provide long-term remissions or even cures in suitable patients, particularly if they are relatively young and in generally good health.

Age and Incidence

By and large, CML is a condition that happens in adulthood and the later years. It can occur in the thirties and forties, though it is more common in the fifties and older.

Causes

In the great majority of cases there is no known cause. It has been known for several decades that CML is associated with an abnormality of the chromosomes. An abnormal chromosome called the **Philadelphia chromosome** is seen within the malignant granulocytes in most cases of CML, but we don't know exactly how it came to be there or what caused it. In other words, we know that CML is almost always associated with a primary problem in the genetic material of the cells. (That is true of most cancers, except that we rarely see an obvious chromosomal problem in the other cancers.) We also know that **this genetic problem does not seem to be passed on to other family members**, so the relatives of anyone with CML are at no higher risk than the rest of the population. Although CML is one of the conditions that is more common after radiation exposure (such as after a nuclear accident), in the majority of cases there is no known exposure.

Symptoms or Problems That You May Notice

As with CLL, it is quite common for patients with CML to have no symptoms caused by the condition when it is first diagnosed. Later on—again, as with CLL—there may be symptoms caused by interference with the normal functioning of the marrow. Thus CML can cause anemia, low platelets, or low white cells resulting in **tiredness**, **bruising**, **or bleeding** and an increased number or severity of **infections**.

In CML the malignant cells grow in the bone marrow only, not in the lymph nodes, so you will not develop enlarged lymph nodes or experience any symptoms related to nodes. If the CML cells grow rapidly, however, you may experience constitutional symptoms, including night sweats and itching all over the body.

Diagnosis and Tests

The diagnosis of CML is often suspected when a routine blood test shows too many granulocytes in the blood and the ones that are there appear abnormal when seen under the microscope. In the diagnosis of CML, your doctor will almost certainly recommend that a sample of bone marrow (see page 120) be taken, and additional special tests (for the Philadelphia chromosome, for example) may be done on it. You may also be recommended to have a CT scan or an ultrasound of the abdomen because the spleen is quite often enlarged in patients with CML.

The Main Objectives of Treatment

It is usually simple to control CML for a time using standard chemotherapy drugs, often given by tablet or capsules. Eventually, however, the condition no longer responds to therapy. In recent years, therefore, physicians have been using more aggressive therapy early on in an attempt to induce long-term remissions or even potential cures. The most aggressive forms of therapy include **bone marrow transplantation** (see page 228), and in CML this therapy seems to play a useful role, particularly in the younger and fitter patients.

Types of Treatment

Chemotherapy The first drug most commonly used nowadays is the biologic agent **interferon** (see page 232). Because this and other medications, such as **busulphan** and **hydroxyurea**, that may be used in CML have to be monitored very carefully, your doctor will be testing your blood every few weeks (or more often) to check on the white cells, platelets, and red cells.

Bone Marrow Transplantation (BMT) CML is one of the conditions in which there is good evidence that BMT does make a difference to the long-term outcome. Because BMT is an extremely arduous treatment, however, and because many people with CML are in their fifties or older, and may have other preexisting medical problems (such as heart or lung conditions), the procedure of BMT is quite hazardous in this age group. Hence your age and medical condition may make the risks of BMT in your case greater than any potential benefits.

ACUTE LYMPHOBLASTIC LEUKEMIA (ALL)

The Most Important Features of ALL

Acute lymphoblastic leukemia is a leukemia that can occur in children or in adults. For reasons that are not fully understood, it seems to be both more treatable and more curable in children, with the great majority of children gaining remission and more than half being cured. Although the outlook is not quite so favorable in adults, cure is achieved in a large number of cases, and remissions are achieved in more. We are not sure why this is the case. It may be that there are several different types of ALL and that the type or types that occur in children are somehow more responsive to chemotherapy. Because of these differences in treatment and outlook, I discuss childhood and adult ALL separately.

ALL IN CHILDHOOD

Age and Incidence

Leukemia is the most common type of cancer in childhood, and about four-fifths of childhood leukemia is of the ALL type (most of the rest is of the acute myeloid type). The peak incidence is at about three or four years of age.

Causes

Although the precise causes of ALL are not known, there are several situations in which the chance of getting ALL is increased. ALL (and sometimes other leukemias) is more common in people with certain inherited disorders than in the general population. The chromosomal disorder Down's syndrome is one of these, and there are several others as well. It is also possible that exposure to ionizing radiation might be implicated. While it is certainly known that radiation (from nuclear accidents, for example) can cause myeloid leukemias, there is still some uncertainty about whether exposure to radiation can cause ALL. This issue may be resolved with more research.

There is no evidence that viruses play any important role in ALL. At present most specialists feel that the most common cause of ALL in childhood is probably spontaneous mutation (changes in the genetic material) of the lymphoblasts in the marrow during a phase when cell growth is very rapid.

Symptoms or Problems That May Be Caused by ALL

In general, ALL is likely to cause symptoms that happen because the normal bone marrow cells are unable to function properly. That means the child may experience some or several of the following problems: anemia, causing tiredness and lethargy, pale complexion, and shortness of breath; insufficient white cells, causing prolonged or severe infections; or lack of platelets, causing bruising, bleeding, or petechiae (see page 120). In addition, some children have pain in one or more bones or in the abdomen. Occasionally there may be swelling of the salivary glands or of the testes in boys. It should be emphasized that some or all of these symptoms are quite common in everyday childhood illnesses, so do not think that every sore throat your child has is a sign of approaching leukemia. On the other hand, **any prolonged or severe illness that your child has should always be checked by your family's doctor**.

Diagnosis and Tests

The story of your child's illness and a routine physical examination are very important in alerting your medical team to the possibility of ALL. A routine blood test may indicate that ALL is a possibility, but the definite diagnosis is made by taking a sample of bone marrow (see page 120).

Factors That Influence the Treatment and Prognosis

Several factors have a bearing on the outlook in cases of ALL. In general, the higher the number of leukemic cells seen in the bloodstream, the more serious the condition is likely to be. Tests done on the leukemic cells (chromosome tests and others) may identify more serious subtypes, and several blood tests are available that can help predict future behavior. The disease is more likely to be aggressive in children older than ten years or younger than one year, in black children, in boys, and in cases where a mass of lymph nodes is visible in the mediastinum on the chest X ray.

The Main Objectives of Treatment

ALL is curable in the majority (more than half) of children, so the objective of treatment is cure. Even if cure is not achieved, long remissions are frequent.

Types of Treatment

The treatment of ALL usually includes four phases: initial treatment—called **induction**, meaning induction of remission—is followed by **consolidation** or continuation therapy. In addition, **prophylactic** therapy designed to prevent recurrence of the leukemia in certain places, particularly the brain and spinal cord, is also given. In many types of schedules a continuation of therapy, called **maintenance** therapy, is also given.

There are many different ways of giving chemotherapy for ALL, and your specialist will explain to you exactly what is being recommended for your child. In general, however, the treatment of ALL involves many drugs given over a fairly short period of time. The schedule for administering chemotherapy has been shown to be very important, so do make sure that you understand it and that you and your child do not miss any appointments. In general, the drugs that are most commonly used include: **vincristine**, **prednisone**, **daunorubicin** (a drug similar to **Adriamycin**), **L-asparaginase**, and sometimes **mercaptopurine**, **etoposide**, or **methotrexate**. In addition, there will usually be prophylactic treatment to the brain and spinal cord involving injections of methotrexate into the cerebrospinal fluid, sometimes with another drug, **cytosine arabinoside**. In certain circumstances, radiotherapy to the brain and spinal cord may also be recommended.

The role of bone marrow transplantation is still being decided. It is certainly useful if the ALL does relapse, but it is now being investigated as treatment early in the disease if the prognostic factors in a particular case suggest that chance of a relapse is high. If it is recommended, your specialist will discuss it with you in detail.

In every case the effect of the treatment has to be monitored by blood tests and bone marrow samples. I'm afraid there is no substitute for bone marrow samples, so your child will have to have several of these (though not usually very many).

Because children who have had treatment for ALL are highly susceptible to infections, it is very important for you to know and follow the guidelines for reducing the chance of getting an infection (see page 125) and to report any infection or fever at once.

ALL IN ADULTHOOD

Age and Incidence

ALL accounts for about a fifth of all leukemia in adults. It is slightly more common in males than in females and in white people than in black people.

Causes

As with ALL in childhood (see above), in most cases there is no identifiable cause. In a few cases, however, ALL has been found in association with exposure to radiation and with certain congenital or inherited conditions such as Down's syndrome.

Symptoms or Problems That You May Notice

For reasons that are not fully understood, ALL may cause not only symptoms that are like those of childhood ALL but also enlargement of the lymph nodes in some cases, behaving in some respects like an aggressive or high-grade lymphoma (see page 147). It is not clear why adult ALL develops in nodes as well as in marrow. In adults the symptom of pain in a bone (particularly in the sternum or breastbone) can occur, and there may also be headache.

Diagnosis and Tests

As with ALL in childhood, the condition may be suspected after your doctor takes a history and examines you. A routine blood test may show strong evidence of ALL, but this usually needs to be confirmed with a sample of bone marrow.

Factors That Influence the Treatment and Prognosis

The following factors suggest a less good outlook: being older, having a large number of leukemic cells in the bloodstream, and a number of other factors (some of which are determined through tests on the leukemic cells).

The Main Objectives of Treatment

The main objective of treatment is to cure the patient, which is achievable in a third or more of cases. Even if cure is not possible, remissions may be quite long lasting.

Types of Treatment

The treatment of adult ALL resembles the treatment for childhood ALL. Several drugs will be used, often for up to two years. These may include: **anthracyclines** (such as **Adriamycin** or **daunorubicin**), **vincristine**, **cyclophosphamide**, **steroids**, **methotrexate**, **6-mercaptopurine**, **L-asparaginase** (commonly called **asparaginase**), and others. Prophylactic treatment of the brain and spinal cord (with injections of **methotrexate** or **cytosine arabinoside** and radiotherapy) may also be recommended. Bone marrow transplantation (see page 228) may be used in certain circumstances (in certain types of relapse or if the risk of relapse is high).

ACUTE MYELOID LEUKEMIA (AML)

AML and Related Conditions

AML is an acute leukemia (that is, the malignant cells appear very immature) that seems to originate from the cells in the bone marrow that are (or are related to) the granulocyte series of white cells. In fact, there are several different subtypes of AML, some of which may be different conditions, although they behave in a similar way to AML. The important point is that, collectively, they are all quite different from the acute *lymphoblastic* leukemias. For that reason, AML and the leukemias like it are often called the **acute nonlymphoblastic leukemias**, or **ANLL**. For the purposes of this book, it is not as important to know the different subtypes of AML (or ANLL) as it is to understand the group as a whole. For that reason I will call the whole group AML (as many books do), even though technically it is more accurate from a biological point of view to call the group the ANLLs.

The Most Important Features of the Tumor

AML is one of the types of cancer in which the prognosis has improved dramatically over the last two decades. Before the era of modern treatment, AML was regarded as a rapidly progressing fatal condition. Now, although it is regarded as an extremely serious condition, if the patient is in the younger age group (the forties or under) and if high-dose therapy is possible, approximately half of the patients will have a long-term remission and possible cure.

Age and Incidence

AML occurs in adulthood and (as with many cancers) gets more common with age. It is rare before the thirties and becomes steadily more common into adulthood and old age.

Causes

As with so many malignancies, we do not fully understand the causes of AML, and in the majority of patients with AML we cannot identify any particular cause or causes. There are, however, certain circumstances that can precipitate AML. Four situations that seem to make AML more common are the following.

Certain Medical Conditions A group of conditions that affect the bone marrow increase the chance that AML will develop later on. These conditions, the **myelodysplasias**, usually occur in older people. In the myelodysplasias, the marrow fails to produce normal amounts of red cells, white cells, or platelets, even when the person's intake of vitamins or minerals is adequate.

Exposure to Nuclear Radiation People who happen to have been exposed to nuclear accidents (at nuclear fuel-processing or power plants) or to nuclear explosions (survivors of Hiroshima and Nagasaki) have a much higher-than-average chance of later developing AML. Usually the condition takes ten or twenty years to appear. Clearly the granulocytic and related bone marrow cells are in some way sensitive to radiation and can be damaged in a way that can lead to AML.

Exposure to Certain Chemicals A few chemicals can also cause AML to develop. Although most of these chemicals are not likely to be encountered in daily life, in the 1920s it was found that prolonged exposure to **benzene**, for example, increased the chance of developing AML. Certain kinds of anticancer **chemotherapy drugs** can also have this effect. How the drugs are given, and for what purpose, has a lot to do with it. For example, the drug melphalan, when given continuously over a long period for the treatment of multiple myeloma, does definitely increase the risk of AML. When the same drug is given for other conditions, however, and in a different way (in short bursts of a few days at a time), it does not increase the patient's chance of developing AML at all.

Certain Inherited Conditions A few inherited conditions carry a higher-than-average chance of AML. The best known of these is Down's syndrome, in which a chromosomal abnormality causes children to develop with several abnormalities of the face, central nervous system, heart, and growth pattern. People with Down's syndrome (or with one or two other inherited conditions) may develop

AML in later life, although we do not fully understand why or how.

Symptoms or Problems That You May Notice

AML usually comes to light when it causes the bone marrow to be compromised and to fail to function normally. All three lines of bone marrow products (the red cells, the white cells, and the platelets) may be affected. A typical story might be that the patient has been feeling particularly **tired** for several weeks (due to the anemia) and has then developed **infections** (due to the reduced number of normal white cells) such as a bad sore throat that lasts for weeks, accompanied by some bruising or bleeding, particularly in the form of bruises or **petechiae** (little red or purple spots in the skin).

In certain rare circumstances, the early symptoms can be worsened by problems with bleeding (from the gums or at other sites), a symptom likely to be associated with some of the subtypes of AML. Also, in rare circumstances, there may be very large numbers of AML cells, which can clog the lungs and cause **shortness of breath**. This symptom, like serious bleeding, is fortunately rare.

Diagnosis and Tests

In almost all cases the diagnosis will be suspected when a blood test shows immature, nonlymphocyte, white cells in the blood. Almost always the diagnosis will need to be confirmed with a sample of bone marrow (see page 120). The material obtained from the bone marrow will be examined under the microscope, and usually the marrow is seen to be crammed with immature cells of the myeloid (granulocyte or similar) types. These cells are called **myeloblasts**, or **blast cells** for short.

In some cases the blast cells may appear so abnormal and immature that it is very difficult to tell exactly what they are. For that reason, special tests on the marrow sample are often done, including staining the cells for certain types of markers, looking at the cells' chromosomes, and so on. In a few cases, therefore, the specific type of leukemia may not be known for several days. Obviously the delay and uncertainty can cause great anxiety to patient and family. However, the information may be quite important (in distinguishing an AML from an ALL, for example), so it is worth the effort it takes to be patient.

The bone marrow test may be the only test needed to confirm the diagnosis, although routine tests of kidney function and so on will be done and may be important as guides to future treatment.

Factors That Influence the Treatment and Prognosis

AML carries a somewhat better prognosis in the younger age group than with older patients, possibly because younger patients (below the forties or fifties) may be better able to tolerate the treatment. Special tests on the genetic material of the leukemic cells (called **cytogenetic testing**) may also help define the behavior of the leukemia in a particular case.

The Main Objectives of Treatment

The main objective of treatment of AML is to try to cure the patient. Usually that involves giving intensive chemotherapy to see if the leukemia responds and goes into remission (remission, in this case, being defined as having a normal number of blast cells in the marrow). The treatment is usually called **induction chemotherapy**. If the leukemia does respond to the chemotherapy and goes into remission, some patients can be cured.

Types of Treatment

Induction Chemotherapy The drugs most commonly used in induction chemotherapy include the anthracyclines—usually **daunorubicin** or **Adriamycin** or, more recently, **idarubicin**—together with other drugs that usually include **cytosine arabinoside**. Differing combinations of drugs, including **all-trans retinoic acid** in some cases, may be used according to special tests done on the leukemic cells.

Usually two courses of chemotherapy are given (some days or weeks apart), and then a further bone marrow sample is taken to see if the leukemia has responded to the therapy. Along with the chemotherapy drugs, other drugs are often given to make sure that no kidney problems occur during the treatment. Antibiotics and antifungal drugs may also be required for some or all of the time. In addition, regular red cell and platelet transfusions are necessary.

Consolidation Therapy Treatment with more chemotherapy is usually used for some months after the induction therapy.

Bone Marrow Transplantation (BMT)

For more than twenty years now, BMT (see page 228) has been used in the treatment of AML. Since AML is a disease of the bone marrow, the object of BMT is to obliterate the existing (malignant) bone marrow cells with chemotherapy, radiotherapy, or both and then to replace them with bone marrow cells taken from a donor, usually a brother or sister (or other close relative) or occasionally a person identified from a marrow donors' registry who happens to have the same tissue type as the patient. After the transplant has been given, you may need to be on drugs that reduce the chance that the new marrow will cause you problems (called graft-versus-host disease). These drugs must usually be taken for a long time.

BMT is a major undertaking and involves several weeks of intensive care, during most of which the patient is kept in protective isolation to avoid catching any infections while the new marrow is taking hold. You will need to discuss with your doctor what the likely chance of success is (it will depend on your age and medical fitness, among other things) and also what side effects you will experience and for how long.

The therapy (both induction chemotherapy and BMT) for AML is usually quite arduous and almost always makes the patient feel very ill for much of the time. It is important to emphasize, however, that the chance of cure or long-term remission is vastly improved from a few decades ago. The undoubted difficulties may well be worth enduring if there is a reasonable chance of long-term benefit. It is important for you to discuss the details of the treatment and your own particular case with your doctor.

HAIRY-CELL LEUKEMIA

Hairy-cell leukemia is a rare type of leukemia, somewhat similar to CLL, in which the leukemic cells have long filaments apparently growing from the cell surface, hence the "hairy-cell." It occurs in adulthood and older age, and seems to carry a somewhat better prognosis than CLL in the same age groups. The best initial treatment is with a group of drugs called **purine analogues**, usually 2-chloro-deoxyadenosine (2CDA), which is given as an intravenous injection for five days or so consecutively. Often only one or two courses are needed. Hairy-cell leukemia is one of the types of cancer in which the biological agent **interferon** also seems to be useful. As well as these medications, in some patients removal of the spleen—splenectomy—seems to help a lot.

LIVER (HEPATOCELLULAR CANCER)

Number of new cases diagnosed per year in the United States: 19,900

SUMMARY OF THE KEY FACTS IN THIS SECTION

- Primary liver cancer (known as hepatocellular cancer), as distinct from secondaries in the liver from a primary elsewhere, is not very common.
- It generally occurs in people who have long-standing damage to the liver caused by alcohol or (less commonly) continuing damage following an infection with hepatitis B or C.
- It commonly spreads to all parts of the liver, but if this has not happened it may be possible to remove the tumor surgically. If that is not possible, the prognosis is poor.

The Most Important Features of the Tumor

Primary cancer of the liver (as distinct from secondary cancers in the liver from a primary cancer in, for example, the bowel or the breast) is not very common in this country. It usually develops after long-standing damage to the liver, which may be the result of a previous infection with hepatitis B or C or of continuing damage from alcohol or, rarely, some other substance that damages the liver. Primary liver cancer is also known as **hepatocellular carcinoma** or **cancer** (usually abbreviated **HCC**), and I use that term to avoid confusion with secondaries in the liver. (It is also sometimes known as **hepatoma**.)

In a small number of cases, hepatocellular cancer can be cured by surgical removal, but often it spreads—or probably develops—in many areas of the liver, making it impossible for a surgeon to remove it. In those circumstances, cure is very unlikely, although it is often possible to control the symptoms for a time.

What You Really Need to Know about the Liver

The liver is a large organ (in fact, it is the biggest internal organ in the body) and is divided into two distinct lobes, the left and the right. The main bulk of the liver is not supplied with nerves that carry pain messages; in fact, only the outer covering of the liver (known as the capsule) and the large ducts leading out of the liver are sensitive to pain. Thus it is possible for tumors to grow inside the liver for a considerable time before the person is aware

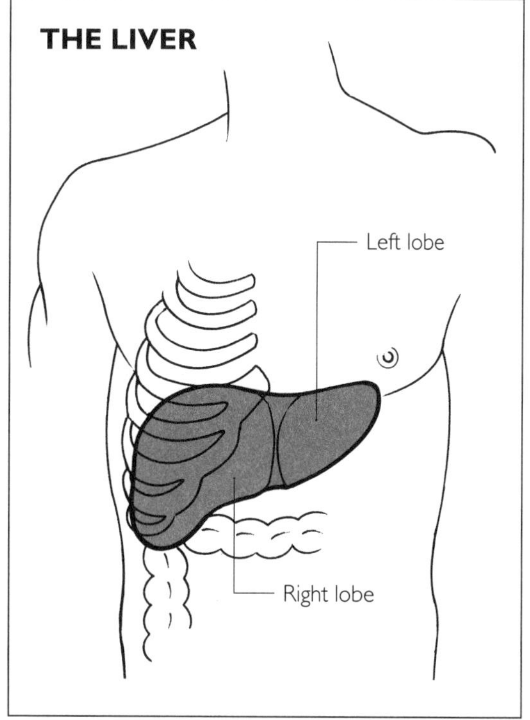

of them. Only when a tumor happens to stretch the capsule or press on a large duct will severe pain be felt.

The liver performs a wide range of functions to do with the control of the internal environment of the body. It regulates many substances in the bloodstream, removing or rendering harmless potential poisons, controlling the way the body stores and transports nutrients, and so on. As a result, it is responsible for providing tissues such as muscle with the appropriate components for growth and repair. If the function of the liver is seriously impaired (as it can be in a bad attack of hepatitis, and in advanced cirrhosis, as well as in advanced cancer), other tissues cannot maintain themselves properly. Hence the person may notice loss of muscle bulk and may become abnormally thin (this is termed **cachexia**).

The liver also processes the end products of red blood cells at the end of their useful life. It degrades the hemoglobin from the red cells and produces the yellowish fluid called bile, which it secretes via the bile duct into the digestive tract. If this function is affected by blockage of the major ducts in the bile duct system, bile spills over from the liver into the bloodstream. This causes **jaundice**, a yellowish discoloration of skin and eyes. Jaundice is a sign that the bile duct system is not carrying bile away from the liver. (It can be caused by other things besides cancer, such as acute attacks of hepatitis, a gallstone in the main bile duct, and so on.)

These three aspects of the liver—the lack of nerve supply, its importance in building muscles, and the excretion of bile—help to explain the symptoms associated with hepatocellular cancer.

Age and Incidence

In this country, hepatocellular cancer tends to be a disease of middle age or later, and the people who are most likely to develop it are those with long-standing liver damage (see below). In other countries—particularly China, other areas of Asia, and Indonesia—it is much more common as a result of widespread infection with hepatitis B and C. In fact, worldwide, hepatocellular cancer is the most common type of cancer and, because there is a vaccine that will prevent hepatitis B, the most preventable.

Causes

Most cases of hepatocellular cancer follow long-standing liver damage, and the most important causes are the following.

Alcohol Long-standing damage from alcohol may result in scarring of the liver, called **cirrhosis**. Probably about one in twenty people with cirrhosis will eventually develop hepatocellular cancer.

Hepatitis B or C Most cases of hepatitis get better completely and do not result in any long-term damage to the liver, and hence do not increase the chance of getting hepatocellular cancer. Some people, however, for reasons that are not fully understood, develop a long-term type of liver damage after an attack of hepatitis B or C. If long-term damage does occur, the risk of later developing hepatocellular cancer is increased.

Other Substances A few other substances can cause liver damage and increase the risk of cancer. By and large, these are solvents and other materials formerly used in some industries. Nowadays exposure to such chemicals is strictly controlled. One point needs emphasis: the birth control pill may be associated with benign (noncancerous) liver tumors, **but there is no evidence that the birth control pill increases a woman's risk of developing hepatocellular cancer**.

How the Cancer Tends to Spread

Hepatocellular cancer tends to spread through the liver or probably develops in several parts of the liver at the same time. Because of this, it is frequently undetectable in the early stages and often involves both lobes of the liver at the time of diagnosis. It may also spread to lymph nodes nearby and around the rest of the abdomen as well, sometimes causing ascites (fluid in the abdomen).

Symptoms or Problems That You May Notice

Because of the lack of nerves that carry pain messages, the early stages of hepatocellular cancer usually cause few symptoms or no symptoms at all. Later there may be a mild **ache** or discomfort, sometimes felt in the upper right-hand part of the abdomen or sometimes in the center. Usually this pain is very mild and similar to indigestion, and, of course, indigestion-type pain is very common and is not, in itself, a sign that hepatocellular cancer is developing. Later stages may cause moderate to **severe ache or pain** in the upper part of the right side of the abdomen, the center of the abdomen, or the back.

More commonly the first symptom is a **mild loss of appetite** and **loss of weight** (particularly loss of bulk in the muscles of the arms and legs), sometimes accompanied by mild **nausea**.

Jaundice (see page 134) can occur if one or more of the tumors blocks part of the bile duct system or if there are many tumors and the liver is unable to excrete enough bile.

In more advanced stages, the liver's ability to regulate many of the chemicals in the bloodstream is lost, a condition that may produce **drowsiness and confusion**, which may later progress to coma.

Diagnosis and Tests

Important clues as to the diagnosis will come from the story of your symptoms, but it may be that examination by your doctor does not reveal any abnormalities. Hence in many cases the diagnosis is made as a result of some or all of the following tests.

Ultrasound or CT Scan of the Liver Both an ultrasound and a CT scan can give important information about the possibility of hepatocellular cancer. Either or both may be recommended. In a few circumstances, an MRI scan may add some further information. However, in themselves the scans can only suggest that there is a tumor in the liver and may not distinguish with certainty between, say, secondary cancers in the liver (which are more common than primary hepatocellular cancer) and a primary. Hence other tests may be required as well.

The AFP Blood Test and Other Tests Hepatocellular cancer cells often produce a substance called **AFP** (**alpha-fetoprotein**), which acts as a marker of hepatocellular cancer in approximately two-thirds of cases. (AFP is also produced in other tumors, particularly germ-cell tumors). Other blood tests can give information about the functioning of the liver and also whether the person has a past history of hepatitis infections and is carrying particles of the hepatitis virus in the bloodstream.

If the patient is in the right age group and has a history of liver damage, further tests to confirm the diagnosis may not be needed. Otherwise a biopsy may be suggested.

Liver Biopsy A biopsy may be done with a fine needle under local anesthetic. The procedure does not require an incision, as the needle is thin and can be introduced into the liver through the skin. It may be done on an outpatient basis or may require a day or so in the hospital.

In some circumstances a liver biopsy may be done under general anesthetic and may require an operation in which an incision is made through the skin.

The biopsy may be used not only to diagnose the hepatocellular cancer but also to determine the severity of any liver damage.

Factors That Influence the Treatment and Prognosis

The main feature that determines the future is whether or not the cancer can be removed. In a few cases the cancer may be confined to one area or one lobe. Unfortunately, it is more usual for the cancer to have spread to all areas of the liver at the time of diagnosis. If so, then surgical removal may not be feasible.

The Main Objectives of Treatment

If the cancer can be removed surgically, the objective is cure of the patient. If it cannot be removed, the objective of treatment is to control the symptoms as long as possible.

Types of Treatment

Surgery In general, removal of a hepatocellular cancer means removing the entire lobe in which it is situated. That is a considerable undertaking, and much depends on the general medical condition of the patient and the capacity of the remaining liver tissue to perform all the functions of the liver (which may not be possible if there is severe cirrhosis, for example). Hence any operation will require very detailed discussion with your surgeon about the possible aftereffects, the risks and hazards, and of course the chance of cure.

Radiotherapy Radiotherapy can be used to control symptoms if removal is not possible. Radiotherapy to the liver is an arduous treatment and may cause moderate to severe nausea and lethargy. It is important to discuss the potential benefits and side effects with your radiation oncologist.

Chemotherapy Generally speaking, hepatocellular cancers are not sensitive to chemotherapy, although some combinations of drugs (and some combinations of drugs with radiotherapy) are being investigated. If a trial of a newer therapy is recommended to you, be sure to discuss the potential benefits and hazards with your doctor.

Other Therapies Several other types of therapy have been tried in hepatocellular cancer. In particular, the use of monoclonal antibodies carrying doses of radioactive isotopes has been investigated with some success. This treatment is available in only a few centers and is suitable only in selected cases. Some centers have also investigated the use of drugs introduced directly into the liver through the hepatic artery. It is possible that this procedure may be more effective than giving the drugs through a vein. In certain centers, liver transplantation may be performed in a few selected cases, and cryotherapy (freezing areas of tumor at surgery) may also have a role.

Screening Screening for liver cancer may be of increasing importance in the future. It is likely that large-scale screening programs (using the AFP blood test or ultrasound scans or both) may be studied for use in high-risk populations, including people who are (or are likely to be) carriers of hepatitis B or C.

LUNG

Number of new cases diagnosed per year in the United States: 177,000

SUMMARY OF THE KEY FACTS IN THIS SECTION

- There are two major types of lung cancer, small-cell and non–small-cell.
- Smoking is the major cause of the great majority of cases of lung cancer.
- Surgery, radiotherapy, or both are important in the treatment of non–small-cell lung cancer, and chemotherapy (and in certain situations radiotherapy) in the treatment of small-cell cancers.
- Control of the disease is often achievable, although cure is not very common.

The Most Important Features of the Tumor

Although we always talk of lung cancer as if it were a single condition, there are actually two main types of lung cancer. The types behave rather differently from each other, and each is treated with a different approach. Lung cancers are classified on their histologic appearance (that is, what they look like under the microscope) and are divided into those called **small-cell lung cancers** (sometimes also called **oat-cell** lung cancers) and the others, which are usually grouped together as the **non–small-cell lung cancers**. The *non*–small-cell lung cancers (which together make up nearly three-quarters of all lung cancers) grow moderately slowly and spread to the lymph nodes in the chest before spreading to distant parts of the body. The *small-cell* lung cancers grow more rapidly and often spread to distant parts of the body even if the lymph nodes in the chest are not involved. The two types of lung cancer also respond differently to treatment. By and large, small-cell lung cancers are responsive to chemotherapy (and to radiotherapy as well), although the response may last for only a limited amount of time. Non–small-cell lung cancers are are less responsive to chemotherapy, and both surgery and radiotherapy are important methods of treatment. In both cases, complete surgical removal, and sometimes cure, is occasionally possible, although usually it is not feasible.

Age and Incidence

Lung cancer is currently the most common form of cancer in men and is now the second most common one in women. It is relatively rare below the age of forty, and the incidence rises rapidly above the age of fifty, the average age of onset being sixty.

Causes

The primary cause of lung cancer is (I am not going to be preachy about this) cigarette smoke. Depending on the type of the lung cancer, up to 96 percent of sufferers are smokers, and probably most of the nonsmokers who develop lung cancer have spent large amounts of time in the company of smokers, inhaling their smoke (known as passive smoking). Thus a nonsmoker married to a heavy smoker (someone who smokes a pack a day or more) or working in close proximity to a smoker every day has an increased risk of lung cancer. Other factors can be contributory causes of lung cancer. In certain occupations, most of which have now been rendered safe (such as uranium mining or working with asbestos), lung cancer is or used to be much more common than in the general population. Even among workers in high-risk occupations, however, cigarette smoking further increases the risk of lung cancer by a factor of ten or so.

Of course, there are exceptions. In rare cases, a person develops lung cancer who has not smoked cigarettes and has not been exposed to second-hand smoke.

NON-SMALL-CELL LUNG CANCER

How Non–Small-Cell Lung Cancer Tends to Spread

Non–small-cell lung cancers tend to spread methodically and somewhat predictably. Usually they spread first to the collection of lymph nodes in the middle of the chest cavity. This space between the lungs and the heart is called the **mediastinum**, and the **lymph nodes** in it are called mediastinal lymph nodes. It can also spread to lymph nodes low down in the neck, just above the collarbones.

Very occasionally a lung cancer may cause a blockage to the big veins in the mediastinum, leading to rapid **swelling of the face, arms, or upper chest**. If that happens (and it is not very common), immediate treatment is necessary.

At a later stage the cancer can spread to distant parts of the body, including the liver, brain, and bones.

Symptoms or Problems That You May Notice

In some cases a lung cancer may first be detected by a routine chest X ray done for some other reason, and it may not be causing any particular problems or symptoms at that time. In most cases, however, there will be some symptoms. The main factor making the early diagnosis of lung cancer difficult is that most of the symptoms caused by the cancer are symptoms that many smokers experience from time to time anyway. These include **shortness of breath** and a **reduction in the amount of exercise that you can do** (for example, being able to climb only one flight of stairs without stopping

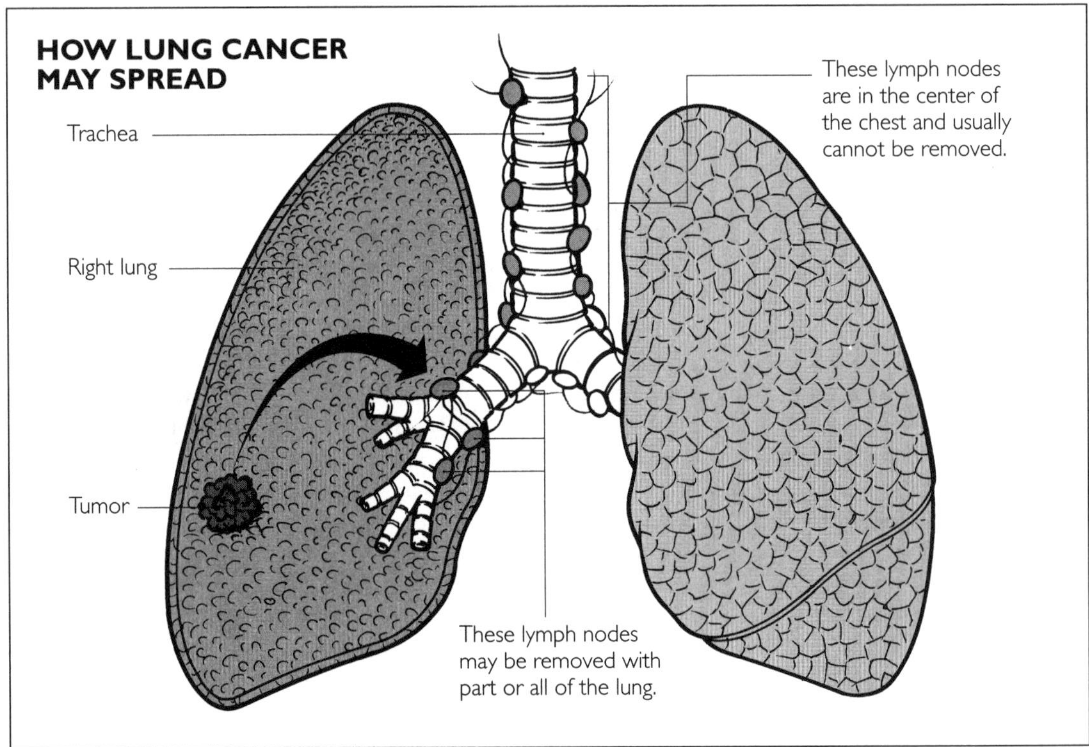

where previously you could manage two). In many cases, therefore, it is not possible to distinguish the symptoms of lung cancer from the symptoms caused by smoking.

Other symptoms are more specifically suggestive of cancer of the lung. One sign in particular is a marked and **persistent pain in the chest or upper back**, particularly if it remains in one place and is continuous or nearly continuous for many days or a few weeks. Among the other symptoms, the most important are: a **persistent cough** that will not go away and that lasts a long time when you haven't got bronchitis, **coughing up blood**, or a **sudden and severe shortness of breath** (or sudden and severe worsening of any shortness of breath you may already have). Sometimes the tumor can cause fluid to build up in the chest around the lungs (the medical term for this is a **pleural effusion**), a condition that can also cause a marked shortness of breath, persistent cough, and sometimes a pain in the side that gets worse when you breathe in. Also, if the tumor happens to be blocking a major airway, it can sometimes cause an infection in the part of the lung behind the blockage, that is, a **pneumonia**. The usual symptoms of a pneumonia include a **fever**, with a **cough and yellow sputum**, plus a sudden increase in **shortness of breath**, and often some pain. If someone who has smoked heavily gets a pneumonia, the doctor might well want to check to see whether a cancer has caused it.

These are the symptoms related to the lung itself. In addition, the cancer can cause constitutional symptoms, such as **loss of weight**, **loss of appetite**, and a general feeling of lethargy and tiredness, or "just **not feeling well** at all."

Factors That Influence the Prognosis and Treatment

The most important factor that affects both the prognosis and treatment is whether or not the tumor has spread to the lymph nodes in the center of the chest. If it has not, surgery may be feasible; however, if the nodes are involved, surgical removal is probably not feasible.

Diagnosis and Tests

After your doctor has taken your history and examined you, he or she will almost certainly order a chest X ray. In many cases, this will be followed by a **bronchoscopy** in which a thin flexible telescope is gently put down the airways of your lungs, after which a biopsy of any suspicious areas is performed. Sometimes, if the X ray suggests that one or more of the mediastinal lymph nodes is involved, a **mediastinoscopy** may be recommended instead of a bronchoscopy. The procedure is very similar to bronchoscopy, except that a thin telescope is inserted through a small incision in the neck (made under anesthetic) instead of through the airways. This procedure may be very important in finding out whether the lymph nodes are involved and hence whether surgery is feasible or not. In some situations other types of biopsy or fine-needle aspirate (see page 328) may be recommended.

In addition to (or sometimes instead of) these tests, your doctor may recommend a CT scan and other tests, including a liver ultrasound or a bone scan. Almost always a series of blood tests is recommended because the cancer occasionally causes disturbance of some of the salts in the blood (particularly the calcium), a condition that may require additional treatment.

The Main Types of Non–Small-Cell Lung Cancers

It is possible to subdivide the non–small-cell lung cancers based on their histological appearance. The two commonest types of non–small-cell lung cancer are the types called **adenocarcinoma** and **squamous carcinoma**. The third main type is called **large-cell carcinoma** or **large-cell undifferentiated carcinoma**. These different groups seem to blend in with each other to a certain extent; for example, it is thought that the large-cell group may consist of some types of adenocarcinoma that have become undifferentiated and perhaps some squamous cancers that have done the same. In any event, the subtype does not affect the behavior of the tumor very much (although it does have some effect).

The Main Objectives of Treatment

In a few cases the tumor may be small and may not have spread to the lymph nodes in the chest. In those cases your surgeon may be able to remove the entire tumor in an attempt to cure the cancer. If that is not possible, treatment is aimed at trying to reduce or prevent symptoms. If the tumor is partly obstructing a major airway, it may be possible to prevent it from closing the airway completely by giving radiotherapy. Radiotherapy is also used for reducing pain. If the tumor is bleeding and causing you to cough up blood, that may be controllable either with radiotherapy or by using laser light (via a bronchoscopy) to seal the ulcerating surface of the tumor and control the bleeding for a time.

Types of Treatment

Surgery If the tumor is located in the outside part of the lung, away from the center, and if it has not spread to lymph nodes in the mediastinum, it may be possible to remove it surgically. If surgery is technically feasible, you will be evaluated before the operation to estimate how much shortness of breath you will experience after the operation. Your surgeon may remove one part or lobe of the lung along with the tumor (a **lobectomy**), or sometimes the entire lung on that side may have to be removed (a **pneumonectomy**). If the lung on the other side is working quite well, you may experience little disturbance of your breathing. The preoperative assessments are important in determining that. This kind of operation is major surgery, comparable to major abdominal surgery. Hence you and your doctor should discuss what you are likely to experience after the operation and how long it will take for you to start getting back to normal (usually a number of weeks).

Radiotherapy Radiotherapy is the other major method of treatment in non–small-cell lung cancer. It can be helpful and in a few circumstances may be curative. It is particularly useful if the cancer is encroaching on a major airway or is causing moderate or severe pain. A thorough discussion with your radiation oncologist is essential because it is very important for you not to have unrealistic expectations of the treatment.

Laser Therapy A laser is like a very sharp, accurate knife, except that it uses a thin, very intense beam of light instead of a metal blade and it seals the wound it makes. In the treatment of cancer of the lung, a laser can be used to control bleeding from the surface of the cancer (a condition that causes blood in the sputum). The operation is done by a bronchoscopy, using a special bronchoscope that has a laser light inside it. It does not need an incision, and so recovery is relatively quick. It may be useful in some selected cases but in most cases of lung cancer does not offer any advantage over the other methods.

Chemotherapy The exact role of chemotherapy in the treatment of non–small-cell lung cancers is still unclear. Some types of chemotherapy—including drugs such as the **platinum** drugs, **etoposide**, **vinblastine**, **vinorelbine**, and **Taxol**—may cause partial remissions and improve the quality of life, even if they do not prolong survival. However, chemotherapy has many side effects (which vary depending on the drugs used), so you will need to discuss the potential risks and benefits with your doctor before deciding whether to go ahead with this type of treatment.

SMALL-CELL LUNG CANCER

Small-cell lung cancers behave somewhat differently from non–small-cell lung cancers. In particular, they have a high tendency to spread to distant parts of the body at a relatively early stage. However, they very often respond to chemotherapy and radiotherapy.

How Small-Cell Lung Cancer Tends to Spread

We do not know precisely why, but small-cell lung cancers are more likely than the non–small-cell type to spread to other parts of the body at a relatively early stage in their progress. In particular, the liver, the bone marrow, and the brain may be involved at quite an early stage.

Symptoms or Problems That You May Notice

Local and Generalized Symptoms Small-cell lung cancer may cause the same types of symptoms as non–small-cell lung cancer (see above) and some other problems as well. Like non–small-cell lung cancer, it may cause shortness of breath, discomfort or pain in the chest, blood in the sputum, a pleural effusion with cough or pain, and (not often) blockage of the big veins in the mediastinum with swelling of the face and arms. Sometimes a small-cell lung cancer may also cause constitutional symptoms such as weight loss, loss of appetite, and feeling generally unwell.

Symptoms Due to Hormone Production Some small-cell lung cancers cause additional problems resulting from their ability to manufacture imitations of some of the body's hormones. In part, they can do this because they seem to be derived from certain cells in the lung that are part of the body's hormonal (endocrine) system of glands. These cells (we presume), once they have settled down in the lungs, switch off their ability to make hormones. In some cases, however, when these cells become cancerous, they are able to switch on their previous ability and start to manufacture one or several hormones in large quantities. A number of different things may happen as a result (although some of these problems are very rare indeed). Three problems are fairly common. First, the cancer cells may secrete factors that release steroid hormones. Excess steroid hormones may cause the patient to become obese, with a rounded, moon-shaped face, and to have high blood pressure. The cancer may also produce hormones that interfere with the body's ability to handle various salts, including sodium and calcium. If the tumor interferes with sodium, the patient may become very faint and possibly go into a stupor or even a coma. If the tumor interferes with calcium, the patient may experience nausea, generalized aches and pains, and also possibly go into a stupor or coma. Some extra treatment may therefore be needed to counteract the effect of excess hormones. Your doctor will explain the details of any treatment that is needed.

Diagnosis and Tests

After taking your history and examining you, your doctor may recommend tests, first, to assess the extent of the primary cancer in the lung and, second, to find out whether it has spread to any other parts of your body. Thus you will almost certainly be recommended to have a bronchoscopy or mediastinoscopy to assess the primary tumor and take a biopsy.

In addition, you will probably be recommended to have a CT scan of your chest. This test may give useful information about the size and location of the cancer and also whether any of the mediastinal or other lymph nodes are involved.

After routine blood tests have been done, your doctor may also recommend a bone scan, a CT scan of your abdomen, and (in some circumstances) a brain scan or a sample of your bone marrow.

Main Objectives of Treatment

Small-cell lung cancers are generally less likely to be cured by surgery because of their tendency to spread. It is therefore quite common to start therapy with chemotherapy, hoping to control any cancer cells (even if they cannot be detected) that may have spread to other parts of the body.

Types of Treatment

Chemotherapy Chemotherapy is usually the first type of treatment used in small-cell lung cancers.

Most commonly a combination of drugs is used. A number of different drugs are quite effective in small-cell lung cancers, including **cis-platinum**, **vincristine**, **Adriamycin**, **etoposide**, **cyclophosphamide**, and others. There are different ways of combining the drugs, and your doctor will explain the details of the recommended treatment and discuss with you any side effects such as nausea, possible hair loss, and so on.

Usually the treatment will be given every three or four weeks for a specified number of times (often around six or so). There is substantial evidence to show that continuing the therapy for longer periods of time does not do any good and may be detrimental in the longer term.

Radiotherapy Small-cell lung cancers are generally responsive (or "sensitive") to radiotherapy. Radiotherapy is used where the problems or symptoms are localized, that is, confined to one area of the body. If there is a tumor in, say, the back or the hip that is causing pain or may cause a fracture, your doctor may recommend that you be assessed by a radiation oncologist. In certain situations, radiotherapy can also be given to the brain (to the whole brain rather than one part of it) in order to treat any secondaries or sometimes to prevent possible future secondaries.

Surgery In most cases of small-cell lung cancer, surgery is not useful because the chance of spread means that it is not helpful to remove the primary tumor. In a few situations, however, it may be possible or advisable to perform surgery. If this is true in your case, your doctor will discuss it with you.

LYMPHOMA (NON-HODGKIN'S LYMPHOMA)

Number of new cases diagnosed per year in the United States: 52,700

SUMMARY OF THE KEY FACTS IN THIS SECTION

- The lymphomas (also called the non-Hodgkin's lymphomas) are a group of about two dozen different types of cancers of the lymphocytes.
- Some of these are fast growing and, if left untreated, would be fatal in a few months.
- Fortunately, the fast-growing ones are often sensitive to intensive chemotherapy and can be cured in many cases.
- The more slowly growing ones are commonly widespread throughout the body. They are then relatively easy to control with less aggressive chemotherapy, although cure is rare.
- Sometimes the more slowly growing lymphomas are limited to one or two lymph nodes in the body and may then be cured with radiotherapy.

The Most Important Features of the Lymphomas

The lymphomas are a group of more than two dozen types of cancer of the lymphocytes, the most important cells of the immune system. The different types of lymphoma behave in different ways. Some are very slow growing and often fluctuate, sometimes growing, sometimes shrinking. Others are very fast growing and if not treated will cause serious damage in a few months. Still others are intermediate in their speed of progression and the damage they may do. Paradoxically the faster-growing lymphomas are potentially very serious but quite often curable (with intensive chemotherapy with or without radiotherapy). The slow-growing ones cause much less disturbance to the patient. If they are localized to one or two lymph nodes only, they may be curable with radiotherapy. If they are more widespread, however—which they usually are—they are usually controllable for many years with mild chemotherapy but are considered incurable.

What Are Lymphocytes?

Lymphocytes are cells that predominantly live and grow in two places: the lymph nodes and the bone marrow (for more about them, see "What You Really Need to Know about the Bone Marrow and Lymph Nodes," page 120). For reasons that we do not fully understand, some cancers of lymphocytes—the lymphomas—cause trouble mainly in the lymph nodes. Other cancers of the lymphocytes—the lymphocytic leukemias (see page 122) and multiple myeloma (see page 161)—cause trouble mainly in the bone marrow. There is some overlap between problems in the nodes and problems in the marrow, and several types of lymphoma cause problems in both areas. In general, however, it is reasonable to think of a lymphoma as mainly a malignancy of lymphocytes based in the lymph nodes and spleen (see page 122) as distinct from malignancies of lymphocytes based in the marrow. There are exceptions to this general rule, namely, some lymphomas that begin in organs of the body other than lymph nodes, such as the stomach, thyroid, or bowel.

We do not know exactly what happens as lymphomas develop and spread. Some types of lymphoma will start in one place—such as a lymph node or, in some cases, another organ such as the bowel—spread first to nearby lymph nodes, and only later spread to other parts of the body. Other types of lymphoma seem to begin in several areas simultaneously; the technical term for this is **multicentric** origin. In the latter case, the fact that the lymphomas are widespread, involving many areas of the body, does not mean that they were missed or misdiagnosed at an earlier stage.

Terms Used to Describe Lymphomas

The names and terms used to describe lymphomas need some clarification because the way in which the lymphomas have been classified and named can be confusing—to doctors as well as to patients! One type of cancer of the lymphocytes with a very characteristic way of behaving and a distinct appearance under the microscope was first described in 1832 and named Hodgkin's disease after its discoverer, Dr. Thomas Hodgkin. Later on, other types of lymphoma were described and, as a group, were called the **non-Hodgkin's lymphomas**. Nowadays most people simply abbreviate "non-Hodgkin's lymphomas" to "lymphomas," as I am doing in this section. This nomenclature is therefore really an accident of history. The point is that the terms "lymphoma" and "non-Hodgkin's lymphoma" refer to the same group of cancers.

Age and Incidence

Lymphomas occur more commonly with advancing age but can be seen at any age from childhood to old age. In general, the incidence of all lymphomas has been increasing slightly over the last few decades. This seems to be chiefly due to a disproportionate increase in a certain type of lymphoma in the elderly. Nobody knows the reasons for this at present.

Causes

In the great majority of cases, we do not know the cause. In a small proportion of cases, however, four types of factors that may be relevant have been identified.

1. Occupational Exposure In a small number of occupations, primarily related to forestry and agriculture, certain chemicals or substances seem to increase the risk of developing lymphoma.

2. Inherited Conditions In a small number of inherited conditions, the immune system is badly impaired or damaged from birth. People with these rare syndromes (which are in themselves often quite serious) have a higher risk of later developing lymphoma.

3. Certain Medications or Drugs Certain medications may also increase the risk of lymphoma. These include certain kinds of chemotherapy drugs used to treat, for example, Hodgkin's disease. These risks are, in general, slight.

4. HIV and AIDS In the last few years, it has become apparent that people who have HIV and later develop AIDS have a higher-than-average risk of developing lymphoma. Probably this is because HIV itself damages part of the immune system and somehow enables malignancies of the immune system to develop.

How the Cancer Tends to Spread

Lymphomas tend to spread in different ways, depending on whether they are high grade or low grade and depending on whether they begin in lymph nodes or in other organs. In general, the higher-grade lymphomas spread first to other lymph nodes (local or distant) and do not involve the bone marrow until quite late in their progress. Low-grade lymphomas are quite often widespread and frequently involve the bone marrow early in their progress. It is a peculiarity of the lymphomas that the less aggressive types often involve a distant organ such as the bone marrow at an early stage, while the more aggressive types do not. This may be related to the way in which these different types of lymphoma originate and the type of lymphocytes they originate from. At present we do not fully understand the significance of this pattern of spread.

If the lymphoma begins in an organ other than a lymph node (for example, the stomach), it is quite likely to spread to the adjacent lymph nodes first and to distant sites later in its progress.

Symptoms or Problems That You May Notice

In general, lymphomas are conditions that cause two types of symptoms: symptoms related to enlarged lymph nodes and generalized constitutional symptoms.

Symptoms Related to Enlarged Lymph Nodes Most people who develop lymphoma will first go to their doctor because they have noticed some enlarged lymph nodes in the neck, armpit, or groin. It needs to be said that the vast majority of enlarged lymph nodes are not caused by lymphoma but by common everyday infections such as an ordinary virus and will disappear in a few weeks. In some cases, however, the enlarged lymph nodes are quite big—up to three centimeters (an inch) or so—have appeared without any obvious cause such as a virus infection, and are not usually tender when touched. Lymph nodes like this are suspicious and may be caused by lymphoma, although there are several other things that can cause them. Usually nodes like this do not cause any symptoms, although in a few cases they may cause a mild discomfort or ache if they are very large, particularly if they are in an area such as the armpit or neck where they can interfere with movement.

Generalized (Constitutional) Symptoms If there are many lymph nodes involved, lymphoma can cause you to feel **generally unwell** with **loss of energy**, **loss of appetite**, **loss of weight**, **and excessive sweating at night**. In themselves, these symptoms (sometimes called B symptoms because of their similarity to symptoms that occur in Hodgkin's disease) may not affect the prognosis, though (particularly in the more slow-growing lymphomas) they may be a factor in deciding when to start treatment and in the choice of medications.

Diagnosis and Tests

Two factors need to be established with every person who has lymphoma: the **type** of lymphoma (see below) and the **stage** (that is, how widespread it is).

Lymph Node Biopsy Usually the type of lymphoma is established by a biopsy, examining a piece of a suspicious lymph node. In most cases, this involves a local anesthetic during which the node is removed and sent for examination. The examination includes looking at the specimen under the microscope but may also involve other tests (particularly if the lymphoma is not easy to diagnose from its appearance alone). These tests include various types of staining procedures and some other newer tests, including analysis of the chromosomes and genes of the lymphoma. Because some of the lymphomas are difficult to categorize, a number of tests may be needed, and you may not get the complete results of the biopsy for several days, so try to be patient.

Staging Tests Having determined what kind of lymphoma it is, your medical team will then go on to find out what stage it is, in other words, what other parts of the body besides the lymph nodes are involved. The tests required may include a chest X ray, a liver ultrasound, a sample of bone marrow, and in many cases a lymphogram, a CT scan, or MRI scan. Very occasionally, other tests such as a biopsy of the liver may be needed. At the end of these tests, your doctor will have a fairly clear picture of what type of lymphoma you have and which parts of your body are involved with it.

The Main Types of the Cancer

Site of Origin Most lymphomas begin in lymph nodes and may spread to other lymph nodes, either nearby or in distant parts of the body. Some lymphomas, however, begin within collections of lymphocytes that are situated in other areas or organs, such as the stomach, the thyroid gland, the intestine, or several other sites. Lymphomas that begin in organs other than the lymph nodes are called **extranodal lymphomas**. They often behave somewhat differently from the more common nodal lymphomas and so are treated differently.

Grade and Type In addition to the site of origin, lymphomas are also classified by their type and grade. Both factors have a major influence on the treatment and prognosis.

Factors That Influence the Treatment and Prognosis

The Type and Grade of the Lymphoma The most important aspect of lymphoma that determines what happens next, and what happens in the long term, is the type of the lymphoma. A great deal of research on an international scale has gone into the classification of the lymphomas. Some years ago a committee of specialists divided the lymphomas into thirteen different types based on their histological appearance. The particular names given to those thirteen types are not particularly important for understanding the lymphomas. What is important is that the types were divided into three groups: low grade (sometimes called "indolent"), high grade, and intermediate grade (sometimes called "aggressive").

To a certain extent, knowing the type and grade of the lymphoma helps your medical team predict how aggressive the tumor is going to be. They can thus, to some extent, base the treatment on the grade of the lymphoma and on the stage it is at, taking into consideration any symptoms that you may be experiencing and your general medical condition.

Because the objectives and types of treatment for the low-grade lymphomas are quite different from those for the intermediate and high-grade ones, I deal with the two broad groups separately in the next two sections. I then briefly discuss the extranodal lymphomas.

THE LOW-GRADE LYMPHOMAS

How Low-Grade Lymphomas Behave

If the low-grade lymphoma is limited to one lymph node group or two lymph node groups adjacent to each other, it can often be cured with radiotherapy. Unfortunately, most low-grade lymphomas are not like this but are widespread or generalized throughout the body at the time of diagnosis (see above). In most cases the generalized low-grade lymphomas are slow growing, and quite often lymph nodes involved with low-grade lymphoma fluctuate in size. In other words, it is quite common for lymph nodes to get larger and then to get smaller over periods of weeks or months without treatment. The idea that a cancer can actually come and go, often of its own accord, surprises most patients. In general, cancers do not behave in this way, but such fluctuations are a very common feature of these particular tumors.

Although the generalized low-grade lymphomas grow slowly, they are almost always incurable. The symptoms may fluctuate and may disappear from time to time, but the disease progresses steadily, usually over many years. Thus treatment has to be tailored to what is actually happening at the time.

The Main Objectives of Treatment

Generalized low-grade lymphomas may cause constitutional symptoms, and occasionally some of the lymph nodes may cause local problems such as discomfort. For much of the time, however, people with low-grade lymphoma may have no symptoms at all. Because the condition has been basically incurable, and because the symptoms are intermittent, the usual policy in treating low-grade lymphoma is to give chemotherapy or radiotherapy when the patient experiences symptoms and to stop treatment once those symptoms have been controlled. Currently there are research studies going on to see if early or aggressive therapy is of benefit.

Types of Treatment

No Treatment For much of the time, people with low-grade lymphoma may not need any treatment at all. This often causes surprise and sometimes concern. It's quite difficult to accept that there is a type of cancer that does not require treatment. Nevertheless, many studies have shown that this is the best approach to low-grade lymphoma, and so far there is no proven benefit from using very aggressive therapy early in the disease.

Chemotherapy At some point, either the constitutional symptoms or symptoms related to nodes will probably require some treatment. The first line of treatment of low-grade lymphoma usually requires oral medication only. The most commonly used drugs are the chemotherapy agent **chlorambucil** with or without the steroid **prednisone**. Other drugs commonly used are **cyclophosphamide**, **vincristine**, or sometimes **melphalan**. Often one or more of these drugs will be given for a week or two weeks at a time (depending on the exact schedule) for a few months. In some centers, the biologic agent **interferon** (see page 214) may be given for a time after chemotherapy. The treatment will be stopped when the nodes or the symptoms have subsided and will be started later when the nodes or symptoms start causing problems again. Quite often treatment can be given when needed in this way over a period of several or many years. After several courses, however, the tumor usually becomes resistant to these gentler agents, and the treatment may have to be changed. At that point, combinations of other more aggressive chemotherapy drugs are usually used, some or all of which may have to be given by injection. Usually combinations of drugs, including **Adriamycin**, will be recommended, or other drugs such as

etoposide may be used. These drugs are very useful when the gentler drugs have stopped being effective.

Radiotherapy At times there may be symptoms related to a group of lymph nodes in one particular area, say, the neck or armpit. If the symptoms are particularly annoying and if the patient feels well otherwise, it is sometimes helpful to use radiotherapy on the particular area that is causing difficulty. In other circumstances, if a lymph node appears likely to cause trouble—say, by blocking the bile duct—radiotherapy can be used to stop trouble from developing. If it is recommended in your case, your oncologists will discuss the full details with you.

THE INTERMEDIATE AND HIGH-GRADE LYMPHOMAS

How Intermediate and High-Grade Lymphomas Behave

The intermediate and high-grade lymphomas progress more rapidly than the low-grade ones and also do not fluctuate in their progress but advance steadily. Left untreated, they will usually cause marked deterioration in a year or so. In a large number of cases, however, they can be cured with intensive therapy.

The Main Objectives of Treatment

As some of the intermediate and high-grade lymphomas will be cured by intensive therapy, the objective of treatment is to try to cure the patient, if the patient is able (physically and psychologically) to undergo the therapy.

Types of Treatment

Chemotherapy Regimens Often a combination of chemotherapy drugs, sometimes four to eight different drugs or even more, is used. There are many different ways of giving the drugs: some require weekly injections, and some require injections every three or four weeks, for example. A small number of courses may be recommended as part of the treatment of localized intermediate-grade lymphoma, or a longer duration of more intensive therapy may be recommended for the higher grades. Your doctor will explain the exact schedule recommended, but all are intensive and arduous. Side effects are common and include nausea, weight loss, tiredness, low white-cell counts (and susceptibility to infection), anemia and low platelet counts (sometimes requiring transfusions of blood or platelets), hair loss, mouth ulcers, and several other types of less common problems. Two important points should be kept in mind. First, these lymphomas can be cured in a fair number of cases, so the arduous therapy may well be justified. Second, the effects of the therapy, especially the fatigue, continue for many weeks or even a couple of months after the chemotherapy. Don't be too hard on yourself if you find that you are still feeling exhausted some weeks after the treatment.

Radiotherapy Radiotherapy is often used in conjunction with chemotherapy in the treatment of the more localized types of intermediate and high-grade lymphomas. This is especially true if there is one particularly large area affected.

CNS Prophylaxis Certain types of lymphoma have a high tendency to spread to the central nervous system, particularly to the meninges (the membranes covering the brain and the spinal cord). In a few circumstances, therefore, treatment may be recommended to destroy any lymphoma cells that may be lurking there, even if there is no definite indication of their presence. Because this type of treatment is given to prevent future problems rather than to treat existing ones, it is called preventive therapy, or **prophylaxis**. In the treatment of lymphoma, prophylaxis to the central nervous system (CNS) is given by a series of injections into the fluid inside the brain and spinal cord, by radiotherapy to the brain and spinal cord, or both. If injections are required, they are usually given by thin needles inserted at the lower part of the back (lumbar puncture and instillation), though other methods may sometimes be used. If CNS prophylaxis is recommended in your case, your doctor will explain why and will discuss the particular method to be used in your case. CNS prophylaxis is used only for those few types of lymphoma that have a high propensity to spread to the CNS, so do not feel that your treatment is incomplete if you are not receiving it.

TREATMENT OF EXTRANODAL LYMPHOMAS

The initial treatment of extranodal lymphomas may differ from that of lymphomas that begin in lymph nodes. For example, if the lymphoma begins in the bowel, it is often necessary to remove part of the bowel and then to give chemotherapy afterward. If the lymphoma occurs in the stomach, removal of the whole stomach may not be needed, and a biopsy may be sufficient, followed by chemotherapy. In other areas of the body, it may not be feasible to remove the primary tumor, and in those circumstances, chemotherapy may be used first and may be followed by radiotherapy. Situations like these are not very common, and the exact form and type of treatment does vary from case to case, so you should discuss the recommended treatment fully with your specialist.

TREATMENT OF LYMPHOMA IF IT RECURS

Lymphomas are unusual compared to almost all other types of cancer in that, if they recur, they can still be controlled for a time in many cases and even cured in some cases. A number of different types of treatment are being investigated and used in such cases, so your doctor may discuss several options with you. These may include the following.

Bone Marrow Transplantation Bone marrow transplantation (see page 228) has been used for many years now in the treatment of leukemias and lymphomas, and there is a great deal of data now accumulated on the use of BMT and on the treatment's success rate in different circumstances. Depending on the reasons for using BMT and on whether the patient's own marrow is involved with the lymphoma, the marrow used may be the patient's own marrow (this is called autologous bone marrow transplantation) or a donor's. In each of these circumstances, the chance that the treatment will succeed does vary, so you will need to discuss the chances of success in your own case. In all settings and in all circumstances, bone marrow transplantation is a considerable undertaking, so be sure that you understand from your doctor precisely what the objectives are in using it, what are the anticipated chances of success, what side effects will be expected from the therapy, and how long they will last.

Other Types of Therapy Many newer agents are being investigated for use in lymphoma. These include **biologic agents** (see page 231) such as the **interleukins**, which activate certain cells in the immune system, **interferons**, or **monoclonal antibodies**. If any of these newer types of therapy show promise in treating your particular type of lymphoma, your doctor will discuss the pros and cons with you in detail.

MELANOMA SKIN CANCER (MALIGNANT MELANOMA)

Number of new cases diagnosed per year in the United States: 38,300

SUMMARY OF THE KEY FACTS IN THIS SECTION

- Melanoma (also called malignant melanoma) is a type of skin cancer that begins in the cells that make the coloring, or pigment, of the skin.
- A major factor in causing melanoma is sunlight.
- It is very much rarer than the other types of skin cancer (which are actually very common).
- In some cases, melanoma may be a very aggressive type of cancer with a high tendency to spread to distant parts of the body.
- Despite its potentially aggressive behavior, a majority of patients can be cured by surgery, if it is diagnosed when it is at an early stage and has not spread deeply into the skin or to the lymph nodes.
- The behavior of a melanoma is often very difficult to predict. Unfortunately, it may in some cases recur many years after the first skin lesion is removed.
- Because sunlight is an important contributory cause, prevention (using sunblocking creams and avoiding sunburn or deep tanning) is a real possibility.

The Most Important Features of the Tumor

Most of the skin consists of layers of flattish cells, the skin cells, which give the skin its tough protective capability. Some of the cells in the skin (the melanocytes) manufacture a brownish pigment (melanin) that absorbs ultraviolet light and protects the skin against damage from sunlight. If these cells become cancerous, that cancer is called a melanoma. It is much less common than the ordinary forms of skin cancer (see pages 187–190) and in some cases has a much higher tendency to spread to distant parts of the body. The most important consideration with a melanoma is how deeply it has penetrated into the skin. The ones that do not penetrate deeply can almost always be cured by surgical removal. If a melanoma has penetrated quite deeply into the skin or has spread to lymph nodes, the chance of cure is much lower. As regards

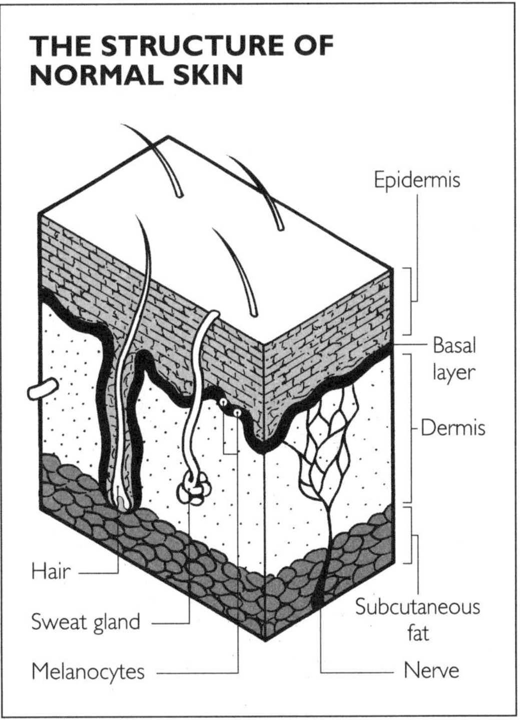

the causes of melanoma, sunlight is a major factor, particularly if you have skin that is easily susceptible to sun damage (for example, people with red hair and people with many freckles) or, more important, have had damage to the skin in the form of sunburns in childhood. Hence prevention by using sunblocking creams and avoiding sunburn or deep tanning is a real possibility.

What You Really Need to Know about the Skin

Function The skin consists of two main layers, the outer **epidermis** and the supporting **dermis** beneath it, and is quite well designed to resist insults from the outside world, to repair and renew itself, to keep moisture inside the body, and to perform several other functions such as cooling the body (by producing sweat) and helping to control salt levels. In addition, the skin contains cells that produce a brown pigment called **melanin**, which is important in protecting the skin against damage from ultraviolet light in sunlight. In Caucasians, Asians, and other light-skinned people, the amount of melanin pigment in the skin is relatively small. The lighter the skin, the more easily it will be damaged by sunlight. In black-skinned people, the melanin is packaged differently, to give the skin its color and also ensure far better protection against damage from sunlight. Hence dark-skinned people have a lower chance of developing problems associated with exposure to sunlight (including melanoma), except in the areas of the skin that are not deeply pigmented such as the palms and the soles.

Structure The top layer of the skin is the epidermis, and it is this layer that protects the body from damage. Each day, millions of dead skin cells are lost from the top of the epidermis as part of the normal wear and tear of daily life. (In fact, most of the dust that accumulates in our houses consists of those dead cells shed normally from our skin!) This loss of cells requires a high rate of repair and renewal, and that function is carried out by cells in the bottom part of the epidermis called the **basal layer**. (Because that layer is at the junction between the epidermis and the dermis below it, it is sometimes referred to as the **junctional area.**) The process by which skin cells are lost and replaced is well understood. Skin cells are produced in the basal layer of the epidermis and steadily work their way to the surface as new cells are produced below them. As the cells work their way upward, they become flatter and gradually fill up with a tough chemical called **keratin**, which gives the skin its resilient, protective abilities. By the time the cells reach the surface, they are filled with keratin. At that point they die, and the dead cells are then shed from the surface. The epidermis, therefore, is basically a layer of protective cells that are constantly being scuffed off from the surface and replaced from the bottom. This is the process by which the skin performs its major function of protection.

Below the epidermis is the dermis, and this is a supportive layer, the foundation on which the epidermis is laid. It is made up of connective tissue, a fibrous tissue that is tough and elastic.

The dermis and epidermis contain many other structures such as hair follicles, sweat glands, sebaceous glands (which provide some lubrication and waterproofing for the skin), and of course nerve endings, which allow us to feel things that touch or influence our skin.

While the skin protects the structures underneath, it also needs some protection of its own, particularly from ultraviolet light. That protection is provided by another group of cells produced in the basal layer of the epidermis which produce the pigment melanin. Melanin is dark brown, and if it is packaged in a certain way within the skin, the skin will appear dark brown. This feature of your skin is partly genetically controlled, which is why the human species has both dark-skinned and light-skinned people. The **melanocytes** normally live low down in the epidermis near the basal layer. Unlike the majority of skin cells, they do not usually move upward to the surface in large numbers.

Quite frequently, however, small areas of the skin will have more melanin than the surrounding skin. There are two types of such areas: freckles and moles.

What You Really Need to Know about Freckles and Moles

Usually the melanocytes are spread evenly throughout the skin (and therefore the melanin is too). This gives the skin an even color. Many people also have some areas where melanin has collected to create dark brown spots. These areas are called **freckles**. As everyone knows, more freckles appear in the summer after exposure to sunlight, and those that are already there often become slightly darker. This is the normal response of the melanocytes to sunlight. Freckles are flat (if you run your finger over your freckles, you won't feel anything like a bump or a lump).

The melanocytes may also create other colored lesions called **moles**. Two features of moles are relevant here. First, in a mole the melanocytes collect and move *downward* into the upper part of the dermis, forming a little bump in the dermis. Thus moles (unlike freckles) can be felt if you run your finger over them. Second, moles do not come and go with the sunlight; they are permanent, and they usually appear by the time you are three years old. I should stress that **the vast majority of moles on the skin are completely innocent and do not carry any increased risk of cancer (melanoma) whatsoever**. A few unusual types of moles do carry a higher risk, and these are described below, but again, please remember that **the vast majority of moles are completely benign**.

Age and Incidence

Although melanoma is not very common, it is more common than most people think. It is extremely rare in childhood and infancy, and in fact it reaches its peak incidence in the forties. It affects males and females equally. Dark-skinned people do not get melanomas of the dark areas of the skin, but they may get melanomas in light areas, such as under the fingernails or toenails, in the lips, or in the eyes.

Causes

Although we don't know all the causes of melanoma, we do understand most of the factors that put people at increased risk for developing it. There are basically two types of risk factors: external factors (which in practice means sunlight) and factors that are inherited or present in the skin at birth.

Sunlight Sunlight is by far the most important preventable risk factor for melanoma. Unfortunately, there is no level of sunlight that causes no damage whatsoever. In theory, therefore, any amount of sunlight will cause some damage. Furthermore, we all need *some* sunlight because, as it happens, sunlight is one of the essential ingredients that allows our skin cells to manufacture vitamin D. Without any sunlight, we would all eventually become deficient in vitamin D and develop rickets. Hence prevention of melanoma is a matter of balancing the risk of excessive sun damage against our need for sunlight and enjoyment of it. Fortunately, it is possible to draw up sensible practical guidelines that can minimize the risk of melanoma. These are given in the "Prevention" section below. It is important to note that the main risks seem to be suffering a bad sunburn before the teen years or adolescence and (perhaps) constant exposure with a "year-round deep tan." Although the latter may be very desirable cosmetically and socially, it may be very unhealthy for the skin, contributing to both melanoma and wrinkles.

Certain (Rare) Kinds of Moles or Skin Lesions Quite often a melanoma can develop from a particular type of mole. The correct name for this type of mole is a **dysplastic nevus**. A dysplastic nevus tends to be flat or only slightly raised and when seen from above is often irregular in shape. It is also usually darker than an ordinary mole and larger, often more than five millimeters (one-fifth of an inch) in

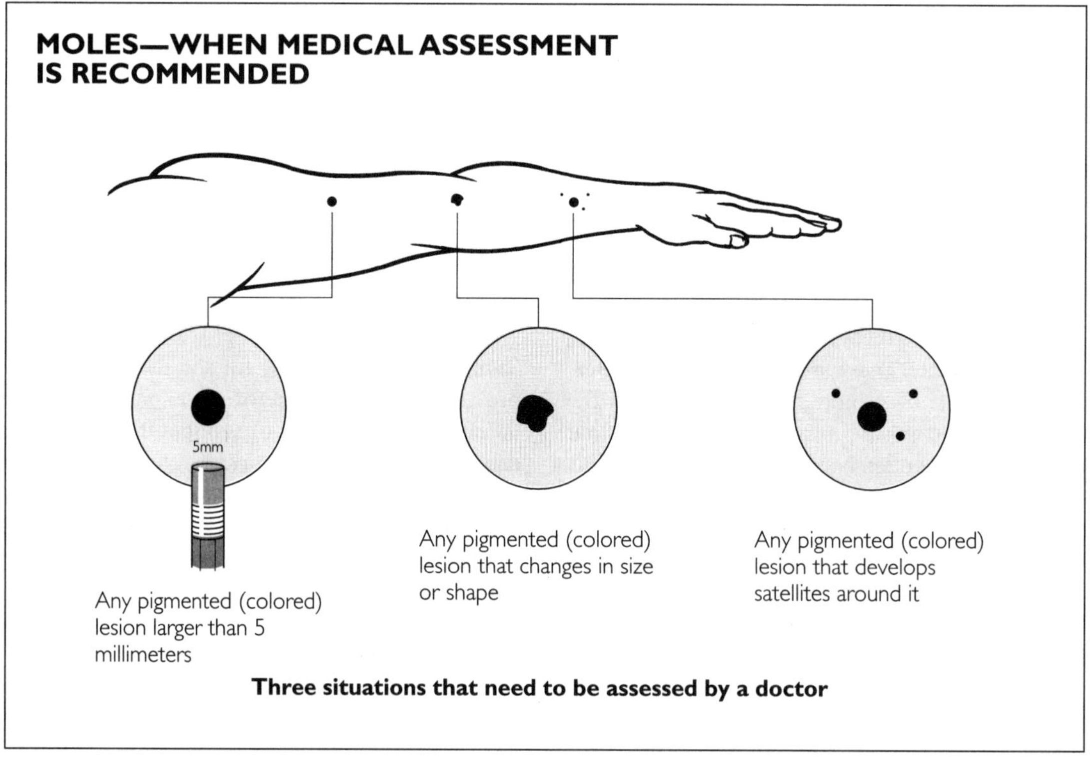

Three situations that need to be assessed by a doctor

diameter. (Although size in itself is not a danger sign, it is important to have larger moles assessed by a doctor.) By contrast, the ordinary type of mole is usually round (or almost round) and is usually raised. The most important danger sign, however, is evidence of **change in a mole**, that is, if a mole that has been present for a long time starts becoming **irregular**, or if it is **larger than five millimeters**, or starts **enlarging** noticeably, or starts developing little **satellite lesions** around it.

If you happen to be born with one or more very large moles of other types, you may also have a slightly increased risk of melanoma from those. The risk from the smaller types of congenital moles is probably nil.

Family Members with Melanoma If a member of your close family has or has had melanoma, or has or has had dysplastic nevi, your risk of melanoma is increased somewhat.

A Previous Melanoma If you have had a melanoma in the past, there is unfortunately an increased chance that you may develop a second one.

How the Cancer Tends to Spread

Local Growth Melanoma tends to grow in two directions. It may spread **along the skin**, for which the medical term is **radial growth**, or it may grow downward into the deeper layers of the skin. For the most part, growth along the skin suggests relatively nonaggressive behavior, while growth deep into the skin seems to indicate more aggressive behavior.

Distant Spread Melanoma may spread to other areas of the body, in many cases going first to the lymph nodes in the area (say, in the groin, if the first tumor was on the leg). Melanoma is often unpredictable, however, and it may spread to other distant areas of the body even if the lymph nodes have not been involved. These areas include the liver, the lungs, and also the brain.

Symptoms or Problems That You May Notice

As mentioned above, the possible signs of a melanoma are: (a) a **new skin lesion** that is colored **blue-black** or is **patchily colored** with brown, black, and purplish areas in it; (b) changes to an **existing mole** such as **becoming larger**, becoming **irregular**, bleeding when you touch it or scratch it, or developing smaller **satellite lesions** around it.

Diagnosis and Tests

Usually the diagnosis of a melanoma is made by a biopsy. When a skin lesion looks as if it might be a melanoma, it is customary to remove the skin lesion entirely (excise it). Thus the biopsy of a suspicious skin lesion is usually called an **excisional biopsy** (because the lesion is excised completely). If the lesion is found to be a melanoma, a further operation is usually needed (see page 154). This is the usual method of doing things; the need for an additional operation does not mean that the initial biopsy was done wrongly. Definitive treatment may sometimes mean a second operation after the diagnostic biopsy.

If the lesion is a melanoma, some blood tests, X rays, or scans or all three may be recommended. There is also a technique that is often used in which the lymph node nearest to the tumor is identified by a special dye injection (for example, the node may be in the groin if the melanoma is on the leg). That node is then removed to see if the tumor has spread. This is called **sentinel node sampling** and may be of use in determining the prognosis.

The Main Types of the Cancer

The type of the melanoma as seen under the microscope does not affect the outlook so much as the way in which the melanoma is growing, which is a strong predictor of the depth to which it has penetrated. Thus the form of the tumor is important because it may predict, to some extent, the depth of the tumor. There are four main types, or patterns, of melanoma.

Superficial Spreading ("Flat") Type This is the most common type of melanoma; about seven out of ten melanomas are of this type. It grows mostly along the skin, penetrating deeper only late in its progress. It usually starts with a colored mole on the skin that, after remaining the same size and shape for many years, begins to change, sometimes quite rapidly. Characteristically, this type of melanoma is irregular in its shape or pattern and is colored in an uneven, patchy way, so that parts of it may appear brown, while other parts appear black, pink, or even white.

Nodular Type This type is more aggressive than the superficial spreading type and often appears in the skin without a preceding pigmented patch or mole. A nodular melanoma is often first detected as a lump or a bump that is usually blue-black in color. This type (for reasons we do not understand) is more common in males than in females. In general, a nodular melanoma behaves more aggressively than the superficial spreading type.

Acral Melanoma (the "Palms and Soles" Type) This type of melanoma occurs on the palms or the soles or under the nailbeds. In light-skinned people, acral melanomas make up only a small percentage of all melanomas, but in dark-skinned people, for whom melanomas in the rest of the skin are very rare, acral melanomas make up between one-third and two-thirds of melanomas.

Lentigo Maligna Melanomas This type of melanoma is commonly found on the faces of elderly people who have had a great deal of exposure to sunlight.

Melanomas can also occur in the eye—at the back of the eye (the retina) or in the iris—or around the mouth, the anus, or the vagina.

Factors That Influence the Treatment and Prognosis

Depth The most important factor in determining the outlook is how deeply the melanoma has spread into the skin. The depth is carefully assessed by the pathologist looking at the melanoma under the microscope. Currently two methods of assessment are used.

Thickness The depth is simply the thickness of the melanoma measured by the pathologist using a special device on his or her microscope. The melanoma can be assessed as: (a) less than three-quarters of a millimeter (less than 0.75 mm), that is, about three hundredths of an inch or about three or four times the thickness of an average human hair; (b) between 0.76 and 1.5 mm; (c) 1.51 to 4 mm; and (d) thicker than 4 mm.

Melanomas thinner than 0.75 mm are relatively common. In fact, about four out of every ten melanomas are in this favorable group; many more are less than one millimeter and have a low chance of recurrence.

Level This is a way of describing how deep the melanoma has spread relative to the layer of the skin: into the epidermis, the various layers of the dermis, or the subcutaneous structures below the dermis. This system was first defined by Dr. Wallace Clark, so you may hear your medical team talking about "Clark Level I" or "Clark Level II."

Because the thickness of the various parts of the skin varies from place to place, being very thin on the eyelid and quite thick on the sole, the two systems of assessment are both useful, and usually the melanoma will be assessed using both methods.

Stage If it happens that the melanoma has spread to the lymph nodes, the prognosis is less favorable and the chance of cure is smaller.

Histology The type of the melanoma as it appears under the microscope (histology) does not usually predict its behavior.

The Main Objectives of Treatment

If the lesion is located in a place where it can be removed, the objective is to remove the melanoma completely with as little disturbance to function and the cosmetic appearance of the area as possible. If the original melanoma was thin, complete removal offers a very high cure rate. Even with thicker lesions, the cure rate is still reasonably good.

Types of Treatment

Surgery Surgery is really the mainstay of the treatment of melanoma and is the only treatment that offers a high chance of cure. As I mentioned above, the initial operation done under local anesthetic may be all that is required. If further surgery is required, your surgeon will be trying to remove a margin of normal skin around the place where the melanoma was, while at the same time trying to minimize the disturbance to function or appearance that the operation may cause. The details of the surgery depend on the size, depth, and position of the melanoma. It is important to understand that the objective of the operation is to reduce the chance that the melanoma will recur locally, which is why usually a margin of normal skin needs to be removed. If needed, it is possible to do skin grafts or other cosmetic surgery to reduce the deficit, although this is rarely necessary.

Radiotherapy In the case of melanoma, radiotherapy is not very useful as a primary treatment and is usually used in the treatment of recurrences or metastases. It can be used effectively to shrink individual lesions if they are causing pain or other symptoms, and it can also be used in other areas of the body if there are secondaries. It is particularly likely to be used with secondaries in the brain or spinal cord.

Hyperthermia Hyperthermia (used in a few centers) is a form of treatment in which an area or part is heated. There are several ways of achieving this, but it has been found that hyperthermia is generally most useful when the lesion is in the skin or is very superficial. Often hyperthermia, if given, is used in conjunction with radiotherapy. At present, hyperthermia (with or without radiotherapy) does not appear to cure any tumors, but it may contribute to the control of tumors for a time in certain circumstances.

Adjuvant Therapy As I mentioned at the beginning of this section, melanoma is generally difficult to predict. If the lesion is thin, the chance of cure is very high. If the lesion is thicker, in some cases the patient will be cured by surgery; in others the melanoma can recur even many years after diagnosis. Thus there have been many attempts to identify treatment that may decrease the chance of recurrence if given after initial surgery (known as adjuvant therapy). If there is a high risk of recurrence, the standard treatment consists of the biologic agent **interferon** (see page 232). In addition, other approaches are being investigated, including **tumor vaccines (antibodies)** (see page 232).

Chemotherapy Although for the most part melanomas are not very responsive to chemotherapy drugs, combinations of chemotherapy drugs can be used in advanced melanomas and do produce a response in some cases. If you have advanced melanoma and this treatment is recommended, you should discuss the potential benefits and side effects with your doctor.

Biologic (also called Biological) Therapy There are two biologic agents with established anticancer activity in patients with advanced melanoma: **interferon-alpha** and **interleukin-2 (IL-2)** (see page 232). Both of these may produce responses, in some cases lasting years. Their use is also being investigated in conjunction with tumor vaccines and also in combination with chemotherapy.

Other Therapy In some cancer centers, a means of giving chemotherapy exclusively to the involved area is being investigated. This is called **isolated limb perfusion** and may be used when a melanoma is on a limb. The chemotherapy is given into the artery supplying that area of the limb. More specific details of this treatment will be explained to you by your specialist.

Screening and Early Diagnosis

The best way of diagnosing any skin problem early is to inspect your skin carefully and repeat the inspection every few months or so, so that you will know if anything new develops. Do look at your whole body surface in a mirror regularly, including your soles, fingernails, and toenails. The problem with skin, as a patient once put it, is that so much of it is on your back and out of sight. If you have a mole on your back or in some other inaccessible place, you should get your spouse or a family member or friend to have a look at it every so often, or use a second mirror to look at your own back. If you have any moles that are particularly large, it is worth seeking medical advice; your family doctor can tell you if consultation with a specialist is advisable. Often that may mean that you will be assessed once a year or so by the specialist. If that is recommended, do try to keep all your appointments. Also, if **any mole changes, bleeds, or develops satellite lesions**, or if a **new mole develops** after the age of forty or so, you should seek medical advice within a week or two.

Prevention

Not only is a bit of sunlight necessary for our vitamin metabolism, but a suntan is a socially desirable asset and is zealously acquired and maintained by many people. Sad to say, however, a suntan is not a very healthy experience for the skin. To reduce the chance of developing a melanoma, **everyone,**

TABLE 4.6: DECREASING THE RISK OF GETTING SKIN CANCER

1. **Sunlight** is a major factor in the cause of all types of skin cancer.
2. The greatest danger from sunlight is **damage to the skin at a young age**, before the age of twenty and particularly before the age of ten.
3. People with **fair skin and red hair are at greater risk** than others because their skin is less protected with the skin pigment melanin.
4. A **blistering sunburn before the age of ten** doubles a person's chance of getting skin cancer later. **So the best and most important time for protection is childhood**.
5. If you have **three blistering sunburns before the age of twenty**, your risk of melanoma skin cancer may be increased fivefold.
6. Sun exposure between mid-morning (around 11:00 a.m.) and late afternoon (4:00 p.m.) is the most dangerous, so plan to **stay in the shade during those hours**. Don't forget, though, that the early morning sun and evening sun can still be dangerous if you are unprotected.
7. **Always use a sunblock of at least SPF 15** and, even more important, make sure your children do the same every time they go out.
8. **Shirts and wide-brimmed hats** provide excellent protection.
9. There is no evidence that suntanning in salons is truly safe.
10. From your skin's point of view, there is no such thing as a healthy tan. A deep tan is a sign of accumulated exposure and therefore of skin damage, and it causes wrinkles!

particularly children, should avoid actual burning of the skin (in other words, letting the skin become red) at any time and should avoid acquiring a **deep brown tan**, even if the skin has never actually been burned in the process (see Table 4.6). People with very light skin (a characteristic often accompanied by red hair and blue eyes) burn more easily, so if you have light skin, you need to take even more care and use sunblocking agents with greater-than-average blocking power.

All these precautions are particularly important for children. In summer, children's skin should be completely protected with a sunblocking cream of at least sun protection factor (SPF) 15 while they are outside. Also, remember to reapply the cream after the child has been swimming. In addition, try to get your child to wear a T-shirt or undershirt and a sunhat when playing outside. This goes against most children's inclinations, so start the educating process early and persevere with it despite the child's protests! Research shows that this can make a great deal of difference.

MOUTH (ORAL CANCER AND ADJACENT AREAS)

Number of new cases diagnosed per year in the United States: 11,300

SUMMARY OF THE KEY FACTS IN THIS SECTION

- "Oral cancer" is the term given to cancers arising in any of the components of the mouth and the oral cavity, including the lip, the tongue, the floor of the mouth, the lining of the cheeks, the tonsils, and the gums.
- Oral cancers are mostly caused by tobacco (smoking cigarettes or chewing tobacco) or a combination of tobacco and alcohol.
- If treated in the early stages, oral cancers may be cured in the majority of cases, by surgery. Radiotherapy and chemotherapy may be used in certain cases.

The Most Important Features of the Tumor

Oral cancers are common and can be diagnosed at a relatively early stage because the mouth area is easily examined by a doctor or dentist. Oral cancers tend to grow and spread in a fairly predictable way, and if detected and treated at an early stage, they can be cured in the large majority of cases. The appropriate method of treatment depends on exactly where the tumor is, how it has progressed or spread, the general medical condition of the patient, and some other factors as well. In general, if feasible, the cancer should be removed by surgery or treated with radiotherapy, chemotherapy, or both, depending on the individual situation.

What You Really Need to Know about the Mouth Area and Where Cancers May Occur

The mouth is basically a boxlike cavity with the lips at the front and the esophagus (gullet) and larynx at the back. The sides are, of course, the cheeks, and the mouth cavity contains the tongue, the gums, the tonsils, and the teeth (which do not develop cancer but may contribute to irritation of the gums or cheeks). All these organs and tissues are exposed to everything we eat and breathe, and they are all (except the teeth) covered with a lining that is designed to withstand a high degree of chemical and mechanical insult. Sometimes, however, the lining cannot withstand very high levels of chemical or mechanical irritation and one or other of the parts listed may develop a cancer.

Age and Incidence

Oral cancers are predominantly conditions that develop in the fifties and sixties, though they sometimes occur a little earlier. They affect men more than women because the main factor that contributes to

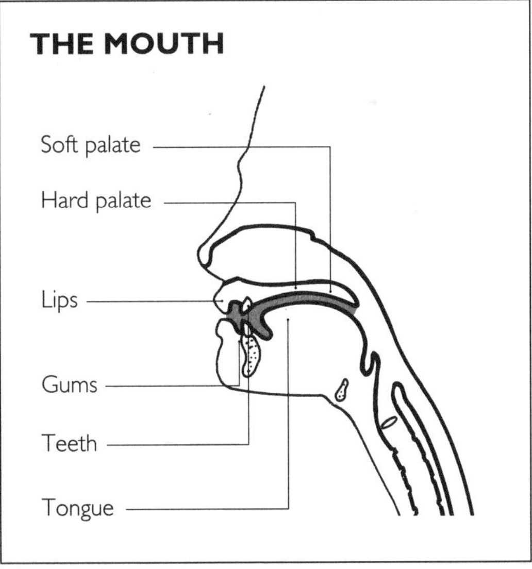

MOUTH

their development is cigarette smoking. At the moment, in this country, men are affected twice as often as women by oral cancer. Because of changes in smoking patterns in recent decades, however, the proportion of women with oral cancer is expected to continue increasing. It is also important to note that people who have developed an oral cancer are at higher risk than average of later developing another tobacco-related cancer (such as cancer of the lung).

Causes

Five main types of factors contribute to the cause of oral cancers. The most important of these are tobacco, alcohol, and (in cancer of the lip) exposure to sunlight.

Tobacco Tobacco contains a large number of chemicals, of which the most important ones that damage the tissues are known. Some of these chemicals are found in the tars and the tarlike components of tobacco. These can contribute to the development of oral cancer whether the tobacco is smoked or chewed. For reasons that we do not fully understand, the chance that a cancer will develop is further increased by consumption of alcohol.

Alcohol Although alcohol causes many medical problems, it is associated with only two areas of cancer: cancer of the liver (which is relatively rare in this country) and cancer of the mouth and esophagus (including cancer of the larynx, pharynx, and other adjacent areas). We do not fully understand what alcohol does to the lining of the mouth to exacerbate the damage done by tobacco, but it does noticeably increase the chance of oral cancer in smokers and people who chew tobacco regularly.

Sunlight As with the rest of the skin, the lips can be damaged by sunlight. The component that causes the problem is the ultraviolet part of sunlight, which is of the right wavelength to damage living tissues. Heavy and prolonged exposure to sunlight over many years causes cumulative damage to the covering of the lips and may contribute to cancer.

Chronic Irritation People who have particularly bad teeth or very ill-fitting dentures have an increased chance of developing oral cancer. Usually the cancer develops at a place in the mouth where there is long-term and severe irritation, say, by a broken tooth with a jagged edge that the owner has neglected for many years. Nowadays this is not a common cause of oral cancer. Cancer of the tongue does sometimes develop in young adults who are nonsmokers, and the reason for this is unknown.

Other Factors In some areas of the world, certain uncommon vitamin deficiencies and some infections may play a role in causing mouth cancer as well as some other cancers.

How the Cancer Tends to Spread

Precancerous Changes Changes in the lining of the mouth cavity may be important early warning signs of cancer. These usually begin as white patches (called **leukoplakia**) or red patches (called **erythroplastic lesions**).

Invasive Cancer If a true, invasive cancer develops, it usually spreads in two directions: **along** the surface of the mouth lining, and also more **deeply** into the tissues underneath the lining. If untreated, it can spread deeper and into such bony areas as the jawbone. It can also spread to lymph nodes in the neck. If it progresses still farther, it can later spread to distant parts of the body, particularly the lungs.

Symptoms or Problems That You May Notice

Two points need to be emphasized. First, oral cancer often causes the same sort of problems that occur in the mouth anyway—**sores** or **ulcers**—but with cancer they **do not heal** or disappear after two weeks or so. Second, these areas are very often **painless**. Hence it is important to make sure that any lesions in the mouth that do not heal are assessed by your doctor.

Sometimes oral cancers can also cause such symptoms as: difficulty in swallowing, difficulty in speaking clearly, pain in the cheek or side of the face, pain in the ear or side of the head, a lump that can be felt in the neck, episodes of choking, or episodes of bleeding. Any symptoms like these should be assessed by a doctor, even though cancer is not the only possible cause.

Diagnosis and Tests

In many cases the first person to draw attention to a suspicious area is a **dentist**, who may see a suspicious lesion when he or she checks the teeth. Because the mouth cavity is so easy to inspect and examine, a lot can be determined during the clinical **history and examination** by your doctor or specialist. The examination may include looking at the far back of the throat using a small mirror or a thin fiberoptic device (a nasopharyngoscope). If there are any suspicious areas, your doctor may suggest a **biopsy**. Usually done under local anesthetic, this procedure involves taking a small piece of the suspicious area to send for microscopic examination. Often an **endoscopy** may be recommended to look at any or all of the esophagus (when it is called esophagoscopy), the stomach (gastroscopy), the back of the throat area (nasopharyngoscopy), or the airways and upper parts of the lungs (bronchoscopy). Any combination of these (sometimes the four are called a quadroscopy) may be appropriate in your particular case, and biopsies are often taken during the procedure. The tests are extremely important for obtaining an accurate assessment of how big the tumor is and which structures are involved in it.

Further tests—usually **CT scans** of the head and neck or **MRI scans**—may be needed as well, in order to see exactly where and how deep the tumor is. Other tests, such as special X rays or bone scans, may be needed in a few cases. Blood tests are also used, and sometimes tests of lung function are required.

The Main Types of the Cancer

In almost all cases the type of cancer is called the **squamous type**, meaning that the cells of the cancer appear flattish, rather like cells of skin. In general, the appearance of the cancer under the microscope does not affect the prognosis or the treatment very much.

Factors That Influence the Treatment and Prognosis

The three most important factors in deciding what type of treatment is best and what the outcome is likely to be are: the **position** of the tumor (that is, on the lip, gum, tongue, the floor of the mouth, and so on), the size and extent of the tumor (whether it involves neighboring structures), and the general **medical condition and the preferences** of the patient (for example, whether the general medical condition of the patient will allow extensive surgery and how important any disability or cosmetic defect caused by the treatment will be in the patient's life). The type of treatment will be selected after detailed discussions of these factors with your specialist.

The Main Objectives of Treatment

As many cases of oral cancer can be cured if they are treated in the early stages, the main objective is to try to cure the patient if that is feasible. Obviously both patient and doctor want the aftereffects of treatment to allow life to be as normal as possible for the patient afterward.

In some cases, cure may not be possible, and in those circumstances treatment is designed to minimize the impact of the condition on normal functioning such as eating and talking.

Types of Treatment

Surgery Surgery is often the mainstay of the treatment of oral cancer. The nature of the operation needed will vary considerably depending on the site and the extent of the tumor. A small tumor on the lip or tongue might be removed with very little detriment to function or appearance, whereas surgery on larger tumors may produce greater effects. If other structures are involved, a larger amount of tissue may need to be removed. For instance, if the tumor is in the gum, the teeth above and adjacent to it will need to be removed as well. In some circumstances, removal or sampling of lymph nodes in the neck may also be recommended. With any of these operations, it may be essential to consider reconstructive surgery. Your surgeon will explain what can be done to minimize any impairment in function or appearance. It is quite common to use a team approach and to involve specialists from several different disciplines in planning the surgery. These may include experts in dental prosthetics, facial prosthetics, speech therapy, and nutrition.

In terms of cure, the success rate, if surgery is feasible and appropriate, is very high indeed. The decision to go ahead with surgery depends on balancing the likelihood of success against the effect that the surgery may have on function (speech, swallowing, facial movement) and appearance. The discussions between you and your surgical team, and their discussions with the medical and radiation teams in a multidisciplinary setting, are therefore very important.

Radiotherapy Oral cancers may also be treated with radiotherapy (see page 216) and are usually responsive to it. Because the radiation can be directed toward virtually any part of the head, radiotherapy is ideal if the tumor is in an inaccessible area and would otherwise require very mutilating surgery to remove it. The treatment itself is relatively easy to tolerate and usually consists of external-beam radiotherapy sometimes with additional brachytherapy. Depending on where and how it is given, you may experience dryness of the mouth, changes in taste, or sometimes reddening of the skin, soreness in the mouth, or other effects during the treatment. Again depending on exactly where the tumor is, the success rate may be as high as surgery or it may be lower. As with surgery, detailed discussion between you and your radiation oncologist about the success rate and any aftereffects will be extremely important.

Chemotherapy Chemotherapy may be used in the initial treatment of oral cancer in combination with radiotherapy or surgery.

The drugs most commonly used in the treatment of oral cancer include **etoposide, methotrexate, platinum drugs, 5-fluorouracil, ifosfamide,** and **Taxol.**

Laser Therapy In a few circumstances, laser therapy may be useful. The laser is rather like a very sharp and accurate knife that seals as it cuts. Only in rare cases in oral cancer does laser therapy have a proven advantage over the treatments mentioned above. If your doctor feels that something may be gained with this treatment, however, he or she will discuss it with you.

MYELOMA (MULTIPLE MYELOMA)

Number of new cases diagnosed per year in the United States: 14,400

SUMMARY OF THE KEY FACTS IN THIS SECTION

- Multiple myeloma is a cancer of one particular type of white cells in the bone marrow called plasma cells.
- It may cause symptoms by interfering with the normal function of the bone marrow and weakening the body's resistance to infection.
- Myeloma may also weaken the bones, and it can also sometimes interfere with the function of the kidneys or other organs.
- It is usually a slow-growing form of cancer, and in the majority of cases can be controlled for long periods of time with chemotherapy.

The Most Important Features of the Tumor

Multiple myeloma, usually just called myeloma, is a relatively rare type of cancer affecting one particular group of white cells in the bone marrow called **plasma cells**. The malignant plasma cells (usually called **myeloma cells**) tend to stay in the bone marrow inside the bones. They cause problems in three ways. First, by multiplying excessively, they may crowd the marrow and reduce the ability of other marrow cells to function normally. Because the plasma cells are part of the body's immune system, when a group of them becomes malignant, the body's ability to fight infection can be compromised. Thus people with myeloma have an increased chance of getting infections. Second, myeloma cells attack and weaken the surrounding bone, causing pain and sometimes fractures. Third, myeloma cells can cause an upset in the balance of certain salts in the bloodstream, notably calcium, and can also interfere with the normal function of other tissues such as the kidneys and nerves.

Myeloma cells are usually sensitive to chemotherapy, and with the careful use of intermittent courses of chemotherapy the disease may be controlled for a long time, often for many years.

What You Really Need to Know about the Bone Marrow and Plasma Cells

The basic facts about the bone marrow are given in the section of this chapter on the leukemias. It should be emphasized, however, that myeloma is not considered a type of leukemia. In theory, because it is a cancer of a type of white cell, and because the white cells that are affected by it spend most of their time in the bone marrow, it *could* be classified with the leukemias; and in practice it has certain resemblances to chronic lymphocytic leukemia (the slowest-growing and most easily controllable of the leukemias). The hallmark of the leukemias, however, is the movement of the malignant white cells into the bloodstream, and this happens only very rarely in myeloma. Myeloma is therefore classified as an entity by itself rather than as a type of leukemia.

In the bone marrow, the plasma cells are mainly responsible for producing **antibodies**. Antibodies are substances produced specifically to counteract certain types of infections, particularly bacteria and viruses. In daily life, we have millions of different "families" of plasma cells producing (or being ready to produce) antibodies to help deal with the various infections and other problems that we encounter. In myeloma, one family of plasma cells (the medical term is **clone**) gets out of control and multiplies excessively. As that family or clone multiplies, all the cells that are members of that clone continue to produce that one antibody.

Eventually they produce so much antibody that it can be detected and measured in the bloodstream, urine, or both. We call that substance the **monoclonal** (one clone) **protein**, or **M protein**, or **M band**, or **spike**. In practice, as the myeloma cells are killed by treatment, the amount of the M band decreases, allowing doctors to monitor the effects of treatment. The M band is therefore called a **marker** of the myeloma. When the M protein is detected in the urine in some patients, it is named (after the person who first described it) **Bence Jones protein**. You may find it useful to know the meaning of these terms, as you will hear them used by your medical team.

Age and Incidence

Myeloma is predominantly a condition of late middle age and older, and the incidence rises from the fifties onward. It can occur in the forties or a bit younger but is rare in that age group. For reasons that are not understood, it affects males slightly more frequently than females, and black people more frequently than other races.

Causes

The causes of myeloma are unknown. It does not seem to be related to any environmental substances or occupational exposure and is not associated with smoking or any other lifestyle habits. As far as we can tell, myeloma just happens to the immune system in the bone marrow as it grows older (which is why the condition becomes more common with age).

How the Cancer Tends to Spread

Myeloma is a condition that usually remains in the bone marrow and therefore affects the areas in which adults have bone marrow, such as the spine, the pelvis, the ribs, the skull, and the upper arms and legs. Very rarely it may spread outside the bones and cause collections of myeloma cells to form in the soft tissues of the body. Again very rarely, it can spread through the bloodstream.

Symptoms or Problems That You May Notice

Myeloma may cause three types of problems. First, it may interfere with the normal functioning of the bone marrow. It may cause problems in the bones themselves, weakening them and causing areas of collapse or sometimes fracture. It can also sometimes disrupt the balance of salts (mainly calcium) in the bloodstream.

Problems Due to Interference with the Function of the Marrow The marrow produces three types of cells: red cells, which carry oxygen; white cells, which deal with infection; and platelets, which control bruising and bleeding. As the myeloma cells in the marrow increase, they reduce the ability of normal marrow cells to perform these three functions. The most common effect of the myeloma cells is to suppress the red cells, causing an **anemia**, which is initially quite mild. This may cause you to feel **tired** and **lacking in energy** and sometimes **short of breath**. Interference with the white cells causes an **increased susceptibility to infections**. Also, once you get an infection, it takes a bit longer to shrug off than usual. Interference with the platelets is less frequent but can cause little purple spots below the skin (**petechiae**) or bigger bruises. In addition, there may be some **bleeding** from the gums or nose or, occasionally, in other parts of the body.

Problems Due to Weakening of the Bones Unlike most other types of white cells, myeloma cells produce a substance that dissolves the area of bone around them. If there are many myeloma cells and they produce a lot of this substance, they can weaken the bone and eventually cause collapse of that area of bone or sometimes fractures. In myeloma, **back pain** is quite common as a result of small degrees of collapse of the spine. **Pain** in the **ribs** or the **pelvis** is also quite common. Occasionally a bone may **fracture**, and this is most likely to happen in the hip or thigh, though it can also happen in ribs or arms.

Other Problems There may sometimes be generalized symptoms with myeloma, such as **fever** or **weight loss**. In some cases, the myeloma cells may also cause an upset in the balance of the **calcium** salts in the bloodstream. This probably happens when the myeloma cells cause small areas of bone to be dissolved (as mentioned above), allowing calcium to be released. The symptoms of excessive calcium in the bloodstream are **nausea** (sometimes with vomiting), **increased pain** in many areas of the body, **thirst** accompanied by passing an **excessive amount of urine**, **constipation**, and later **disorientation** and **confusion**, which can progress to drowsiness or even **coma**.

In addition to causing calcium problems, myeloma can affect the normal function of the **kidney**, reducing a person's ability to get rid of waste products in the urine and causing substances called **urea** and **creatinine** to accumulate in the body and the bloodstream. The presence of abnormally high amounts of those substances indicates that the myeloma is affecting the function of the kidney. In turn, impairment of kidney function causes further problems. Myeloma may also (by various methods) **interfere with nerve function**, causing **numbness**, **tingling**, or **weakness** or **paralysis** of a limb or an area of the body.

Diagnosis and Tests

Three main types of tests are used to establish a diagnosis of myeloma.

Blood and Urine Tests for M Bands The serum (liquid component of blood) can be tested to see if there is an M band present. M bands can occur in many conditions other than myeloma, so in itself an M band does not mean the person definitely has myeloma. The test will also be done on the urine, and the result is quite significant, because an M band component in the urine is very rare in conditions other than myeloma. If there is any suspicion of myeloma, a bone marrow sample will also be recommended in the great majority of cases.

Bone Marrow Sampling This test is almost always required (see page 120). Malignant plasma cells (in other words, the myeloma cells) present in large numbers in the marrow are usually easy to recognize, although occasionally identification can be quite difficult.

X Rays In about half of all cases of myeloma, X rays show little holes in the bones where the myeloma cells have dissolved some bone. In the other half of cases, the holes are probably too small to be detected by the X rays.

Factors That Influence the Treatment and Prognosis

The three most important factors that may influence the outlook with myeloma seem to be kidney function, anemia, and general mobility. If tests show that a person has normal kidney function and is not anemic, and if that person is able to function normally or almost normally (in terms of walking and doing daily tasks), the prognosis is good. If, on the other hand, the kidney function is poor, there is anemia, and the person is severely limited in mobility (for example, bedbound or chairbound for most of the day), the outlook is less promising.

The Main Objectives of Treatment

In myeloma the objective is usually to try to control the condition for as long as possible. In all cases, that usually means chemotherapy. If there are bones that are particularly painful, radiotherapy can be used for rapid pain relief as well.

Types of Treatment

Chemotherapy The mainstay of treatment in myeloma is chemotherapy. Because the tumor is slow growing, and because myeloma is very sensitive to chemotherapy in most cases, it is often possible to use short courses of chemotherapy drugs, often given by tablet. One of the most commonly used drugs is **melphalan**. The drug is usually given for a few days at a time, often with **steroids** as well. Courses are given typically every four weeks, and the patient's situation is monitored closely. Usually the M band is measured regularly, and if the treatment is working, the amount of the M band will decrease. It is customary to stop treatment when the M band stops falling and levels off or disappears completely. At that time, some centers may recommend the use of the biological agent **interferon**. Usually treatment with melphalan is started again only when the M band starts rising or symptoms develop.

In general, the side effects of these drugs are very slight. When given by tablet, there is little or no nausea and little hair loss. At a later stage in the disease, it may be necessary to use larger doses of stronger chemotherapy drugs, including intravenous injections with drugs such as **Adriamycin** and others. If that happens, nausea and vomiting are more common, as is hair loss.

Radiotherapy Myeloma cells are also sensitive to radiotherapy, which may be recommended if you have one area or a bone that is particularly painful or has sustained a fracture.

Surgery Orthopedic surgery may be needed if a fracture occurs that is unlikely to heal on its own.

High-Dose Chemotherapy In certain unusual circumstances, high-dose chemotherapy may be recommended. This may be given with a bone marrow transplant or stem-cell rescue (see page 233). The circumstances in which this would be considered are being evaluated, and you will need to discuss the exact details, including the objectives and potential side effects, with your doctor.

Other Therapies Other types of therapy, including biological response modifiers, have been used in myeloma and may be successful in certain situations where standard therapies do not work or have stopped working. There are several different types of treatment and methods of giving it, so you will need to discuss the details of your own case with your doctor.

Related Conditions

Occasionally a collection of myeloma cells may occur outside the bone marrow and form a tumor in another part of the body. These tumors are called **plasmacytomas** and, because they occur outside the marrow, are usually referred to as **extramedullary** (outside the marrow) **plasmacytomas**. They most often occur around the nasal passages and upper airways. They may be treated with radiotherapy, chemotherapy, or both. They may be cured in some cases but have a tendency to recur in others.

Another related condition is a type of lymphoma that arises from cells that are very much like plasma cells. It produces a different type of M band and is called **Waldenström's macroglobulinemia**. In its behavior and treatment, it most closely resembles a relatively slow-growing (low-grade) lymphoma.

OVARY

Number of new cases diagnosed per year in the United States: 26,700

SUMMARY OF THE KEY FACTS IN THIS SECTION

- Cancer of the ovary starts in one or both ovaries and may spread to other parts of the abdominal cavity.
- Because the ovaries are situated deep within the pelvis, the early stages may cause no symptoms, so that ovarian cancer is frequently diagnosed when it is in the later stages.
- The most important factors affecting the outcome are the stage of the tumor, its grade, and whether or not it can be completely removed by surgery.
- The earlier stages may often be cured by surgery, usually with chemotherapy afterward.
- In more advanced stages, chemotherapy is effective in prolonging control of the disease and sometimes curing it.

Introductory Note: The Main Types of Ovarian Cancer

There are three main types of cancer of the ovary, two of which are not very common. The most common type is **epithelial cancer of the ovary** (so named because it seems to begin in the covering or epithelium of the ovary). When you hear the phrase "cancer of the ovary" with no further details about the type, it is this type that is meant. The other two types are the **germ-cell cancers** of the ovary and the **stromal tumors** (often also called **sex-cord stromal tumors**) of the ovary. These two types of ovarian cancer are relatively rare, but they are important because they behave very differently from the usual epithelial type. I shall therefore deal with them as separate subsections. The first subsection deals with epithelial cancers of the ovary only.

EPITHELIAL CANCER OF THE OVARY: THE MOST COMMON TYPE

The Most Important Features of the Tumor

Cancer of the ovary is a relatively common type of cancer. Because the ovaries are so well protected inside the pelvis, it is quite easy for the tumor to grow and spread before it is detected. The tumor is rather unusual in that it spreads around the abdomen in most cases and doesn't invade outside the abdomen until quite late in its development. Cancer of the ovary is relatively sensitive to treatment after surgery (that is, it often will respond to both radiotherapy and chemotherapy). Some patients will be cured by surgery alone, and more will be cured with treatment after surgery. Unfortunately, however, recurrence is still quite common in this condition.

What You Really Need to Know about the Ovaries

The ovaries are two organs situated deep within the pelvis on either side of the uterus. Each ovary is approximately the size of a walnut (about two inches [5.8 cm] long). The ovaries have two major functions. First, they act as the "storage" system for the ova (or eggs) that are released one at a time each month, providing the first step in fertility and reproduction. Second, they secrete sex hormones (particularly estrogens) and are part of the system that regulates the monthly menstrual cycle.

The physically sheltered position of the ovaries is advantageous in some respects because it means that the whole reproductive system, including the developing fetus during pregnancy, is shielded from accidents and trauma by the bones of the pelvis. If

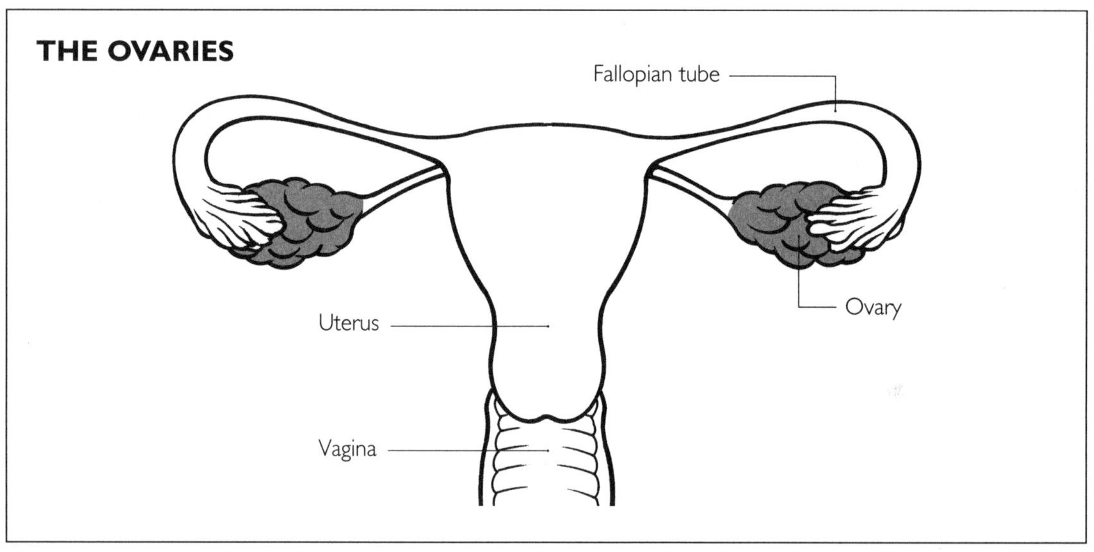

a tumor starts growing in an ovary, however, the ovary may enlarge to several times its original size before any symptoms become apparent, and even then the symptoms are usually mild and rather vague. In other words, early changes in the ovary usually do not cause any problems and may actually be quite difficult to detect even during a pelvic examination by a physician. This aspect of the ovaries explains why, unfortunately, ovarian cancer is often detected after it has spread outside the ovaries.

Age and Incidence

Ovarian cancer can occur at almost any age but generally occurs at over the age of fifty or so. It becomes slightly less common after the mid-seventies.

Causes

As with many of the most common cancers, the exact causes of ovarian cancer are not known, although in a small proportion of cases we know that heredity has something to do with it (see below). Like several other common cancers, it seems to be associated with the Western lifestyle and is relatively rare in developing countries. We also know some things that seem to *decrease* the chance of getting it. Several studies have shown that women who have taken oral contraceptives for some years have a lower chance of getting ovarian cancer than those who do not, as do women who have children in the early twenties or before (compared to women who have not had children or who had children at a later age) and also women in whom the menopause occurs earlier than average. These observations may one day prove to be very important in our understanding of the causes of ovarian cancer. At the moment we do not fully understand what they mean. We can speculate that in some way oral contraceptives, childbirth, and early menopause "rest" the ovary, and that in some way they decrease the amount of time that ovaries spend ovulating. We can further speculate that as a result of having to do less work (in terms of releasing ova), the ovaries are less likely to go wrong and less likely to allow a cancer to develop. At present, however, all we know is that the hormonal environment created by oral contraceptives, pregnancies, and early menopause makes it more difficult for ovarian cancer to start.

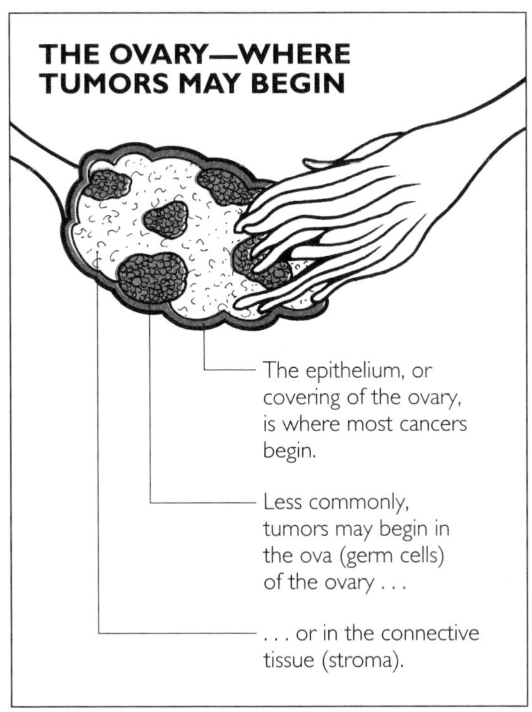

With regard to factors that *increase* the chance of developing cancer of the ovary, we now know that in a small proportion of cases (probably less than one in ten) there is some inherited factor at work. Recent research has shown that in some families there is a genetic predisposition and that any woman who has two or more first-degree relatives (mother, sister, or daughter) who have had ovarian cancer has a significantly higher chance of getting it than the average woman. It also seems that some families have a predisposition not only to ovarian cancer but also to breast cancer at an early age. We think that families in which there are three women with either ovarian or breast cancer may have genetic predisposition. The recently discovered genes BRCA1 and BRCA2 seem to be important in this context, and more information on how they are involved will undoubtedly emerge in the next year or so (see "Recently Identified Genes Called BRCA1 and BRCA2" in the section on breast cancer).

How the Cancer Tends to Spread

For reasons that we do not fully understand, ovarian cancer very often spreads around the inside of the abdomen (the abdominal or peritoneal cavity) quite early in its progress and spreads outside the abdomen relatively late. The cancer often makes small secondary tumors (sometimes called **seedlings**) around the lining of the pelvis (on the outside of the uterus and fallopian tubes) and around the peritoneum (the covering of the intestines) and may create fluid in the abdomen (**ascites**). The cancer may also spread to the lymph nodes in the abdomen and to the outside covering of the liver and to the diaphragm. It may sometimes spread to the inside of the liver as well. Later, spread outside the abdomen can also occur, sometimes creating fluid in the chest cavity (a **pleural effusion**). The tumor can also spread to lymph nodes in the neck and, very occasionally, to other areas of the body as well. More than two-thirds of patients will have cancer that has spread to the abdomen or beyond at the time of diagnosis, while about one-third will have cancer limited to the ovaries or to the pelvic area.

Symptoms or Problems That You May Notice

There may be no symptoms at all in the early stages. If there are symptoms, they are usually vague and often quite mild to begin with. There may be a slight **dragging sensation** in the pelvis or a **mild discomfort**. There may also be a feeling of **bloating** or **distension** in the abdomen, accompanied by **flatulence**. In some cases there may be a **vaginal discharge**.

In some cases the cancer in the ovary may irritate the nearby normal ovarian tissue, which may respond by manufacturing abnormal amounts of sex hormone. That in turn may cause **irregularities in the menstrual cycle**, in particular, unusually heavy periods or bleeding between periods.

Other problems that can occur may include a buildup of fluid (ascites) in the abdomen, which may lead to a considerable and relatively **rapid enlargement of the abdomen** (a change in girth of several or many inches over a small number of weeks, so that clothes which used to fit a month ago are now several sizes too small). Usually this accumulation of fluid is relatively painless, causing a feeling of bloating or discomfort rather than severe or acute pain, which again means it is often noticed later rather than earlier.

Because of its high propensity to spread around the abdomen, the cancer may interfere with the normal function of the bowel. The seedlings over the inside of the abdomen can be "sticky," and parts of the bowel may become attached to them. That may cause the bowel to become suddenly kinked and then blocked because of the kink in it (the medical word is **obstructed**). The first sign of trouble, then, can be **sudden**, **severe**, **colicky pain** (intermittent coming-and-going pain) in the abdomen, sometimes accompanied by **nausea** and **vomiting**. Anyone who experiences such a sudden onset of severe abdominal pain together with vomiting should seek medical attention urgently.

In addition, if the tumor causes a pleural effusion, the fluid around the lung can cause **shortness of breath** or a **persistent cough** without sputum.

Apart from ascites, a pleural effusion, or an emergency caused by obstruction of the bowel, many of the symptoms of ovarian cancer—such as mild discomfort, dragging sensations in the pelvis, menstrual irregularities, and feelings of bloating and flatulence—are widely found among women who do not have the cancer. If you have such symptoms, do not assume that they indicate cancer. Nevertheless, persistent symptoms should definitely be reported to your doctor, and an annual pelvic examination by a specialist (such as a gynecologist) is strongly recommended.

Diagnosis and Tests

As with all medical problems, your doctor will go over your story in detail and then examine you. In almost all circumstances, a pelvic examination will be done. In many cases, however, early problems in the ovary cannot be detected by a pelvic examination alone, so that further tests are almost always required. The tests are usually of two types: scans or X rays and blood tests.

Three types of scans or X rays may be recommended. Usually the ultrasound scan is the easiest. Ultrasound scans are often very effective in detecting problems deep in the pelvis (sometimes more effective than a CT scan). However, you might need a CT scan as well, not only to get another view of the pelvis but also to look at other structures such as lymph nodes at the back of the abdomen. In some centers the MRI scan is also used, though at present we do not know whether this is an improvement on the CT scan for ovarian cancer and, if it is, under what circumstances.

Blood tests can also be very important, in particular, a blood test called the **CA-125**. The CA-125 test measures a substance, or marker, that is released from ovarian cancer cells (and by other cells as well, in certain circumstances). If the CA-125 test is abnormally high, there is a higher chance that the diagnosis is cancer (though not invariably ovarian). The test is not 100 percent perfect, so it can be abnormal if there are other types of problems in the abdomen, including some noncancerous benign conditions. By and large, however, the CA-125 test is a very important aid in the diagnosis of ovarian cancer and in assessing response during treatment. If the scans are suggestive of cancer, a high CA-125 result makes the possibility more likely.

Even if these tests make the diagnosis clear, further assessment is often necessary. Further information may be obtained either by looking inside the abdomen with a small instrument called a **laparoscope** (the procedure is called a **laparoscopy**) or by means of a larger operation (in which the abdomen is opened) called a **laparotomy**. A laparoscopy is usually done under a general anesthetic through a very small incision near the umbilicus, or navel. The specialist uses a sort of thin telescope to look around the abdomen and pelvis and take small biopsy

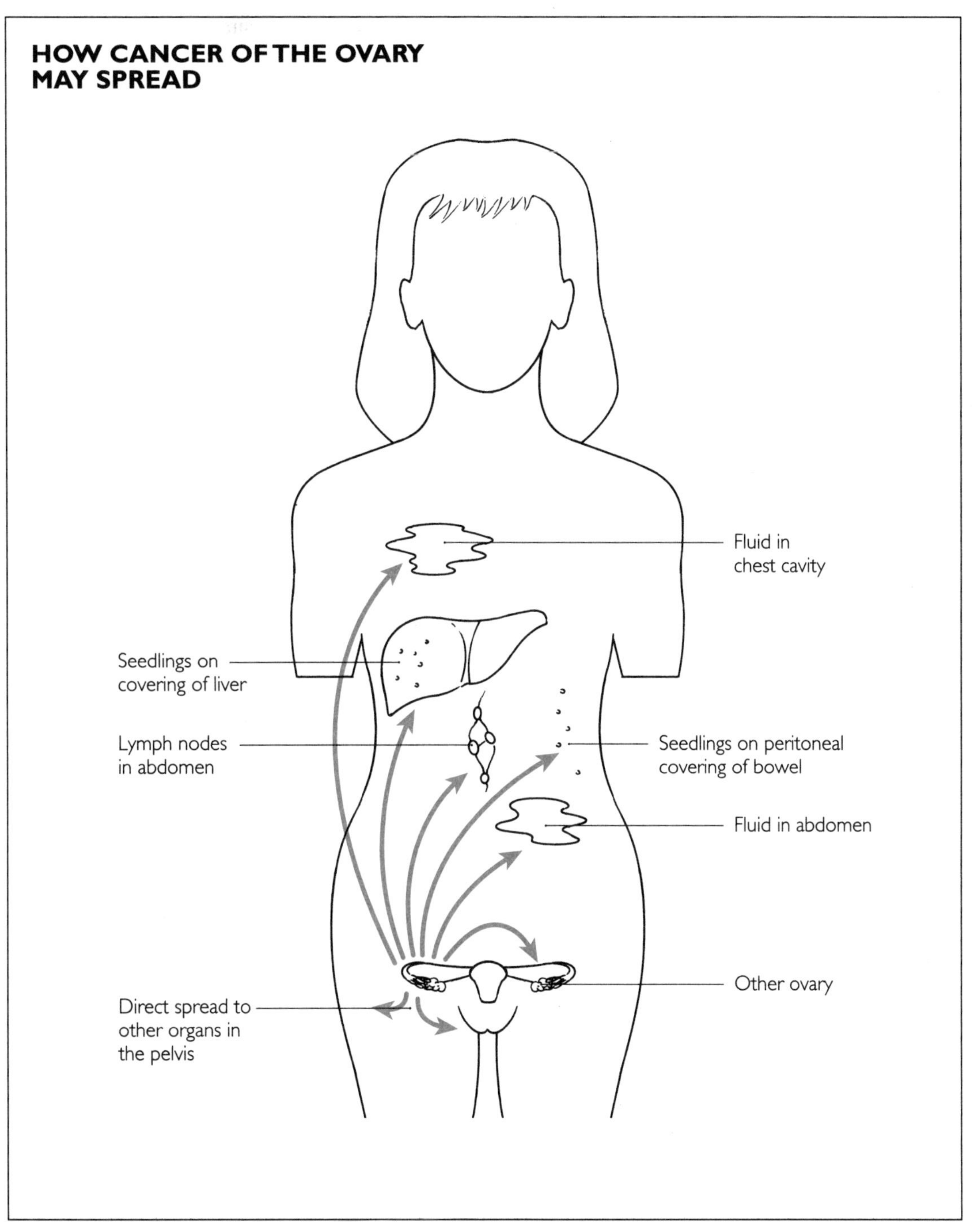
HOW CANCER OF THE OVARY
MAY SPREAD
Fluid in
chest cavity
Seedlings on
covering of liver
Lymph nodes
in abdomen
Seedlings on peritoneal
covering of bowel
Fluid in abdomen
Other ovary
Direct spread to
other organs in
the pelvis

specimens (of tumors, lymph nodes, or peritoneum, for example). A laparoscopy is used exclusively for diagnosis and assessment, not for removing larger areas of tumor.

A laparotomy, on the other hand, is a more extensive operation, with a twofold objective: first, to find out exactly where the cancer has spread to and which parts of the abdomen are involved; and second, to remove as much as possible of the cancer, leaving behind the smallest possible areas of tumor. Because the laparotomy has this dual role in cancer of the ovary—diagnosis and treatment—it is therefore required in most cases of cancer of the ovary. I discuss it in detail in the treatment section below.

Factors That Influence the Treatment and Prognosis

The Stage of the Cancer In cancer of the ovary, a great deal depends on how far the cancer has spread around the abdomen, what it looks like under the microscope, and to what extent surgical removal is possible. If the cancer is limited to the ovaries or pelvis only, it is called early stage (stage one or stage two). If it has spread from the pelvis into the abdomen or beyond, it is called advanced stage (stage three or stage four). In cancer of the ovary, the **stage** of the tumor does make a significant difference to the outlook, so that patients with early-stage cancer have a higher chance of being cured than patients with the advanced stages. However, two other factors are also important: how aggressive the cancer appears to be when seen under the microscope (the **grade** of the tumor); and the **degree to which it was possible for your surgeon to remove all or most of the cancer** at the time of surgery.

The Grade of the Cancer Like most types of cancer, cancer of the ovary can be divided into categories by its appearance under the microscope. Features of the cancer that can be assessed under the microscope include whether the tumor is making mucus or not, whether it has a similar appearance to tissue of the uterus, whether it seems to be making little knobs called papillae, and so on. All these different features allow the pathologist to classify the cancer as either low grade (least aggressive), intermediate grade, or high grade (more aggressive).

One type of ovarian tumor is not quite a true cancer but not definitely benign (noncancerous) either. These tumors, which are called **borderline tumors**, or sometimes tumors of **low malignant potential**, may account for perhaps one in ten of ovarian cancers. Borderline tumors are relatively easy to identify from their appearance under the microscope, but it is not always clear what treatment to recommend. Some borderline tumors can be quite advanced in stage (such as stage three, for example) and yet do not seem to cause trouble even after many years. Others do cause trouble. If your ovarian tumor is one of these borderline tumors, even at a fairly advanced stage, it may not be as serious as the other types of epithelial cancer. The best treatment plan will be discussed with you by your doctor.

The Extent to Which the Tumor Could Be Removed or "Debulked" The third factor that influences the outlook (and the treatment) is the amount of tumor that could be removed at the time of your surgery. Ideally all of the visible areas of cancer are removed and nothing is left behind that can be seen by the surgeon. That is called **complete** or **optimal debulking**. Whether this can be achieved may have nothing whatever to do with the skill of your surgeon! A high-grade, advanced-stage tumor may cause many areas of bowel and other tissues to stick to it, so that it cannot be removed without causing major damage. The amount of tumor removed—the debulkability, or resectability as it is sometimes called—may have much more to do with the nature of the cancer than with the skill of your surgeon.

In summary, therefore, the stage, grade, and debulkability of the cancer are major predictors of its future behavior and of your chance of either a cure or a recurrence. To a large extent, the treatment after the initial surgery will depend on whether the cancer has a low or high chance of recurring.

The Main Objectives of Treatment

The main objective of therapy in cancer of the ovary is to cure the cancer if that is possible. If, after surgery, the chance of recurrence is thought to be very low, no further treatment may be needed. (This applies to early-stage, low-grade cancers that are completely removed. Such cases are generally in the minority.) Most women, however, will require some treatment after surgery. If the chance of recurrence is thought to be moderate, further treatment in the form of radiotherapy to the abdomen and pelvis or chemotherapy may be recommended. If the chance of recurrence is thought to be moderately high or high, or if much of the cancer was left behind after surgery, chemotherapy will be recommended.

Types of Treatment

Surgery In most circumstances a laparotomy will be recommended, either after the diagnosis has been made by a laparoscopy or instead of it. The purpose of the laparotomy is twofold: to establish how much disease there is in the abdomen and where it is and, second, to remove as much of it as possible. During this operation, if it is technically possible, your surgeon will remove both ovaries, the uterus, and the omentum (a fatty apron that wraps around the bowel). In addition, the surgeon will try to remove as much of the cancer as possible and will also take biopsies from many different areas in the abdomen.

This is quite extensive surgery, which is sometimes technically difficult because of the way the cancer sticks to bowel and other structures. A range of surgical procedures may be required during the laparotomy; these will vary from person to person. Your surgeon will discuss the details with you. What can be achieved by surgery will depend on the characteristics of the cancer. Lower-grade cancers are generally less sticky and adherent and so can be removed more easily and more completely. Higher-grade tumors, which may be attached to bowel and other structures, can be difficult to remove completely.

Chemotherapy Cancer of the ovary often responds to chemotherapy. Several drugs may be used, in various combinations. Most commonly a drug called **cyclophosphamide** and one member of the family of substances called platinum drugs are used either in combination with other drugs or (in some treatment plans) alone. In the platinum family of drugs, two are used quite commonly, **cis-platinum** (or cisplatin) and **carboplatinum**. Cis-platinum is, unfortunately, very nauseating, and several antinauseants need to be given with it. Because it can also cause damage to the kidneys, it is given together with several quarts of intravenous fluids, and therefore requires either a short stay in the hospital or three or four hours in the clinic. In some cases it may damage your hearing, and in a few cases it may also cause some damage to the nerves, producing tingling or numbness in the fingers or toes. Carboplatinum, the other platinum drug, is less nauseating and can be given on an outpatient basis.

Another drug that can be of value is the newer drug **Taxol**, which does have some effect in several cases where the cancer has been resistant to platinum, and nowadays is often used in first-line therapy as well. The publicity surrounding Taxol, however, has led many people to expect that it would do much more good than it in fact does. At present, the best way of using Taxol, cis-platinum, and carboplatinum—for example, whether Taxol should be used in first-line treatment—has not been worked out. Your doctor will explain what the standard practice is at his or her center.

In addition to these drugs, other newer agents may be recommended if the tumor recurs or if it is resistant to platinum drugs or Taxol. The details, potential benefits, and side effects will be discussed with you by your doctor.

Intraperitoneal Therapy In some patients, fluid in the abdomen (ascites) can be a problem, and if chemotherapy by intravenous injection does not prove effective, different chemotherapy drugs may occasionally be given by direct injection into the abdomen. Treatment by this method may sometimes be recommended in early-stage disease instead of radiotherapy or chemotherapy and sometimes in the treatment of recurring small nodules of tumor. Various substances can be given in this way: chemotherapy drugs, or substances that are radioactive in themselves, or other agents such as biological agents. If these are recommended in your case, your doctor will discuss the details with you.

Treatment and Sexual Function

Removal of the ovaries will, of course, produce infertility and menopause (if you had not already had your menopause). To decrease the chance of osteoporosis (bone thinning) and heart disease in the future, hormone replacement therapy is usually begun after the surgery. Often, too, sexual function is affected by the treatment. You will need to discuss this aspect with your medical and nursing team and with your partner (see also "Sexuality" in Chapter 10).

"Second-Look Surgery"

In some circumstances, particularly when newer drugs or drug combinations have been used, a second, less extensive operation may be recommended to see how much (if any) of the cancer is left. This operation, called the **second-look**, may be done with a laparotomy or by a laparoscopy. It is no longer used as part of the *standard* therapy in all centers, but it may be important if new forms of therapy have been used or are planned. If so, of course, your doctor will discuss it with you in detail.

Screening and Early Diagnosis

At present, screening for cancer of the ovary is difficult. There are no tests that can be done on the whole population that will reliably detect ovarian cancer or rule it out in people who do not have it. The best recommendation at the moment is that you should have an annual checkup, including a pelvic examination, and that you should report any prolonged abdominal or pelvic symptoms to your doctor. If you have two or more first-degree relatives with ovarian cancer, it is quite likely that you will need more extensive screening (perhaps an annual ultrasound and CA-125). You should discuss this with a specialist in gynecological cancer.

OTHER TUMORS OF THE OVARY

Epithelial cancers of the ovary begin in the covering or epithelium of the ovary. Other cancers can begin in other components of the ovary. Cancers that begin in the tissues that hold the ovary together are called **sarcomas**. Those that begin in elements of the ovary associated with producing ova are called **germ-cell tumors**.

Germ-Cell Tumors of the Ovary

The Most Important Features of the Tumor

Germ-cell cancers of the ovary are relatively rare and behave in quite a different way from the more common epithelial cancers of the ovary. Germ-cell tumors probably arise from elements within the ovary that have, as it were, gone wrong at an earlier stage in development. They occur in a much younger age group, and they are curable in the great majority of cases.

Age and Incidence Germ-cell cancers of the ovary can occur at any age but are more likely in the late teens and early twenties. In general, they account for up to about 3 to 5 percent of all ovarian cancers.

Diagnosis and Tests These tumors usually produce one or two marker substances that can be detected in the blood and that not only assist in diagnosis but also allow monitoring of the tumor during treatment. These substances are the equivalent of the CA-125 test in epithelial cancers but are more sensitive and a more accurate guide to what is happening during treatment. They are beta human chorionic gonadotrophin (βHCG) and the alpha-fetoprotein (AFP).

Types of Treatment These tumors are almost always sensitive to drug therapy and are curable in most cases. The first line of treatment is usually surgery, which is often less extensive than for epithelial ovarian cancer. If, for example, the germ-cell tumor involves only one ovary, the other ovary and the uterus may be left intact and the person can remain fertile. After surgery, drug therapy is usually recommended and usually includes a member of the **platinum family** combined with other drugs, including **etoposide** and **bleomycin**. Usually, too, patients will be followed up after treatment with regular examinations and regular tests checking the markers (the βHCG and the AFP). If you have had a germ-cell tumor and are free of recurrence after five years, you are almost certainly cured, and the chance that the tumor will recur is very low indeed.

Sex-Cord Stromal Tumors

The Most Important Features of the Tumor

Stromal tumors are cancers that arise not from the covering of the ovary but from other cells in it, in tissues that act as padding or support for the germ cells. Whereas epithelial cancers tend to spread inside the abdomen, these sarcomas are very variable. Some have a very low tendency to spread, and some have a moderate tendency to spread but spread very slowly and at a late stage. If the sarcoma is less aggressive (that is, a lower grade of tumor) and if it can be removed completely, there is a high chance that it may be cured by surgery (this applies to Leydig-cell tumors and Sertoli-cell tumors, for example). In other cases, it is much more difficult to predict what will happen, and with some types (such as the fibrosarcoma, for example) spread to distant parts of the body such as the lungs is more likely.

The Main Types There are many different types of sex-cord stromal tumors, which are named according to the cells or tissues from which they appear to have arisen. In fact, deciding exactly what type of tumor is present can be very difficult in this group, and several opinions are quite often needed before a pathologist can say exactly what type it is. A definitive diagnosis may take time, therefore.

Age and Incidence These tumors are very rare before the age at which menstrual periods begin and are most likely to occur in the forties, fifties, and sixties. In total, they account for about 5 percent of all ovarian tumors.

Symptoms These tumors may cause the pelvic or abdominal symptoms associated with epithelial cancer of the ovary (see above) and often cause menstrual irregularities as well, as many of them have a tendency to interfere with the normal hormones of the ovary.

Types of Treatment The treatment of sex-cord stromal tumors depends on the appearance under the microscope and on the extent to which the tumor has been removed. Some will be cured by surgery alone (the Leydig-cell tumors and the Sertoli-cell tumors, for example). In other cases (in granulosa-cell tumors, for example) the prognosis depends on the patient's age (in the younger age group they behave much less aggressively than in adults). In some cases, therefore, chemotherapy may be recommended after surgery, whereas in others it may not be considered necessary or helpful. If chemotherapy is recommended, it may include a member of the platinum family for some types of tumor.

PANCREAS

Number of new cases diagnosed per year in the United States: 26,300

SUMMARY OF THE KEY FACTS IN THIS SECTION

- The pancreas is situated in the upper abdomen. It is possible for tumors to develop in it without causing any noticeable symptoms in the early stages.
- Thus pancreatic cancer is often diagnosed after it has been growing for some time.
- In some cases it is possible to remove the entire tumor surgically. In most cases, however, the objectives of treatment are to reduce symptoms and maintain quality of life.

The Most Important Features of the Tumor

Cancer of the pancreas is a particularly difficult tumor both to detect and to treat. The pancreas is situated behind the stomach and is quite deep inside the upper part of the abdomen, so that a tumor inside the pancreas can grow quite large and still remain undetected. Thus quite often it is not possible to remove a cancer of the pancreas completely. Also, cancer of the pancreas is often resistant to treatment; it does not respond very well to chemotherapy, for example. Fortunately, pain control is now much more effective than it used to be, and a fair degree of comfort can be achieved in many cases by using radiotherapy and analgesics.

What You Really Need to Know about the Pancreas

The pancreas is a slipper-shaped organ that is part of the digestive tract. It makes enzymes that are an important part of the body's ability to digest food. The enzymes made in the pancreas (called, logically enough, pancreatic enzymes) get into the digestive tract by a tube or duct that empties into the duodenum (the part of the digestive tract leading from the stomach into the rest of the small intestine). The pancreas is shaped with a fat end called the head, which, as it were, fits closely into the curve of the duodenum. Because the pancreas is so close to the duodenum, anything that expands the head of the pancreas (such as a cancer) can cause pressure or obstruction to other structures in the same area as the duodenum, particularly the bile duct. The pancreas has another, crucial function. One type of cell inside the pancreas produces insulin, the most important hormone in the control of the body's sugar. Without insulin you develop diabetes. Except in rare circumstances, this particular function of the pancreas is not affected by cancer of the pancreas. If the entire pancreas has been removed in the surgical treatment of the cancer, or if it has been affected by some other condition or therapy, daily insulin injections will be needed as replacement.

Age and Incidence

The incidence of cancer of the pancreas increases with age, and most cases occur after the age of fifty. It is slightly more common men than women.

Causes

The exact causes of cancer of the pancrease are unknown, but in many cases the cancer is associated with cigarette smoking. Not every person who has cancer of the pancreas is a smoker, however, so there must be other factors involved. No obvious reason has been found why the pancreas in particular should be sensitive to the chemicals in cigarette smoke and triggered into developing a cancer. Hence the relationship between cigarettes and cancer of the pancreas is an established fact that currently is not understood.

How the Cancer Tends to Spread

A tumor growing in the pancreas may spread to adjacent structures, including the bile duct and the

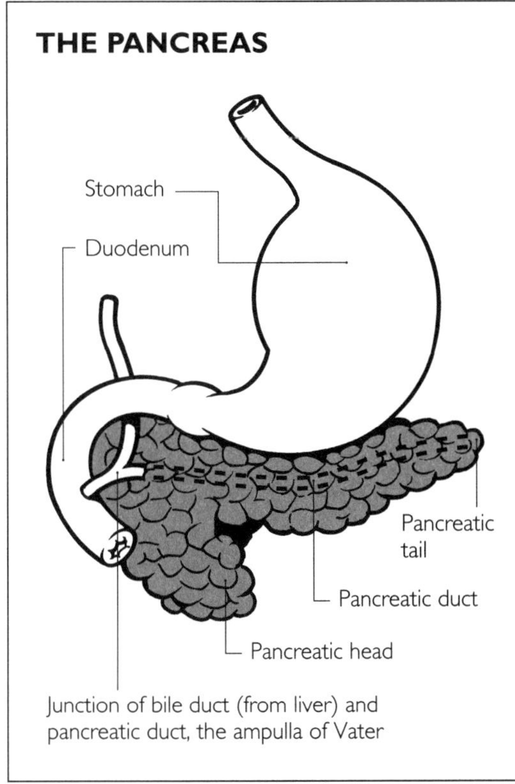

duodenum, to lymph nodes in the area (for example, near the stomach or the small intestine), and across the peritoneal cavity to the colon, small intestine, spleen, or other structures. It may also spread to distant areas of the body, including the liver or the lungs.

Symptoms or Problems That You May Notice

There are often no symptoms at all in the early stages of the disease. The pancreas is situated quite deep inside the abdomen and doesn't have nerves of its own that carry pain messages. If the cancer does cause discomfort or pain, the pain is often an **indigestion-like discomfort** in the upper abdomen, and there is little that reliably distinguishes it from ordinary indigestion or dyspepsia. Occasionally, if the cancer is situated toward the back of the pancreas, you may experience **pain in the back** as well as (or instead of) indigestion.

Apart from pain, the most common symptoms are **loss of weight**, **loss of appetite**, and in some situations **blockage of the bile duct**, causing jaundice. The bile duct is the tube that conducts the yellow-colored digestive juice called **bile** (manufactured in the liver and an important component in digesting food) into the duodenum very close to the pancreatic duct and the head of the pancreas. Problems in the head of the pancreas can block the bile duct, causing the bile to back up first into the liver and then into the rest of the body. When the bile (which has a yellow color) gets into your circulation, your skin and your eyes take on a yellow tinge (the condition known as **jaundice**) and your urine becomes very dark. The position of the pancreas means that it is relatively easy for a cancer in the head of the pancreas to cause jaundice. Sometimes the tumor can reduce the flow of bile sufficiently to interfere with digestion. If that happens, the lack of bile causes **problems with the digestion of fat**, so that the amount of undigested fat in the stool increases. This may make the stools pale in color and bulky. Quite often the stools also smell bad and are difficult to flush away.

Diagnosis and Tests

In general, the most useful tests in detecting cancer of the pancreas are the **CT scan** and ultrasound. Sometimes an **MRI scan** can add further information, and in certain situations your doctor may recommend a special test using an **endoscope**, a thin tube inserted through the mouth into the stomach and then into the duodenum. The opening of the pancreatic duct can be seen when the endoscope is in the duodenum and a dye can be injected (painlessly) into the pancreatic duct. X rays taken when the dye is in the pancreas can show certain kinds of problems. This test is called an **ERCP** (which stands for endoscopic retrograde cholangiopancreatography), and it may be helpful in making the diagnosis or in planning the treatment in some situations.

The Main Objectives of Treatment

In a few cases, cancer of the pancreas can be cured by a surgical operation. In the majority of cases, unfortunately, surgery is not possible because the tumor is often quite advanced before it is detected. Where curative treatment is not possible, the objective of therapy is to reduce symptoms to a minimum and keep the person's quality of life as high as possible for as long as possible. That means that any type of treatment (particularly chemotherapy) has to be discussed in detail with your doctor so that the potential benefits and risks of treatment are fully understood ahead of time.

Types of Treatment

Surgery If the cancer is surgically removable, which occurs in a minority of cases, one of the most common types of operation involves removing the head of the pancreas together with parts of the duodenum and the bile ducts and reconnecting the remainder. The procedure is a major undertaking requiring a highly experienced surgical team and takes several weeks for full recovery.

If the cancer is not completely removable, and particularly if the tumor is already interfering with a bile duct or is about to, the surgeon may create a bypass passage so that the bile can get into the digestive tract by going round the blockage caused by the pancreatic cancer (in some cases this can be done by an endoscope without an actual operation). With both types of surgery, the exact details of the surgery and the aftereffects are very important. Thus you will need to discuss the details thoroughly with your surgeon before proceeding.

Radiotherapy Radiotherapy can be quite useful in controlling pain. The exact site and schedule of the radiotherapy and details of any side effects or aftereffects will be discussed with your radiation oncologist.

Chemotherapy The role of chemotherapy in the treatment of cancer of the pancreas is still uncertain. Quite frequently, cancer of the pancreas is resistant to chemotherapy. That is, in most cases, chemotherapy is unfortunately unlikely to put the cancer into remission or prolong life, although drugs such as **gemcytabine** may improve the quality of life. You should discuss thoroughly the relative risks and benefits of any recommended chemotherapy with your doctor before deciding whether to try it.

PROSTATE

Number of new cases diagnosed per year in the United States: 317,100

SUMMARY OF THE KEY FACTS IN THIS SECTION

- Cancer of the prostate is very common and will affect more than 317,000 males in the United States this year.
- In some cases the cancer may be so small and slow growing that it does not even require surgery when first detected.
- If treatment is required, when treated at an early stage, it is curable by prostatectomy in the majority of cases.
- Even if it spreads to other parts of the body, it may be controlled by hormone treatment for long periods of time.

The Most Important Features of the Tumor

In four important ways, cancer of the prostate is usually quite different from most other types of cancer.

First, the prostate gland's location close to the rectum allows it to be easily examined and assessed by your doctor. Thus regular checkups that include a rectal examination, and perhaps a blood test (see below), offer a possible chance that prostate cancer will be detected at an early stage.

Second, prostate cancer is relatively easy to cure if it is detected and treated before it has spread. That is, if the cancer is small and remains inside the prostate, the prostate gland can be removed by an operation (prostatectomy), which in the great majority of cases results in a cure.

Third, quite often a cancer in the prostate gland is so small and so slow growing that it does not need to be removed at all when it is first diagnosed provided that you can be checked and examined every few months by your specialist. Again, this is unlike the approach to most other types of cancer when detected at an early stage.

Fourth, if the cancer has spread outside the gland, in many cases it can be controlled by hormone treatment or other types of therapy for a long period of time. In this way, too, it is unlike other cancers. Few other cancers that occur in men are so responsive to hormone therapy.

What You Really Need to Know about the Prostate Gland

The prostate gland is a small gland that produces a fluid component of semen. About the size of a walnut, it is situated in front of the **rectum** and underneath the **bladder** and surrounds the **urethra** (the tube that leads urine from the bladder to the penis). It may be helpful to think of the urethra as a tube

THE PROSTATE GLAND

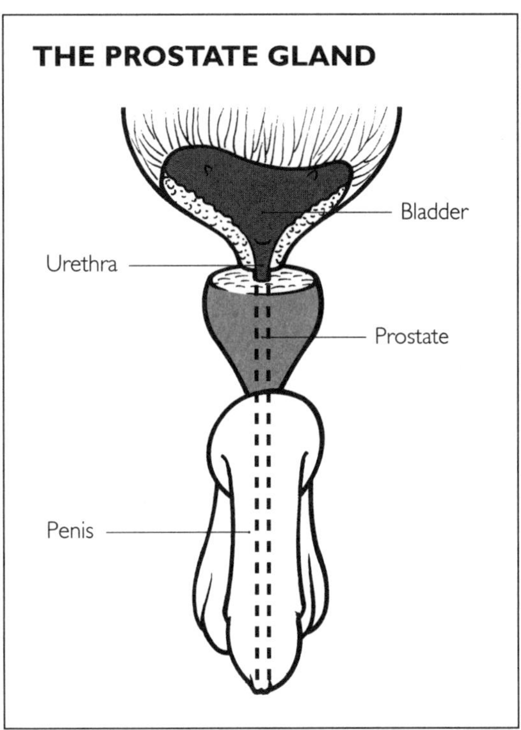

that runs right through the middle of the prostate. As the illustration on page 180 indicates, the back of the prostate is immediately adjacent to the wall of the rectum, making it easy for your doctor to assess the prostate during a rectal examination.

The main function of the prostate gland is to add certain components to the seminal fluid so that the sperm (which originate in the testes) are in the most helpful environment possible and have the highest chance of fertilizing an ovum after the seminal fluid reaches the woman's uterus following intercourse. As befits its role in reproduction, the prostate gland is sensitive to the body's sexual hormones. It matures in response to the male hormones manufactured by the body beginning at puberty. From middle adulthood onward, the prostate gland tends to enlarge (this condition is called **benign prostatic hypertrophy**, or **BPH**), and this enlargement can cause difficulties with passing urine. That is because the urine stream runs through the middle of the prostate, so that as the gland enlarges, it may partially block the urine stream. This ordinary benign enlargement **has nothing whatever to do with cancer of the prostate**. Having BPH (as almost every male does by the sixties and seventies) does not mean you will necessarily develop cancer of the prostate.

Age and Incidence

Cancer of the prostate is very common. In fact, with just over 317,000 cases a year, it is the most common cancer in men and the fourth most common cancer overall. The incidence of prostate cancer rises with increasing age and is quite rare below the age of fifty or so.

Causes

We do not know the causes of prostate cancer, apart from the fact that it is very rare in young adults and becomes increasingly common as males get older. We therefore assume that it is the result of some continuing process of "wear-and-tear" to which the cells of the prostate eventually succumb. At present there are few clues as to which aspects of our lifestyle contribute to the cumulative damage that eventually leads to the cancer. Possible candidates include our diet; in some way the high fat intake that is characteristic of the Western-style diet may play a part in contributing to prostate cancer. It is not certain that dietary fat is the true culprit, however, or, if it is, precisely how it plays a role. It is also known that prostate cancer is more common in black people and less common in Asian people, but again, the reasons are incompletely understood.

How the Cancer Tends to Spread

Prostate cancer, if it spreads at all, tends to spread first to the lymph nodes in the pelvis. In some cases it may spread to distant parts of the body, particularly the bones. Other places, such as the liver, can sometimes be the site of metastases too.

Symptoms or Problems That You May Notice

There are no symptoms that are absolutely specific to cancer of the prostate. In particular, there are no symptoms that distinguish cancer of the prostate from the ordinary enlargement of the prostate (BPH). As the prostate gets bigger with advancing age, BPH commonly causes difficulties in passing urine as, in some cases, cancer of the prostate also does. (Let me repeat that the two conditions have no connection whatever with each other.) Furthermore, cancer of the prostate may cause no symptoms or problems at all in the early stages (hence the value of an annual rectal examination).

Because of the similarity between the symptoms caused by a cancer of the prostate and the symptoms of ordinary enlargement, however, to be on the safe side, **men should have their prostate checked if they have any difficulties passing urine**. Table 4.7 lists the symptoms that may be associated with prostate problems.

If you have or get any of those problems, it is extremely important for you to be assessed by your

TABLE 4.7: SYMPTOMS ASSOCIATED WITH PROSTATE PROBLEMS (which are much more likely to be caused by enlargement than by cancer)

Hesitancy:	having to wait for the urine stream to start
Frequency:	regularly passing urine more often than, say, a year or two ago
Poor Stream:	the urine comes out more slowly and with less force
Urgency:	the desire to pass urine is regularly more urgent than it used to be
Dribbling:	when you have finished passing urine, the urine continues to dribble or drip out
Blood in the Urine:	the urine may contain red blood, or may be smoke colored
Pain in the Lower Abdomen or Pelvis:	without any particular reason for it

doctor, even though in many cases it will be found that there is nothing serious going on.

Diagnosis and Tests

Your doctor will first take the details of your symptoms and then examine you, ensuring that a rectal examination is included. If your doctor feels anything that might suggest cancer, he or she will probably send you for assessment by a specialist (a urologist or a physician with a special interest in urology). Almost certainly, if the specialist is concerned, he or she will do a **biopsy**. This procedure is done with a thin needle, often using ultrasound guidance, and is virtually painless (the wall of the rectum has very few nerve endings that respond to pain). The biopsy produces a small piece of the prostate that can be examined under the microscope to see if there is cancer in it or not.

Blood Tests Several blood tests may also be helpful, some of which may also be markers for the disease and show how the disease responds to treatment later on. Among these, the most commonly used is the **PSA** (prostate-specific antigen).

Other Tests In addition to the foregoing tests, if any cancer is seen in the biopsy specimen from your prostate, your doctor will almost certainly order a **bone scan** because if prostate cancer does spread, it's most likely to spread to bones first. Sometimes a **CT scan** of the abdomen and pelvis or an **ultrasound scan** or both may be of benefit in certain cases.

In a large number of cases, the tests will be normal and will indicate that the cancer has not spread. There is no need to be alarmed when such tests are recommended; they are a routine part of the assessment.

Factors That Influence the Treatment and Prognosis

Three factors affect the treatment and the outlook. First, the **stage** of the cancer is important, that is, whether the cancer has spread or is spreading to the lymph nodes or other parts of the body. The second factor is the **speed of growth**, that is, how fast (or how slowly) the cancer is growing. As I mentioned above, cancer of the prostate in many cases grows very slowly indeed. If it is growing

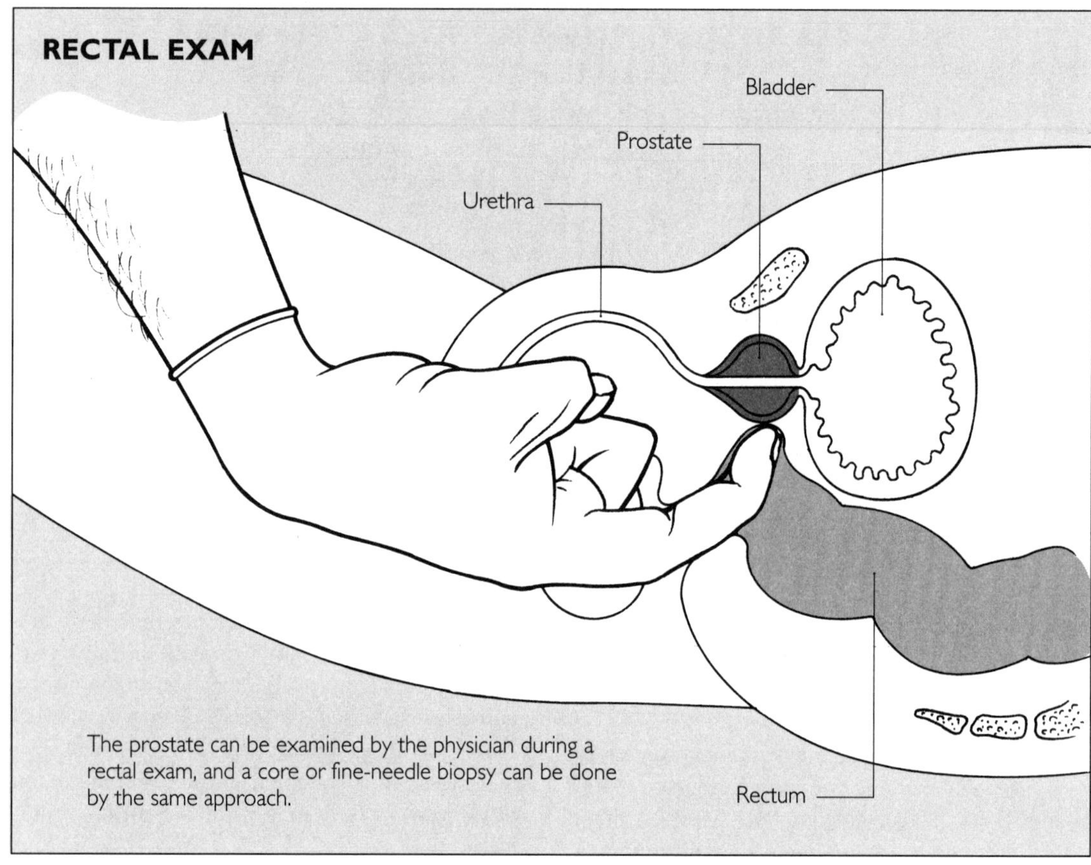

The prostate can be examined by the physician during a rectal exam, and a core or fine-needle biopsy can be done by the same approach.

slowly, the best form of treatment may be to do nothing for the time being. The **grade** of the tumor—its appearance under the microscope—may not give the complete answer to this question, so often if the grade of the tumor is relatively low (that is, it does not appear to be particularly fast growing or aggressive), your doctor may suggest that it be assessed at regular visits every few months to give a more reliable idea of its speed of growth.

The third factor, whether or not the cancer responds to hormone therapy, is important in cases where the cancer has spread or where it comes back after surgery. The medical term is **hormone sensitivity**. If the cancer is hormone sensitive, it may be controlled, often for a very long time, using hormone therapy, no matter where in the body it has spread to.

The Main Objectives of Treatment

Depending on the circumstances, there are three possible objectives of treatment. In many cases the objective is cure, and if the cancer can be removed completely, that should be done. In some cases, however, the cancer may not do you any harm for a very long time (even indefinitely), in which case the objective is accurate monitoring of the tumor. If the cancer has spread, the objective of therapy is to control it by treating both the cancer itself and any symptoms that you may experience.

Types of Treatment

Treatment can be divided into two categories: the treatment required when the cancer is limited to the prostate itself and has not spread elsewhere; and the treatment that may be used if it has spread.

Treatment When the Cancer Has Not Spread

The three possible approaches are as follows.

Surgery One of the most common types of treatment is to remove the prostate gland entirely with an operation called **prostatectomy**. A prostatectomy is usually done through an incision just above the pubic area. In some circumstances the operation may be done via an incision in the perineum (the area around the anus). The prostate gland is removed in its entirety. The lymph nodes in the area may be removed or biopsied at the same time.

This is not the most major surgery, but it is an important operation. You will need to prepare for it by discussing the details with your surgeon.

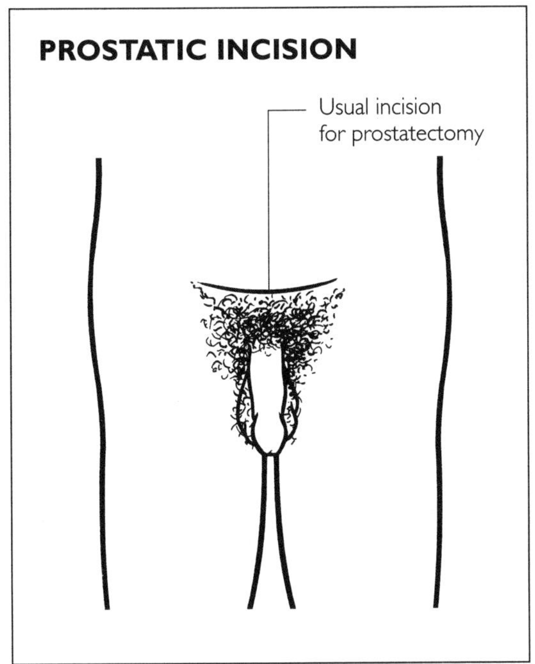

Some aspects of the surgery are relatively standard. First, when you recover from the anesthetic you will have a catheter, a tube in your bladder draining your urine. This is usually kept in for two or three weeks, and it may take some time after it has been removed for you to regain complete control of your bladder, because the muscles become accustomed to having a tube present. In other words, you will have to relearn control of your bladder.

Second, in almost every case, after the prostate gland has been removed, when you have sex and have an orgasm, there will not be any seminal fluid (because the ducts from the testes have been closed and the prostate has been removed).

Third, in some cases, the operation is followed by inability to have or maintain an erection, in other words, impotence. This happens in some cases (a minority), so it is important that you know about it beforehand. Of course, there are many sexual activities that do not require erections, but you need to know about this potential aftereffect so you can discuss it with your partner and perhaps have some counseling and advice about sexual matters. There are treatments (including medications that can be injected into the penis and prostheses that can be implanted) that may be helpful and that you may want to discuss if necessary.

Radiotherapy Radiotherapy is another option and may be used instead of surgery (see page 216). In many cases radiotherapy is easier than surgery because it does not require an incision and you will not need a catheter. The treatment is usually given every day for a few minutes, usually for about four weeks or so. Your radiation oncologist will discuss the details with you.

Side effects are usually relatively mild. During the treatment you may notice mild diarrhea, a slight looseness in bowel movements. Sometimes there may be some reddening of the skin above the pubic area. You will probably notice that you produce less seminal fluid when you ejaculate. It is also important for you to know that radiotherapy may cause impotence. This happens in up to half of cases, so, as with surgery (see page 181) you need to be prepared for the possibility and to discuss the options.

Observation Because in many cases prostate cancer grows very slowly, where an operation or radiotherapy might carry too high a risk, monitoring only may be recommended in the first instance. This option is particularly useful if there is some reason—say, problems with the heart or lungs, or some other medical condition—why a surgical operation would be more hazardous for you than for the average man. When used appropriately—that is, when the cancer is slow growing and easy to assess regularly—this alternative is extremely valuable.

Treatment When the Cancer Has Spread

In some cases the scans, ultrasounds, or X rays mentioned above may show that there is some cancer outside the prostate gland: in the lymph nodes, for example, or in some other location such as in the bones. Or the cancer may have recurred after primary treatment. In either of these situations, the treatment consists of one or more of three options: hormone therapy, radiotherapy, and chemotherapy.

Hormone Therapy In many cases, prostate cancer depends for its growth on male hormones, mostly testosterone. With an adequate supply of testosterone in the bloodstream, most cancers of the prostate can grow; when deprived of it, many of them will shrivel up and, in some cases, may die altogether. Treatment that switches off the supply of male hormones may therefore be recommended.

Three main methods can be used. First, testosterone production may be stopped by surgical castration—removal of the testes. Second, medications can be used that interfere with your body's testosterone production or with the body's ability to use testosterone. Drugs that reduce production include **leuprolide**, **goserelin**, and **cyproterone**; while drugs that block the use of testosterone include **flutamide** and **nilutamide**. Third, treatment may be given using female hormones or substances that behave like female hormones. These include the drug **stilbestrol**.

All these treatments have advantages and disadvantages, and you will need to discuss each of them with your specialist before deciding which of them is most suitable for you.

Radiotherapy Radiotherapy works in the region or the area where it is given and nowhere else. This can be useful if you have a tumor in a bone (for example, your back or hip) that causes pain. Radiotherapy given just to that area will almost always provide excellent relief of the pain.

Chemotherapy Chemotherapy for cancer of the prostate is often quite arduous and is therefore usually recommended only after the other treatments have been tried. Furthermore, chemotherapy does not usually produce a cure; when drugs such as members of the **Adriamycin** family and others are effective, the cancer shrinks but doesn't usually disappear. Hence the potential risks and benefits need to be weighed carefully before going ahead, and again, this is something you will need to discuss with your specialist.

Screening and Early Diagnosis

A screening test should be so good at detecting a disease that it is effective with everybody who is at risk (every man over the age of fifty, or even forty, in this case), even if the person has no symptoms (see page 255). The purpose of a screening test is to detect and treat the cancer at an early stage and, by doing that, to prevent some of the deaths. At present the best candidate for a screening test for prostate cancer is the blood test mentioned above, the PSA. (Several variants of the PSA are also currently being investigated.) We do not yet know, however, if carrying out treatment—such as a prostatectomy—on those cases detected by the PSA test (after confirmation by biopsy) will actually change the outcome. In many cases the prostate cancer grows very slowly and may not need immediate treatment. Research is active in this area, and we may have some of the answers in the next few years.

SARCOMAS OF THE SOFT TISSUES

Number of new cases diagnosed per year in the United States: 6,000

SUMMARY OF THE KEY FACTS IN THIS SECTION

- Sarcomas of the soft tissues are relatively uncommon. They often begin in fat or muscle, frequently in or near a limb.
- Some sarcomas may be very aggressive with a high tendency to spread elsewhere in the body, particularly to the lungs.
- Because of the potentially aggressive behavior of these tumors, surgery should be done to remove the primary cancer completely whenever feasible. With modern surgical techniques, depending on the size and position of the tumor, good function can be preserved and amputation may be unnecessary in many cases.
- Radiotherapy may be required after the operation.

The Most Important Features of the Tumor

Sarcomas of the soft tissues are uncommon cancers that begin in one or other of the tissues that are collectively known as connective tissue (see below). There are several different types of connective tissue—for example, fat, fibrous tissue, and so on—and sarcomas that develop in them are named accordingly: those that arise in fat tissue are called liposarcomas, in fibrous tissue, fibrosarcomas, and so on.

All sarcomas of the soft tissues have certain features in common. The high-grade ones (tumors that appear to be aggressive when seen under the microscope) have a high tendency to spread to distant parts of the body, particularly the lungs. It has been shown that the best chance of cure is to remove the primary tumor completely if it is feasible to do so. If the tumor's location makes such surgery impossible, radiotherapy may be recommended. For reasons that are not fully understood, chemotherapy used after surgery or if the disease is widespread is generally more effective with the sarcomas that occur in childhood than with those in adults, and cure is possible in many cases. The sarcomas that occur in adulthood may be and often are cured by surgery (with or without radiotherapy) if they are localized (that is, in one place) but are, unfortunately, incurable in most cases if they are widespread.

What You Really Need to Know about the Connective Tissues

The connective tissues make up the "packing and padding" of the human body. They include the fat and fibrous tissues that fill in the spaces between other tissues, form the wrappings of blood vessels, nerves, bowel, kidney, and so on, and are also the fundamental components of tendons. They are usually grouped with the other tissues that are derived from the same part of the embryo (the mesoderm). Tissues such as bone and muscle are specialized connective tissues. Thus the term "connective tissue" includes fat, the fibrous tissue around blood vessels and nerves, tendons, muscle, bone, and some other types as well. By convention, malignant tumors of the mesoderm are called sarcomas (whereas the other types of cancers are called carcinomas). Malignant tumors of soft tissues are therefore called sarcomas of soft tissue, and malignant tumors of bone are called osteosarcomas.

Any of the tissues that I've just mentioned—fat, fibrous tissue, muscle, and so on—may give rise to a sarcoma. Sarcomas of bone are dealt with separately under the heading "Bone."

Age and Incidence

A distinct group of sarcomas occurs in childhood, in the first few years of life. A second distinct group occurs from young adulthood onward, through the adult years into old age. There are important differences between these two groups. It is possible that in some way we do not yet understand the sarcomas that occur in childhood are fundamentally different from the ones that occur later.

Causes

In most cases there is no cause that we can identify associated with sarcomas. However, in a small number of cases, there may have been some identifiable cause at work. These (exceptional) factors are the following.

Radiation Exposure Sarcomas (of bone or soft tissue) may occur many years after excessive exposure to radiation: nuclear accidents, for example, or treatment with radiotherapy given many decades ago, before today's stringent safety requirements had been put in place. Because the time interval between the radiation exposure and the development of the sarcoma can be up to forty years or more, such cases are still occasionally seen today, although they are becoming very rare.

Certain Chemicals By and large, safety regulations now prevent exposure to the types of chemicals that have been associated with sarcomas. Certain chemicals in the plastics industry, however, and one or two other substances are known to have caused sarcomas in the past.

Certain Congenital Disorders In a congenital condition called **neurofibromatosis** (formerly known as Recklinghausen's disease), benign tumors of fibrous tissue (fibromas) develop in the sheaths around nerves. These are called neurofibromas. If there are large numbers of them, there is a chance that one may become malignant and turn into a neurofibrosarcoma. One or two other conditions are also associated with an increased risk of sarcomas.

How the Cancer Tends to Spread

Sarcomas can invade the neighboring area and may penetrate quite deeply into tissues surrounding the place where they originate. Thus when surgery is performed it is important for the entire tumor to be removed, including a surrounding margin of normal tissue. As well as invading the neighboring areas, sarcomas have the potential to spread to distant sites via the bloodstream and form cancerous tumors in the lungs. They may occasionally spread to lymph nodes near the area in which they begin.

Symptoms or Problems That You May Notice

The symptoms caused by sarcomas depend on the place in which they start. If the tumor starts on a limb, the most common problem is pain or ache in the area of the tumor, though some tumors may be painless and may be diagnosed as a painless lump. If the tumor begins inside the abdomen, for example, near the back, it may become quite large before it causes any symptoms, which may first be noticed as a mild ache or discomfort in the back.

Diagnosis and Tests

Biopsy The most important part of the diagnosis of a soft tissue sarcoma is a biopsy. Depending on where the tumor is, and whether the diagnosis of sarcoma is already suspected, the biopsy may be an excisional biopsy (in which the whole tumor is removed, together with a surrounding margin of normal tissue). In most cases the first step is removal of a part of the tumor (an incisional biopsy). Whenever possible, the initial biopsy should be performed by the surgeon who will later perform the definitive operation.

CT and MRI Scans Almost certainly a CT scan will be needed to determine the exact extent of the tumor and how far it is invading into neighboring tissues. Depending on the site, an MRI scan may be needed as well, particularly to assess the exact extent of the soft-tissue tumor.

Other Tests A chest X ray and CT scan of the chest is done to see if there is any evidence of secondary tumors in the lungs, and sometimes other staging tests—such as a bone scan—are recommended.

The Main Types of the Cancer

Each of the types of soft-tissue sarcoma is named according to the type of tissue that it appears to arise from. The main types of soft-tissue sarcoma are these (the tissue of origin is given after the name): liposarcoma (fat tissue); fibrosarcoma (fibrous tissue); neurofibrosarcoma (fibrous covering of nerve); malignant fibrous histiocytoma—abbreviated MFH—(primitive mesoderm cell of some type); rhabdomyosarcoma (red muscle); and leiomyosarcoma (white muscle).

Factors That Influence the Treatment and Prognosis

Age Sarcomas in childhood are generally more responsive to therapy and are cured in many cases. We are not sure precisely why this is, but it may be that the types of sarcomas in childhood are fundamentally different from those in adulthood. In particular, the sarcomas are often of the type called embryonal and often respond to chemotherapy (see below).

Whether There Has Been Spread In adult sarcomas it is very important to know whether there has been spread to distant parts of the body. Unfortunately, if the sarcoma has started in a place such as the abdomen where it can grow without causing symptoms, it may have spread before it is diagnosed. Such behavior is a common feature of sarcomas.

Grade The grade is important. If the sarcoma is low grade and has been completely removed, the chance of recurrence and of distant spread is low, and these tumors may often be cured by surgery. Unfortunately, many sarcomas are high grade, with a somewhat higher chance of spread.

Feasibility of Complete Removal The extent of the surgery that can be done is crucial in most cases. If the tumor can be completely removed, the chance of cure is much higher than if it can be only partly removed. Usually this depends on the position of the tumor and how far it has invaded into the neighboring tissues. If a tumor is small and is situated within a large muscle, it may be relatively easy to remove, whereas if it is situated in the abdomen and is attached to neighboring structures, complete removal may not be feasible. Such factors will need to be thoroughly discussed with your surgeon.

Type of Tumor In general, the type of the sarcoma has less bearing on the outlook than the age of the patient, the grade of the tumor, and the other factors listed above. That is, whether a tumor is high grade or low grade is more important than whether it is a leiomyosarcoma or a neurofibrosarcoma.

The Main Objectives of Treatment

The primary objective is to maximize the chances of cure. Depending on the age of the patient and the position and grade of the tumor, surgery with or without radiotherapy may be done, and chemotherapy may also be required. If cure is unlikely, treatment is directed at reducing or preventing symptoms.

Types of Treatment

Differences in Treating Children and Adults

As I mentioned above, there is generally a higher chance of curing the sarcomas in childhood. Chemotherapy may be used after surgery (with or without radiotherapy), particularly for tumors starting in the arms and legs. In general, the use of chemotherapy in the treatment of adult sarcomas is less established, and many cancer centers do not recommend it because the evidence of benefit is not clear.

Surgery The prime objective of surgery is to remove the tumor completely, along with a surrounding margin of normal tissue. If that can be achieved, the chance of cure is increased. Whether complete removal is feasible depends on the position of the tumor, how deeply it has invaded, the size of the muscle or other tissue surrounding it, and so on.

If removal is feasible, your surgeon will design and plan the surgery to minimize any disability the operation may cause. In some cases, it may be necessary to amputate a limb; in others it may be possible to remove the tumor completely without amputation. You will need to discuss the details thoroughly with your surgeon.

Radiotherapy Radiotherapy is recommended after surgery in certain cases and instead of surgery in some cases where the tumor cannot be removed. You will need to discuss the type of radiotherapy, the side effects, and any disability that may result with your radiation oncologist.

Chemotherapy Depending on the age of the patient and the type of the tumor, chemotherapy may be recommended after surgery in some cases. Usually chemotherapy is used more frequently with the sarcomas of childhood. A combination of drugs may be given, among them **ifosfamide** and **Adriamycin** for adults and, in addition, **cyclophosphamide**, **actinomycin D**, **vincristine**, **methotrexate**, and **etoposide** for children. This area is one in which new drug combinations are being investigated, so your medical team may recommend other medications.

Chemotherapy can also be used if the tumor has recurred or has spread and is causing or threatening to cause symptoms.

SKIN CANCERS (EXCLUDING MELANOMA)*

Number of new cases diagnosed per year in the United States: 800,000

SUMMARY OF THE KEY FACTS IN THIS SECTION

- Skin cancers other than melanoma are extremely common. In fact, they are so common and so curable that they are not even included in the cancer statistics!
- There are two main types of skin cancer: **basal-cell cancer** (BCC) and **squamous-cell cancer** (SCC).
- Most skin cancers occur on sun-exposed areas of the skin. Hence they can to some extent be prevented.
- There may often be precancerous areas on the skin called **keratoses**, which may or may not later progress to cancer.
- Treatment depends on the exact position and size of the tumor (or keratoses) and may be by surgical removal, freezing with cryosurgery, destroying the tumor with heat by electrodesiccation, radiotherapy, or chemotherapy in the form of an ointment.

The Most Important Features of the Tumor

There are two main types of skin cancers: **basal-cell cancer** (usually abbreviated **BCC**) and **squamous-cell cancer** (usually abbreviated **SCC**). Both are very common, and both are nearly always caused by sunlight (there are other contributory causes in a few cases). Damage from the ultraviolet portion of sunlight may become worse in the future as a result of the thinning of the earth's ozone layer. Fortunately, both types of cancer very rarely spread, and both types can be cured in the vast majority of cases by local treatment. The local treatment (depending on the position of the cancer and its size) may consist of **surgery**, destruction by heating (**electrodesiccation**), or **radiotherapy**.

In many cases of the squamous type of skin cancer, changes in the skin may be an early warning of possible cancer. These precancerous changes are called **keratoses**; sometimes they look like little white horns or more usually pink, brown, rough patches. They may be treated by freezing, surgical removal, or chemotherapy ointment.

The Main Types of the Cancer

Both types of skin cancer—**basal-cell** and **squamous-cell**—begin in the skin cells of the epidermis (whereas the melanoma type begins in the pigment-producing cells of the skin). In BCC the cancer begins in the basal cells, which are the ones near the bottom of the epidermis. Generally speaking, BCCs are more common than SCCs and are usually slow growing, though they are capable of considerable destruction and mutilation of the normal tissues in the area. They almost never spread to distant sites.

SCCs, the less common type, tend to look slightly different from BCCs. They begin in the cells of the skin that have started to accumulate keratin (the substance that makes skin tough and flaky) and have a slightly higher tendency to spread to distant parts than the BCCs (particularly if they start in skin areas that have not been exposed to sun), although spread is still quite infrequent. There are several other types of skin cancer, arising, for example, from parts of the hair or glands, but these are much less common.

* This section discusses only the common types of skin cancer. Melanoma is discussed in the section called "Melanoma Skin Cancer" in this chapter.

Age and Incidence

BCC Basal-cell carcinomas are becoming somewhat more frequent and nowadays occur more often in people under the age of forty than they used to. This is probably due to changes in suntanning habits and in the future may be increased further by the thinning of the ozone layer.

SCC Squamous-cell cancers occur predominantly in people in their late sixties and early seventies.

Causes

We know some of the factors involved in the causing of both BCCs and SCCs.

Ultraviolet Light Exposure to sunlight—in particular, to the ultraviolet portion of sunlight—is an important factor. People who live nearer the equator have an increased risk of skin cancers, as do people who work in occupations with greater exposure to sunlight and people who have fairer skin and who burn easily. People whose skins tan rather than burn have a lower risk. While it is known that the "B" portion of ultraviolet light is a contributory cause, it is thought that the "A" portion may also contribute. As the "A" portion of ultraviolet light is used in tanning salons and tanning machines, it is possible that people who use tanning salons regularly may have an increased risk of skin cancer.

Certain Chemicals A few chemicals are known to increase the chance of getting skin cancer. These include arsenic (which used to be a component of certain insecticides, chicken feed, and some "nerve tonics" and has sometimes been found in well water) and one or two other chemicals.

Immune Problems There is some evidence that immune suppression may also be a causative factor and that BCCs are more common in, for example, people with AIDS and people who have had transplants.

Chronic Damage SCCs can occur in areas where there has been chronic skin damage. Thus they are known to occur in scars, areas of chronic lupus (a disease that can affect skin), burns, radiotherapy, skin ulcers, and some other lesions.

Genetics The genetic background of the person does play a role in the causing of skin cancers and will become clearer as current research progresses.

Precancerous Changes: Keratoses

Areas of skin that have been damaged by light or heat may develop rough spots or sometimes areas that

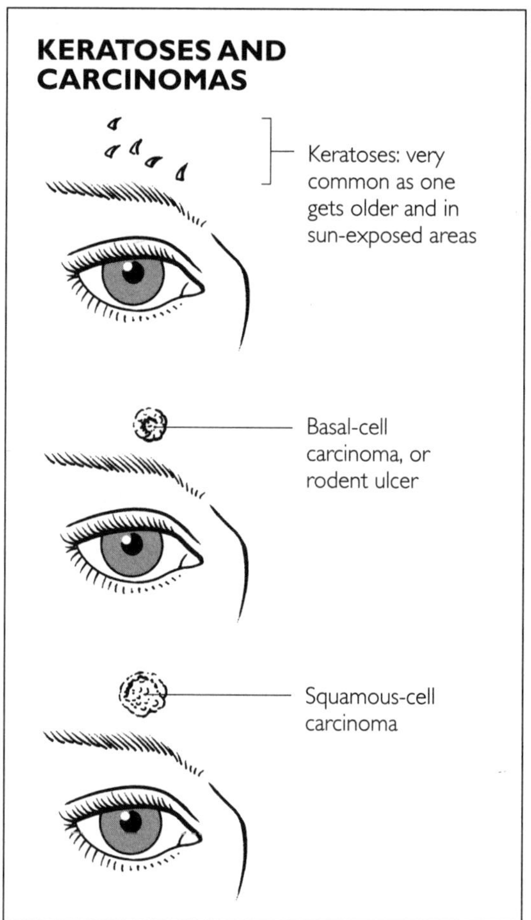

look like little white horns. These are actinic keratoses, and a few of them may later develop into SCCs.

How the Cancer Tends to Spread

In the great majority of cases, BCCs and SCCs do not spread, although they may destroy a great deal of normal tissue in the area if they are not treated. In a few cases, particularly if left untreated, they may spread to lymph nodes and even to distant areas such as the lungs.

Symptoms or Problems That You May Notice

Both BCCs and SCCs usually cause a sore on the skin that is first noticed by the patient. By and large, BCCs cause an ulcerated area with a heaped-up or rolled edge, a rather milky or pearly appearance, and reddish blood vessels visible in the skin nearby. SCCs usually do not have the rolled edge or the pearly appearance and are more likely to appear reddish and scaly. They often occur in areas of previous skin damage. In most cases, with both BCCs and SCCs the area of the skin does not hurt and usually does not bleed.

Diagnosis and Tests

Usually the diagnosis will be made by a biopsy. In many cases, if the appearance of the tumor suggests the probable diagnosis, and depending on where the tumor is and how big it is, the biopsy will be an excisional one in which the whole tumor is removed. Removal may not be possible in all cases.

Factors That Influence the Treatment and Prognosis

Grade The grade of the tumor does have some effect on the outlook. High-grade tumors (those that appear more aggressive when seen under the microscope) have a slightly higher tendency to recur and to spread.

Spread Although spread to other areas is rare, if it has occurred it may influence the outlook. The cancer may still be curable if the other areas (such as lymph nodes) are removed.

Many Other Areas of Damage or Keratoses

If there are many areas of keratoses, they represent further risk of developing new SCCs.

The Main Objectives of Treatment

The main objective of the treatment of BCCs and SCCs is cure. In the majority of cases, this is achievable.

Types of Treatment

Surgery Removing the tumor by surgery is usually possible and has a cure rate in excess of 90 percent. The specific details, and how the area will look and function after the surgery, depend on the location and size of the tumor. You will need to discuss these aspects with your surgeon. In many cases the surgeon uses special surgical techniques (commonly, a technique known as Mohs' surgery, after its inventor) to remove the tumor and take further pieces of tissue until microscopic analysis shows that all of the tumor has been removed. This procedure may require several sessions.

Electrodesiccation In electrodesiccation, heat is used to kill cells in the problem area.

Cryosurgery In cryosurgery (which is used rarely), cells in the problem area are killed by applying freezing to the area using a special instrument. This method is most commonly used for keratoses. Your surgeon will discuss with you how this would be done in your case.

Radiotherapy Radiotherapy can be very useful, with high cure rates, and is often the first choice for areas where surgery would be technically difficult or would have a poor cosmetic or functional result.

Local Medications In some cases (usually with keratoses), ointments containing chemotherapy drugs may be recommended. Again, your specialist will discuss the details with you.

Other Methods Photodynamic therapy (incorporating lasers) may be used in some circumstances. Its role in the treatment of skin cancers is being actively investigated. Injection of the biologic agent **interferon** into the problem area of the skin may also be of benefit.

Prevention

The best chance of avoiding skin cancer is to avoid damage to the skin by sunlight. The standard recommendations are given in Table 4.6 (page 156). It is worth stressing that the chance of developing the sun-damage (actinic) keratoses can be reduced by using sunscreens. If there are areas of extensive actinic keratoses, your doctor may recommend the use of topical chemotherapy in the form of a cream or ointment to reduce the chance of skin cancer developing later.

STOMACH

Number of new cases diagnosed per year in the United States: 22,800

SUMMARY OF THE KEY FACTS IN THIS SECTION

- Stomach cancer is not very common and is one of the forms of cancer that is becoming rarer, probably because of improved techniques of food preparation and preservation.
- It begins in the lining of the stomach and usually causes no symptoms, or only mild and vague ones, in the early stages. As a result it is usually diagnosed when it is relatively advanced.
- If it is detected at a stage when it can be completely removed surgically, there is a chance of cure.
- Stomach cancer is completely different from ordinary (and common) stomach ulcers.
- Nevertheless, after treatment for ordinary stomach ulcers, it is valuable in some cases to check on the ulcer and to make sure that it has healed and was a true benign ulcer and not a cancer.

The Most Important Features of the Tumor

Stomach cancer forms in the glandular lining of the stomach. It progresses in a steady and predictable way, and if treated at an early stage—that is, when it involves only the inner layers of the stomach lining—it can be cured in the majority of cases. Early detection can be difficult, however, because the symptoms in the early stage are very slight and vague.

What You Really Need to Know about the Stomach

The stomach is basically a bag that has a lining that manufactures two important digestive juices: a digestive enzyme called pepsin and hydrochloric acid. After food has been chewed in the mouth and mixed with saliva, it passes down the esophagus into the stomach. The stomach secretes pepsin and hydrochloric acid and then mixes these juices with the food in a churning action. When the food is sufficiently mixed, the muscular ring closing the exit from the stomach (the pylorus) relaxes and opens. The food then passes through the pylorus into the next part of the digestive tract, the duodenum.

The lining of the stomach consists of four layers. The inner layer, the **mucosa**, contains the glands that secrete the acid and the pepsin. The mucosa is supported by the next layer, the **submucosa**. Outside that is the layer that contains the **muscles** needed for the mixing and churning action of the stomach. The outermost layer is a thin smooth layer called the **serosa**. It is in the mucosa that cancerous changes occur.

Age and Incidence

Stomach cancer is one of the few cancers that is steadily becoming less common, that is, its incidence is falling and has been falling for the last two decades or more. Although the reasons for this are not known, it is thought that the decrease is due to an improvement in diet and in particular the way foods are preserved (see below).

Stomach cancer is predominantly a disease of middle adulthood and is relatively rare under the age of fifty. For reasons that are not well understood, it affects men more frequently than women. In fact, the incidence among men is twice that among women.

Causes

Diet It is thought, but not fully proven, that stomach cancer is caused by some form of long-term chemical insult from constituents in the diet. We think that is the case because stomach cancers, as mentioned above, have been decreasing in frequency for many years as standards of food preparation and preservation have improved. Further evidence to support this hypothesis comes from comparisons with other countries. Canada has one of the lowest incidences of stomach cancer among the developed countries. By contrast, Japan has much more stomach cancer, in fact, approximately six times more cases. Moreover, people who emigrate from one country to another early in their lives have nearly the same chance of getting stomach cancer as natives of the country to which they have immigrated. This suggests that long-term exposure, particularly in the first twenty years of life, to something

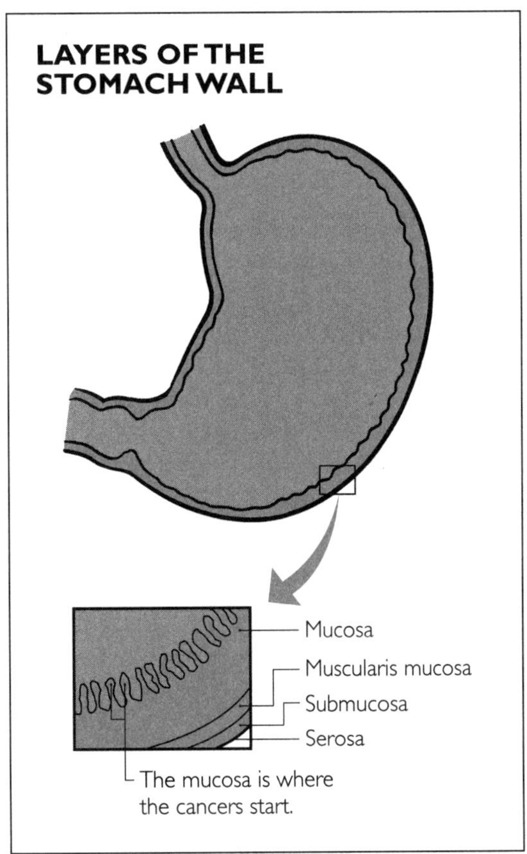

THE DIGESTIVE TRACT SHOWING THE STOMACH

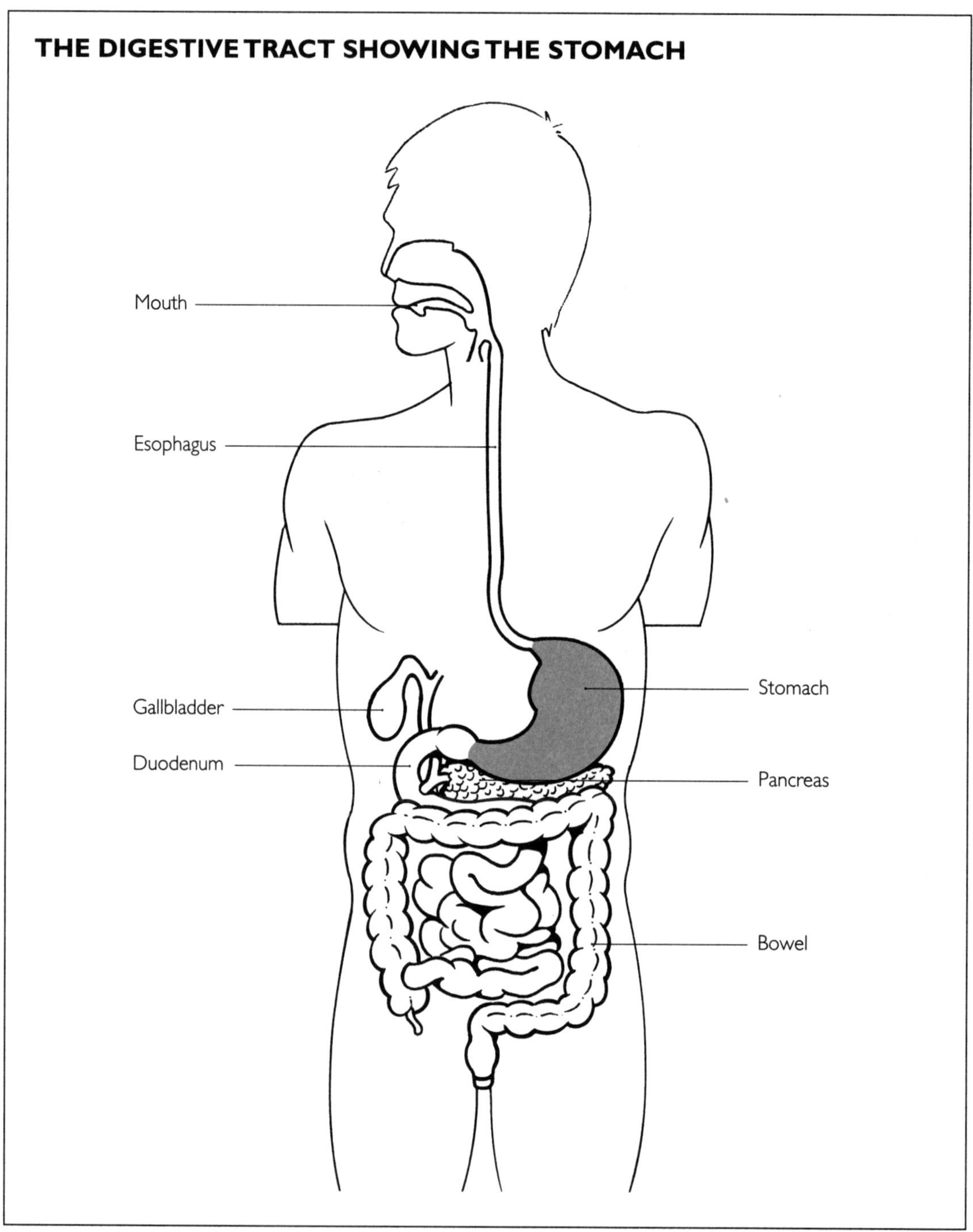

in the lifestyle of the new country is involved in the causation of stomach cancer. Since the stomach lining is exposed to whatever we eat, if there are carcinogenic substances in the diet, long-term exposure increases the risk of cancer. Currently it is thought that the most likely carcinogens in our diet are chemicals called **nitrites** and substances like them. These chemicals are present in food that is badly preserved, so our improving standards of food preparation may have something to do with the decrease in stomach cancer. Similarly, there seems to be a slight increase in stomach cancer in groups that have a lower income and a diet poorer in fresh vegetables and fruit. Thus it is also possible that somehow fresh fruit and vegetables protect the stomach wall against damage from nitrites or similar carcinogens. Recently some research has shown that stomach cancer is more frequent in people whose stomachs contain the bacterium *Helicobacter pylorii,* the bacterium that causes ordinary (noncancerous) ulcers. The exact role of this bacterium in stomach cancer (if any) is not yet fully understood, but there does seem to be some association.

Low Acid Production There is some evidence to suggest that if the stomach wall produces low amounts of hydrochloric acid (or none at all), there is a somewhat increased risk of cancer. People with a condition called pernicious anemia (in which the stomach stops producing acid) may have an increased risk of cancer, as may people who are older and whose production of stomach acid has decreased over the years.

Is There Any Connection between Ordinary Stomach Ulcers and Cancer? The mention of stomach acid brings us to a topic that causes a lot of concern and worry: are stomach ulcers connected in some way to the causing of stomach cancer? The answer in the vast majority of cases is a clear no. If you have ordinary stomach ulcers, there is very little chance (if any) that they will progress to cancer. However, as mentioned above, the bacterium *Helicobacter pylorii* is known to be an important cause of ordinary ulcers and may also play some role (which is not yet understood) in stomach cancer. So there may be a very indirect association between the two conditions, even though one does not progress into the other. From the practical point of view, however, if you have an ordinary ulcer, your doctor may want to check on your ulcer after treatment to make sure that it has healed properly and therefore was a truly benign ulcer (and not a cancer).

How the Cancer Tends to Spread

Stomach cancer begins in the lining of the stomach, the glandular layer on the inside. As it grows, it penetrates more deeply into the stomach wall and then through the stomach wall to the outside of the stomach. If it does so, it may involve adjacent organs such as the pancreas or spleen and may also spread to lymph nodes in the area. Later on, it may spread to other distant lymph nodes (in the neck, for example) and may also spread across the abdominal cavity to other parts of the abdomen. In this way it may cause ascites—that is, fluid that accumulates in the abdomen—or it may cause secondary tumors on the ovaries in women or near the rectum or the umbilicus. It may also spread via the bloodstream to the liver.

Symptoms or Problems That You May Notice

The main difficulty in diagnosing stomach cancer at an early stage is that it may cause no symptoms at all, or may cause very mild and vague "everyday" symptoms. The most common symptom is a **mild ache** in the upper part of the abdomen. In general, this is indistinguishable from the indigestion-type ache or pain, which almost everybody gets from time to time and which may be accompanied by belching or feelings of fullness. Sometimes there are no local symptoms but only generalized symptoms such as **tiredness**, **loss of energy**, and **decrease in appetite**. The problem is that most of us occasionally experience such local or general symptoms, and unfortunately there are no features that identify symptoms as being specifically signs of stomach cancer. In a small percentage of cases, the first sign of stomach cancer may be a major abdominal crisis, such as bleeding from the stomach or obstruction of the bowel.

Diagnosis and Tests

The definitive diagnosis of stomach cancer is done by taking a **biopsy** of the lesion. That is usually done during a **gastroscopy**, in which your specialist will pass a thin tube containing a telescope system down the esophagus into the stomach in order to inspect it and take specimens of anything that appears suspicious. Sometimes the gastroscopy is done as the first investigation or sometimes a special X ray called a **barium meal** is done first. In a barium meal, you will be asked to drink a white liquid which shows up on X rays, and X rays will be taken while it is in your stomach.

As well as some or all of these tests, routine blood tests will be done. If the biopsy does show stomach cancer, your doctor will probably recommend further tests to see if the cancer has spread anywhere else. These tests may include a **CT scan** (or an **MRI scan** if that is thought necessary).

The Main Types of the Cancer

Adenocarcinomas Most stomach cancer arises from the glands in the mucosa and is therefore termed **adenocarcinoma**. (Other types of malignant tumors can occur in the stomach, and these will be mentioned briefly below.) There are four basic patterns of growth commonly seen in adenocarcinomas of the stomach. These patterns of growth do predict, to some extent, how aggressively the tumor is likely to behave. Some cancers grow as a thin spreading layer over the mucosa. They are called **superficial spreading** cancers of the stomach and are the least aggressive type. Some are particularly small and confined to the mucosa and submucosa, and these are often called **early** stomach cancers. (This type of cancer is more common in Japan.) Others form a sharply defined **ulcer** only, though they are not caused by and have nothing to do with ordinary stomach ulcers (see above). Again, these have a better-than-average prognosis. Other cancers grow almost like a cauliflower, with a stalk area and a branched head. They are called **polypoid** cancers (meaning "like a polyp"). If the cancer grows in this pattern, generally its behavior will also be less aggressive. Growth in an **infiltrating** pattern into the stomach wall (often making an ulcer in the center) suggests that the cancer is somewhat more aggressive, and, as it happens, this is the most common type of stomach cancer. Sometimes the cancer grows in a diffuse way throughout the whole wall of the stomach rather than in a specific area or identifiable lesion. This type, **linitis plastica**, is the most aggressive.

Other Malignant Tumors of the Stomach

Malignant tumors of the stomach other than adenocarcinomas are discussed in other sections of this book. For example, **lymphomas** (cancers of the lymphocytes) may originate in the stomach. These tumors behave much more like lymphomas of other parts of the body than adenocarcinomas of the stomach, so the section on lymphomas is relevant (see page 145). The stomach wall can also sometimes give rise to **sarcomas** (cancers of connective tissue). These behave more like sarcomas of any other part of the body, so the section on sarcomas (see page 183) will give you an idea of what the tumor is like and how it is treated.

Factors That Influence the Treatment and Prognosis

The most important factor influencing the type of treatment and the outlook is the **stage**, in other words, how far the cancer has progressed. If the cancer is limited to the mucosa and the submucosa of the stomach wall, the chance of cure is quite high. Cancers of this stage are quite common in Japan (where cancer of the stomach is more frequent and where screening programs are in existence). Unfortunately, in this country there is a higher chance that the cancer will have penetrated more deeply, in which case the prognosis is much more in doubt. To some extent the type of the cancer and the way it is growing (see above) can help predict the stage of the cancer, but the most important features are: whether the cancer has penetrated all the way through the stomach wall or only into the mucosa and submucosa, whether it has involved adjacent organs such as the pancreas or spleen, whether it has spread to the lymph nodes, and whether there is any spread to distant organs.

The Main Objectives of Treatment

In some cases the cancer can be completely removed and the patient has a high chance of being cured. In other cases, cure is less likely but removal of the tumor will reduce the chance of later problems in that area (such as bleeding or obstruction). In other cases it may not be feasible to do surgical removal, and the objective is to try to control symptoms.

Types of Treatment

Surgery Surgery is the most important type of treatment in stomach cancer. The exact extent of the operation depends on where the tumor is and how far it has spread. Usually a large part of the stomach or all of the stomach will need to be removed—a **partial** or a **total gastrectomy**. Depending on whether the cancer involves other structures nearby, parts of the pancreas, liver, or spleen may need to be removed at the same time, if that is feasible. The exact details of the operation will be discussed with you by your surgeon. As with all surgery, it is important to understand that the actual operation may differ from what is planned. Sometimes what the surgeon finds may mean that the operation has to be somewhat more extensive or that what was planned cannot be achieved in practice.

If the tumor cannot be removed in its entirety, it may be possible to remove most of it in order to prevent future problems or to create a bypass channel, using a loop of bowel, so that food can get out of the stomach if the exit is blocked by tumor. Again, details of operations such as these will be discussed with you by your surgeon.

In general, operations on the stomach may have some effect on the amount you can eat at each meal and also on your bowel habit, though the latter is less common. Usually the volume you can manage is lower, leading to a sensation of fullness after a smaller amount of food.

Radiotherapy Radiotherapy can occasionally be of value if a tumor cannot be removed and is obstructing one area of the stomach or digestive tract and causing pain. Radiotherapy may also be helpful if a tumor that cannot be removed is causing continued bleeding.

Chemotherapy At present, chemotherapy drugs produce responses in some cases, but generally the responses do not last for a long time. Several drugs are currently being tested, as are some combinations of drugs. The most commonly used drugs include **5-fluorouracil**, **folinic acid**, **etoposide**, **Adriamycin**, **methotrexate**, and **cis-platinum** or **carboplatinum**. If your specialists recommend you to consider being involved in any of these treatments, including investigational drugs, and also clinical trials of adjuvant treatment, they will discuss with you the full details of the therapy, including potential benefits and side effects.

TESTICULAR CANCER

Number of new cases diagnosed per year in the United States: 7,400

SUMMARY OF THE KEY FACTS IN THIS SECTION

- Cancer of the testicle is a rare type of cancer, usually found in men in their twenties or thirties.
- There are two main types: seminomas and a group called nonseminomas.
- Seminomas are slower growing and are very sensitive to radiotherapy and chemotherapy. They can be cured in almost all cases.
- Nonseminomas are more rapidly growing and have a higher tendency to spread to lymph nodes in the abdomen and to distant parts of the body.
- Fortunately, nonseminomas are also sensitive to therapy and are curable with chemotherapy in a very high proportion of cases, even if there is spread to distant parts of the body.

The Most Important Features of the Tumor

Testicular cancer is not very common. Because it tends to affect men in their twenties or thirties, however, it is the most common cancer in that age group. These cancers originate in a type of cells, the **germ cells**, that have the potential to grow and develop into large numbers of different tissues and organs. It is thought by some authorities (but not universally accepted or completely understood) that there are two basic types of germ cells. One group will eventually end up producing **sperm**. Sperm, of course, have all the information necessary to produce an entire new human being when they meet and fertilize an ovum. We believe that germ cells of the *other* main type are descendants of the cells that originally produced the whole person from an embryo. In other words, they are torchbearers descended from the primitive cells that in the early stages of the growth of the embryo gave rise to all the other various types of cells and tissues that make up the entire person. Cancers of these torchbearer cells are sometimes called **embryonal** cancers for that reason.

The two types of germ cells, many medical authorities believe, may account for the two main types of testicular cancer: **seminomas** (cancer of the sperm-producing cells) and **nonseminomas** (cancers of the embryonal type of cells), of which there are several subtypes. Seminoma is a slower growing tumor and is very sensitive to radiotherapy. It is cured in almost all cases either by radiotherapy alone or sometimes by radiotherapy followed by chemotherapy. There are several types of nonseminomatous cancers of the testicle, and the names are a little confusing, but they include the **teratomas**, the **embryonal cancers**, and the **mixed germ-cell tumors**. In practice, some tumors also seem to have features of both seminomas and nonseminomas.

Age and Incidence

It is likely that the events that start off a testicular cancer occur during fetal life, that is, when the patient is himself an embryo. It takes two or more decades for the cancer to develop and become detectable. Hence testicular cancers are usually detected in young adulthood. The seminomas tend to appear ten years later, on average, than the nonseminomas.

Causes

The causes of testicular cancer are unknown. The incidence of the cancer has risen slightly over the last two or three decades. It is also somewhat higher in whites than in blacks and in higher-income groups than in lower-income groups. We do not yet know whether that means that a lifestyle factor plays a role in the causation of testicular cancer.

It is also known that a testicle that does not descend into the scrotum (as normal testicles do) before the child reaches the age of seven or so is at higher risk of developing testicular cancer than a normal descended one. We assume this means that testicular tissue requires the cooler external atmosphere of the scrotum as it matures and that a testicle that is retained inside the body at a higher temperature is in some way more prone to developing cancer.

Another important factor is a prior testicular cancer. In other words, if there has been one testicular cancer, the remaining testicle is at greater risk of developing a cancer.

There is also a slight increase in the risk if a close family member has had testicular cancer. Whether this means there is some inherited factor at work, or whether it is a shared environmental factor, we do not know.

How the Cancer Tends to Spread

Both seminomas and nonseminomas tend to spread to lymph nodes in the abdomen, seminomas late in their progress, nonseminomas earlier. Nonseminomas may also spread to the lungs and, less often, to the liver or the brain. Even if spread has occurred, there is still a very high chance of cure.

Symptoms or Problems That You May Notice

In most cases, cancer of the testicle is first detected when the patient himself discovers a **lump on the testicle**. The lump is almost always painless and is usually discovered while the patient is showering or bathing. Usually there are no other symptoms. Very occasionally, with nonseminomatous cancers, the testicular lump may be small and remain unnoticed, and the first noticeable symptom may be a **lump in the neck**, pain or **discomfort in the back**, or **shortness of breath** due to metastases in the lungs.

Diagnosis and Tests

The essential step in making the diagnosis is to remove the tumor, and with it the testicle on that side, for examination under the microscope. This operation is called **orchiectomy** and generally speaking is done under a general anesthetic so that certain procedures can be done at the same time to reduce the chance that the cancer will spread. There are several different approaches, and you will need to discuss the exact details of the planned surgery with your surgeon.

Markers Almost all testicular cancers produce one or more abnormal substances called markers, which can be detected in the bloodstream of the patient. These substances, which cause no difficulties or symptoms in themselves, are very useful in providing a reliable measure of how much cancer there is in the body and whether the treatment is working.

The two markers most commonly detected in blood tests in testicular cancers are **alpha-feto-protein** (usually abbreviated **AFP**) and **beta human chorionic gonadotrophin** (abbreviated **βHCG**). With both AFP and βHCG, the amount of the substance in the blood is a useful and almost always reliable guide to the amount of the cancer still present. They are important in confirming a diagnosis of testicular cancer and later on in monitoring the effects of treatment.

Thus, as treatment proceeds, the medical team watch the results of the blood tests for AFP and βHCG very carefully to make sure that the treatment is working, that the cancer is being eliminated and, in some cases to confirm or determine the exact point at which it is safe to stop treatment.

Other Tests In testicular cancers—particularly with the nonseminomas—other tests, to see if the cancer has spread elsewhere, are also very important. A chest X ray will certainly be recommended. Depending on the circumstances, CT scans of the abdomen or chest, a lymphogram, an ultrasound scan of the liver, and sometimes some other tests may also be recommended. In a few cases an IVP (intravenous pyelogram) X ray of the kidneys may also be recommended.

Factors That Influence the Treatment and Prognosis

Testicular cancers are curable in the great majority of cases, with the treatment required to achieve cure varying with the type of the tumor and the stage. As stated above, the differences between the two main types (seminomas and nonseminomas) are important. Thus they are considered under separate headings below.

The Main Objectives of Treatment

The primary objective of treatment is complete cure. The amount of treatment required to achieve cure varies depending on the type and extent of the cancer. Because cure is achievable, it is very important for you to complete all the recommended treatment.

Treatment of Seminomas of the Testicle

Seminomas of the testicle are almost always very sensitive to radiotherapy, and in most cases radiotherapy is the only treatment required. The exact details of the radiotherapy vary from case to case. Your radiation oncologist will discuss the specifics of your treatment with you.

In some cases the tumor may be at such an early stage that the chance of cure following the initial surgery is very high. In those cases, no treatment may be required after surgery, provided that you are carefully monitored and regularly checked by your oncologist. The monitoring approach is used in a few but not all cancer centers.

Sometimes the tumor may recur after initial treatment, or there may be a great deal of tumor present at the time of diagnosis, or there may be some reason why radiotherapy cannot or should not be used. In those cases, chemotherapy (in conjunction with radiotherapy or by itself, depending on the circumstances) may be recommended. Several chemotherapy drugs are very useful in this context. The most commonly used are **etoposide**, **bleomycin**, and the **platinum** drugs, but others can be and often are used.

Treatment of Nonseminomatous Types of Testicular Cancer

Three types of treatment are common for the nonseminomas (which include malignant teratomas, embryonal carcinomas, and others).

If the cancer is at an early stage, and if the markers (see above) are normal after surgery, no further treatment may be recommended apart from regular checking and monitoring by your oncologist. The monitoring is important because small recurrences that are detected and treated early may be cured in most cases.

If the tumor is more extensive (for example, if it has spread to lymph nodes in the abdomen), usually surgery will be recommended, with the objective of removing all areas that are clearly involved with tumor. (This may have been done already, depending on the exact details of your case.) After the surgery, chemotherapy may be recommended, though in some circumstances chemotherapy is given before the surgery. Among the drugs most commonly used in the treatment of nonseminomas are **etoposide**, **bleomycin**, and the **platinum** drugs. Several courses of these drugs are given (typically fewer than six). The full details will be discussed with you by your oncologist.

If the disease has spread to other areas of the body (for example, the lungs), chemotherapy will be used as the first treatment option.

Two other points are worth emphasizing about the nonseminomas. Sometimes after chemotherapy an abnormality may still be seen in the chest X ray or perhaps in one of the lymph glands in the abdomen. Quite often this residual lump will be removed, so that future follow-up is not complicated by the appearance of that lump on the X rays or scans. Almost always these lumps prove to be benign scars left after all the malignant tissue has been killed by the treatment. Removal tends to be standard practice in most cancer centers.

Second, in the nonseminomas, any recurrence is likely to happen in the first two years after diagnosis. If you were diagnosed more than two years ago and there is no sign of recurrence, the chance of recurrence later is very small indeed.

Fertility

Depending on what is being recommended to you, treatment may make you infertile and unable to start a pregnancy. For that reason, you may be recommended to give a sample of your sperm for **sperm banking** before the treatment begins. The sperm will be preserved at very cold temperatures and remain viable (alive) for many years, probably decades. One caution, however: quite often, patients with testicular cancers have very low sperm counts even before the treatment is started, probably as a result of the body's response to serious illness (it happens in other types of cancer as well). Thus your sperm may be unsuitable for banking even before treatment. I mention this point only to guard against too great disappointment if things work out that way.

If your sperm count is satisfactory after treatment—as it may well be—you will be able to start a pregnancy, and there will be no long-term risks to the fetus such as increased risk of miscarriage or malformation of the fetus.

Related Conditions

In some unusual circumstances, tumors that are similar to the nonseminomas of the testicle may appear in other areas of the body. This may happen inside the chest in the mediastinum or occasionally in the brain. It is uncertain why or how this happens, although it is thought that perhaps some remnants of embryonal cells have by chance ended up in that area and have later become malignant. The treatment of these types of cancer is very similar to that mentioned above, except that radiotherapy is likely to be used as part of the therapy if there is tumor in the brain. Sometimes, too, different combinations of chemotherapy drugs may be given. Such occurrences are relatively rare, and the exact details of each case will need to be discussed with you by your oncologist.

THYROID

Number of new cases diagnosed per year in the United States: 15,600

SUMMARY OF THE KEY FACTS IN THIS SECTION

- Cancer of the thyroid is not common and is curable in most cases.
- It usually starts as a nodule in the thyroid gland in the middle area of the neck.
- It is often slow growing and in many cases can be cured completely by surgery, particularly in the younger age group.
- In many cases, treatment with radioactive iodine may be required after the surgery.

The Most Important Features of the Tumor

Cancer of the thyroid is not common. In most cases, thyroid cancer is slow growing and can be treated by removing part or all of the thyroid gland. In some cases, surgery is the only treatment required, and the patient will be cured by the operation. In many circumstances, however, treatment with radioactive iodine will be recommended after the operation. The radioactive iodine is taken up by any remaining thyroid cells and usually kills them. In a small number of cases there may be recurrence of the tumor, and treatment with further radioactive iodine, radiotherapy, or chemotherapy may help control the disease at that stage. Curiously, although the thyroid is a very important gland in controlling the body's metabolism, its function is not usually upset by the cancer. If the gland is completely removed, however, you will have to take tablets of thyroid hormone for the rest of your life to replace the natural hormone that your thyroid was producing.

What You Really Need to Know about the Thyroid Gland

The thyroid gland is situated in the middle of the neck and is shaped a bit like a large butterfly. It sits in front of the piece of cartilage that forms the Adam's apple. Normally, you cannot see the thyroid gland or feel it. The gland produces a hormone—thyroxine or thyroid hormone—that regulates the body's metabolism. This hormone contains iodine, and the thyroid gland is very good at collecting iodine from the bloodstream. This feature of thyroid cells can be used in treatment, as many thyroid cancer cells retain their ability to take up iodine and can be killed by treatment with radioactive iodine.

The Main Types of the Cancer

There are four types of thyroid cancer. The three most common types begin in the thyroid cells that

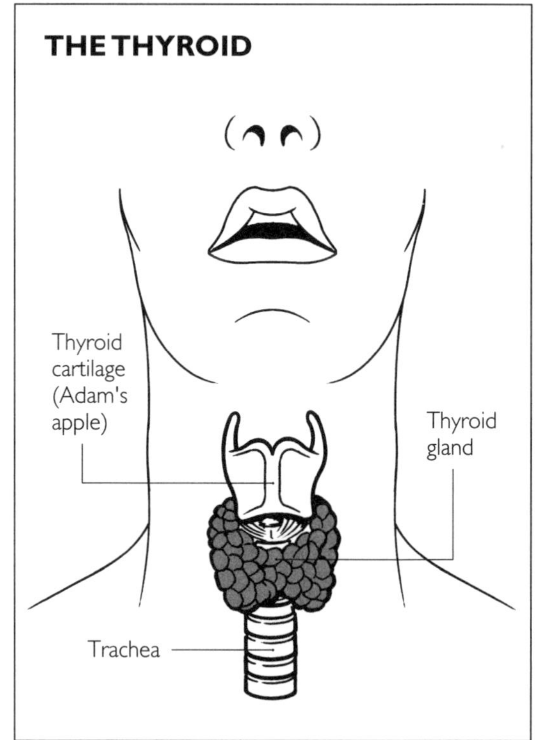

produce thyroxine and are named by their appearance under the microscope: **papillary**, **follicular**, and **anaplastic**. Anaplastic carcinoma is a fast-growing type of cancer and is fortunately very rare. The fourth type, which is more unusual, begins in other cells inside the thyroid and is sometimes associated with problems in other glands in the body. It is called **medullary carcinoma of the thyroid**, and in some cases the tendency to develop it may be inherited.

Age and Incidence

In general, thyroid cancer can occur at any age and so is seen in young adults and even in teenagers. The anaplastic type is more common in later adulthood.

Causes

In most cases there is no identifiable cause of thyroid cancer. In a few cases it may be associated with previous radiation exposure. This seems to apply particularly to the papillary type of thyroid cancer if the radiation exposure occurs early in life. Another factor that may be significant is iodine deficiency. In parts of the world where there are lower amounts of iodine, the chance of getting thyroid problems, including a slight increase in cancer, appears to be higher. In most areas of the developed world this is not a problem, as table salt has iodine added to it to prevent iodine-deficiency problems.

As I mentioned above, the tendency to develop the medullary type of thyroid cancer (the type associated with other glandular problems) may be inherited in some cases.

How the Cancer Tends to Spread

Cancer of the thyroid usually spreads slowly and predictably. In most cases it grows slowly, over years, and the primary tumor usually remains within the gland and does not invade out of the gland into neighboring tissues. Later it may spread to lymph nodes in the neck and in some cases to other parts of the body via the bloodstream. The anaplastic type is somewhat more aggressive than the other types and has a higher tendency to spread.

Symptoms or Problems That You May Notice

Usually the first, and often the only, sign of a problem is a lump in the thyroid gland in the middle part of the neck which can be seen and felt by the patient. I should stress that most lumps in the thyroid gland are not cancer. Even so, **all thyroid lumps need timely and careful assessment** by a specialist. Usually these lumps are painless and are not tender (in fact, if a lump causes pain, it probably is not thyroid cancer).

In addition, thyroid cancer does not in itself cause any upset or change in the ability of the thyroid to produce normal amounts of thyroxine.

Diagnosis and Tests

The first step, and a very important one, is for your doctor to get the full details of the lump from you and to examine your neck carefully.

Scan and Ultrasound Because nodules or lumps in the thyroid are quite common, and most are not cancer, usually there will be either a **thyroid scan** or an **ultrasound** test of the thyroid. In most cases, both tests will be done. The thyroid scan (which uses an isotope that behaves in the same way as iodine) shows whether the nodule is actively taking up the isotope, and the ultrasound will show whether the nodule is hollow, that is, whether it is a cyst or not. By and large, cysts in the thyroid are not cancerous and need only be kept under observation.

Biopsy In many cases, some type of biopsy will be recommended. Usually this is done with a thin needle under local anesthetic and is called a **fine-needle aspirate**. If there is evidence or suspicion of cancer, this test will be followed either by a surgical biopsy or a more extensive operation.

Other Tests If there is evidence of cancer, a CT scan of the neck may be recommended to assess the exact extent of the tumor and whether or not there are any lymph nodes involved.

Factors That Influence the Treatment and Prognosis

The more aggressive types of thyroid cancer tend to occur in the older age group. The types that occur in adolescence and young adulthood (even when they have spread to lymph nodes) are curable.

The Main Objectives of Treatment

Thyroid cancer is curable in most cases, particularly in the younger age group, so the first objective of treatment is cure. In the older age group, if the cancer has spread, treatment is directed at controlling it for as long as possible.

Types of Treatment

Surgery Because thyroid cancer is slow growing in many cases, particularly in the younger age group, surgery is often curative. The whole thyroid or part of the thyroid may need to be removed. The details of the surgery will be discussed with you by the surgeon. Skin in the neck area heals very well, and the scar of thyroid surgery very often becomes invisible after a time. If most or all of the thyroid has been removed, you will need to take thyroxine tablets for the rest of your life (see below).

Radioactive Iodine and Radiotherapy In most cases, a dose of radioactive iodine will be recommended to kill any cancer cells that may be left behind (and normal thyroid cells as well). This treatment is not painful, but because of the safety measures associated with all radioactive substances, it needs to be done very carefully. You will need to be in the hospital for a few days in a special room (so that your neighbors do not get exposed to radiation), and the nursing staff will take special precautions when disposing of your urine and so on. You need to follow instructions carefully so that the radioactivity does not affect anyone else. Most patients say that the procedure is not unpleasant, though a few find it boring!

In addition, radiotherapy given by external beam may also be recommended. If it is, your radiation oncologist will explain the full details to you.

Other Therapy In some cases, particularly in the elderly, the cancer may spread. Depending on the age of the patient and other factors, further treatment with radioactive iodine, radiotherapy, and even chemotherapy may be recommended. There are several options here, and some new medications are being evaluated. You and your doctor will need to discuss precisely what is being recommended in your case.

Thyroid Hormone (Thyroxine) Replacement Treatment If all of the thyroid has been removed, or if the amount remaining is insufficient to produce enough thyroxine for your body's needs, you will need to take thyroxine tablets for the rest of your life. There are no side effects from these tablets. It is, however, essential for you to take the tablets every day and not miss any doses. You also must have the levels of thyroid-stimulating hormone in your bloodstream checked regularly to ensure that your dose of thyroid hormone is correct, so please make sure that you keep all your appointments for follow-up. If you are taking too little thyroxine, you may start gaining weight, feel tired and lethargic, and notice the cold weather more than you used to.

Medullary Cancer of the Thyroid Because the tendency to develop medullary cancer of the thyroid may be inherited, if that is the type you have, your specialist may recommend that other members of your family be tested. A blood test called a calcitonin test may help in early detection of this particular type of thyroid cancer.

RARER CANCERS IN CHILDHOOD

A Brief Note about This Section

Because there are more than two hundred types of cancer, it is not possible in this book to discuss all of them in as much detail as those in the preceding sections. I therefore summarize the most important features of some of the less common tumors in a paragraph or two. The fact that these tumors are discussed less extensively is not intended to suggest that they are less important in any way. Any diagnosis of a cancer is a major concern, probably the biggest that anybody will ever face, and that concern is no less major because a cancer is rare. The summaries that follow are intended to provide an overview that you can use as a basis for discussions with your doctor. As I stress throughout, your relationship with your doctor is a major part of your treatment, and even the most detailed discussions in a book are no substitute for it.

The Most Important Features of the Childhood Cancers

The types of cancer that occur in childhood are unusual in three important respects. First, they are uncommon; and because they are unexpected and rare, they are often psychologically much more painful for the parents. Second, childhood cancers are in general more curable than adult cancers. Although the reasons for this are not understood, the chance of cure—even though the treatment may be hard on the child and on the family—is quite high. Third, in most types of childhood cancer we have no clues as to the cause. The most likely explanation of some childhood cancers is that there is a built-in fault or flaw in a group of cells. In other words, it is not caused by anything that the parents or the child has done or taken or been exposed to; it is purely a matter of bad luck. In some cancers—particularly the tumor of the eye, retinoblastoma—*we know* that the cancer is caused by a genetic fault and therefore is *definitely* a matter of mischance and not caused by anything that could have been avoided. In the case of many other childhood cancers, we know that there are some inherited conditions that increase the risk of developing that cancer. It is likely that in the future we will have more information about the causes of more of the childhood cancers, and it may be found that most, if not all, are caused by built-in errors in cell growth and not by anything that anybody has done.

The Main Types of Childhood Cancer

In childhood the commonest types of cancer are leukemias, tumors of the brain and spinal cord, lymphomas, and sarcomas of bone or soft tissues. There are specific sections dealing with each of these cancers. The most common type of **leukemia** in childhood is acute lymphoblastic leukemia, and you will find the section on that cancer starting on page 127. Other types of leukemia in childhood are relatively rare, but information in the relevant section may be helpful. Tumors of the **brain** and **spinal cord** in childhood are dealt with in the section starting on page 60. **Lymphomas** will be found on page 142. Cancers of **bone** (osteosarcoma and Ewing's) can be found starting on page 41, and **soft-tissue sarcomas** are in the section beginning on page 183. In addition to these types, several other cancers can occur. It is not possible to deal with all of them, but three are summarized briefly below: Wilms' tumor of the kidney, neuroblastoma, and retinoblastoma of the eye.

WILMS' TUMOR OF THE KIDNEY

Wilms' tumor is an embryonal (see page 196) cancer of the kidney, and most cases are diagnosed when the child is between one and five years old. In some cases the cancer is associated with congenital abnormalities, and in a small number of families the tendency to develop the tumor is inherited. In some cases there is a tumor on each kidney (left and right).

Symptoms

In most cases the first symptom is a swelling or mass in the flank noticed by the parent or by the child. There is often some pain in that area, usually moderate but occasionally severe.

Diagnosis and Treatment

CT scans, ultrasounds, and other tests will be recommended to assess the tumor mass and to find out if there has been any spread. Surgery is almost always the first treatment used, and the objective is to remove as much of the tumor as possible and to assess the abdomen accurately to see if there has been any spread. As well as the surgery, chemotherapy will be given in almost all cases, usually after the operation, but some centers use the chemotherapy before surgery. The drugs most commonly used include: **vincristine**, **actinomycin D (dactinomycin)**, **Adriamycin**, and sometimes **cyclophosphamide** or **ifosfamide**, **platinum drugs**, or **etoposide**. Full details of the exact treatment recommended for your child will be explained by the specialists. Although the treatment may be somewhat arduous, the chance of cure is very high. It should also be emphasized that with Wilms' tumor—unlike many other tumors—if the tumor later recurs, it can sometimes be cured with further treatment.

NEUROBLASTOMA

Neuroblastoma is a cancer of a group of cells (called neural crest cells) that are related to the development of certain types of glandular tissues and part of the nervous system known as the sympathetic nerves. There are many peculiarities about the way neuroblastoma develops and behaves. For example, there is some evidence that tissue that looks like neuroblastoma can be found relatively often in young infants, and yet the actual cases of neuroblastoma that later develop are much less frequent. This suggests that neural crest cells may perhaps form lesions that look like neuroblastomas but that after a period of time usually turn into normal mature tissue. In some cases, it seems, this maturing process does not happen, and a true neuroblastoma is the result. At present, however, this is speculation. About half of all neuroblastomas will be diagnosed in the first two years of life.

Symptoms

Neuroblastoma tumors can develop anywhere where there is tissue of the sympathetic nervous system. In general, that means the back of the abdomen, in the adrenal glands above the kidneys, at the back of the thorax, and occasionally in other areas. Most commonly the patient has symptoms of swelling or mass in the areas, accompanied by some pain. Often the tumor will have spread to lymph nodes or to bone or other areas at the time of diagnosis.

Treatment

If the tumor has not spread, it will be cured in most cases by surgery. If the tumor has spread, chemotherapy will almost certainly be recommended. Neuroblastoma responds to chemotherapy in many cases. In general, the prognosis is related to the child's age at the time of diagnosis, and the younger the child, the better the outlook. Research is going on to find the factors that predict the outcome (and that may help in the selection of treatment).

RETINOBLASTOMA

Retinoblastoma is a rare cancer of the retina (the back of the eye) and is curable in the great majority of cases. One type of retinoblastoma is inherited (see page 26), and the other form (which makes up most cases of retinoblastoma) occurs without a genetic basis to it.

Symptoms

Usually the first sign of a retinoblastoma is a change in the appearance of the child's eye, often first noted by the parents, usually before the child is three (and only rarely after the age of six). The pupil may appear milky or white. There may also be a squint, and sometimes the child may notice difficulty with vision or there may be pain.

Diagnosis requires expert assessment under an anesthetic.

Treatment

Nowadays, depending on the individual circumstances, it is often possible to treat the retinoblastoma in a way that preserves, or partially preserves, vision. Radiotherapy is often used, as is treatment of the retina with laser (photocoagulation) or with other methods. If the tumor has not spread into the nerve at the back of the eye, the chance of cure is very high.

Because there is a possibility of the tumor being inherited, anybody who has been cured of retinoblastoma and also wants to start a family should have genetic counseling to discuss the situation in detail.

RARER CANCERS IN ADULTHOOD

A Brief Note about This Section

Because there are more than two hundred types of cancer, it is not possible in this book to discuss all of them in as much detail as those in the preceding sections. I therefore summarize the most important features of some of the less common tumors in a paragraph or two. The fact that these tumors are discussed less extensively is not intended to suggest that they are less important in any way. Any diagnosis of a cancer is a major concern, probably the biggest that anybody will ever face, and that concern is no less major because the cancer is rare. The summaries that follow provide an overview that you can use as a basis for discussions with your doctor. As I stress throughout, your relationship with your doctor is a major part of your treatment, and even the most detailed discussions in a book are no substitute for it.

ANUS

The anus is the muscular ring at the end of the rectum. The term "anus" includes not only the ring itself but the two centimeters (three-quarters of an inch) or so above it (that is, the final two centimeters of the bowel). Cancer of the anus is not common but can be cured in the majority of cases, particularly in the early stages. Most cancers of the anus are of the squamous type and are more likely to occur when there has been long-standing irritation to the anal region. If the tumor is small and has not spread, the treatment—with surgery or radiotherapy (usually with chemotherapy as well)—has a high chance of success.

Cause

In general, anal cancer is more common in people who have long-standing problems in the anal area.

The most common problems that are likely to predispose to cancer are: infections including genital warts, chlamydia, herpes, gonorrhea or Trichomonas, the human papilloma virus (HPV, see page 82), being HIV-positive or having AIDS, and longstanding anal problems such as a fistula or a fissure. Anal cancer is more likely to occur in people who practice anal intercourse, but this may be because of infections transmitted by that method. Common anal problems such as hemorrhoids or skin problems around the anus do slightly increase the chance of anal cancer, which is why examination of the anal area and a rectal examination should be part of the annual medical checkup.

Symptoms

There may well be no symptoms at all in the earliest stages, but usually an anal cancer will at some stage cause either bleeding from the anus or discomfort on defecation. Although both these symptoms are also common with simple noncancerous problems such as hemorrhoids or a fissure, because of the possibility that the symptoms may be caused by cancer, **it is very important for anyone with anal bleeding or discomfort to get a medical assessment**.

Diagnosis

The diagnosis is usually based on your doctor's examination and then a biopsy. Further tests may then be recommended to find out if there has been any spread of the cancer. Usually these will consist of CT scans of the pelvis or abdomen and ultrasound scans (which may include a rectal ultrasound in which the ultrasound image is produced by introducing the probe into the rectum). An MRI scan may or may not be recommended as well.

Factors That Influence the Treatment and Prognosis

The size of the tumor and whether it has spread (for example, to local lymph nodes) are important factors in determining the type and extent of treatment.

Treatment

Surgery If the tumor can be removed entirely by surgery, and if it is a small tumor, that should be the first choice of treatment. The cure rate for small tumors that are removed entirely is very high. Depending on the exact location and the size of the tumor, it may be possible to remove it without affecting the function of the anus, that is, the person's ability to defecate in the normal way. If the tumor is too large or is situated in an area that makes limited surgery impossible, your surgeon may recommend removal of the tumor and the anal sphincter together with some of the rectum. In that case, usually you will require a colostomy after the operation and will therefore pass stool via the colostomy rather than via the anus. These aspects of the planned surgery and the effect on your life afterward are clearly very important, and you will

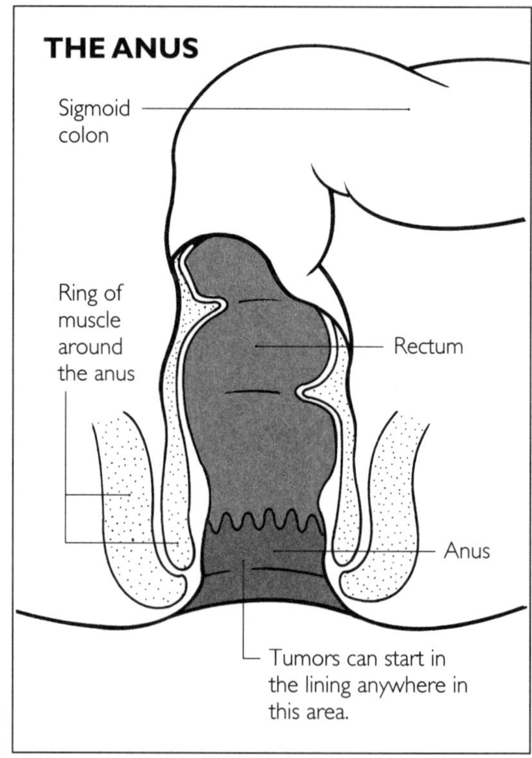

want to discuss exactly what is planned with your surgeon. (There is more about living with colostomies in Chapter 10.)

Radiotherapy Radiotherapy can be used in addition to surgery (before or after) or, in certain circumstances, instead of surgery. In some cases, radiotherapy may also be given to the lymph nodes in the groin. The exact details of the radiotherapy treatment will be explained by your radiation oncologist.

Chemotherapy In general, anal cancer is moderately sensitive to chemotherapy, particularly to drugs such as **5-fluorouracil** and **mitomycin**. The optimal way to use chemotherapy is still being investigated; at present it is usually given after surgery and with radiotherapy.

BILE DUCT

Cancer of the bile duct is a rare cancer that occurs within the bile duct system of the liver.

Cause

In most cases the cause is unknown (unlike cancer of the liver where long-term liver damage is a known contributory factor). In other parts of the world, damage to the bile duct system from such things as parasites is a known risk factor but is rarely applicable in this country.

Symptoms

Because of the position of this cancer, it is likely to obstruct the excretion of bile and therefore cause jaundice at an early stage. It spreads along the bile duct system and into the neighboring liver tissue.

Diagnosis

Diagnosis is usually based on some or all of the following tests: ultrasound scans of the liver, CT scans, cholangiogram (in which dye is injected and X rays are taken as it passes through the bile duct system), and biopsy.

Factors That Influence the Treatment and Prognosis

The feasibility of removing the cancer completely is the most important factor affecting the outlook. If it can be removed, the prognosis is better, although the chance of recurrence with this particular cancer is quite high. If it cannot be removed entirely, the outlook is less good.

Treatment

Surgery If the tumor can be removed in its entirety, surgery is the treatment of choice. If removal is not possible and if obstruction of the bile ducts is causing jaundice and other symptoms, in some circumstances it is possible to bypass the obstruction by a procedure in which a tube is inserted into the bile duct system. This may be done using an endoscope or under X-ray vision. The other end of the tube is placed in the bowel or, if that is not possible, leads to a bag outside the body. If the procedure is not technically feasible using an endoscope or under X ray, a surgical operation may be recommended. The exact details of the surgery will vary

THE BILE DUCT

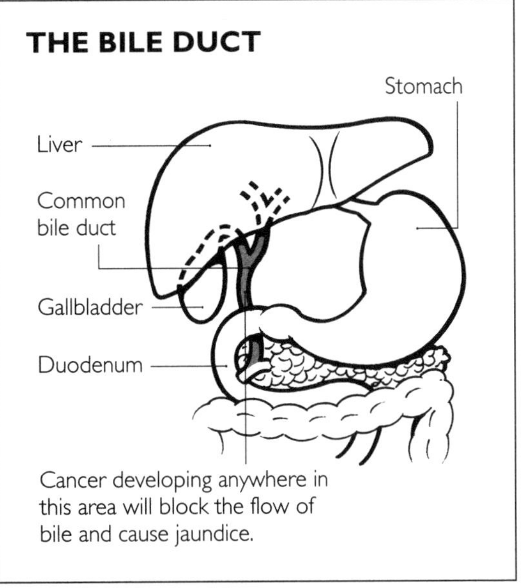

Cancer developing anywhere in this area will block the flow of bile and cause jaundice.

from situation to situation, and your surgeon will discuss them with you.

Radiotherapy Radiotherapy may be used instead of surgery for certain tumors in certain situations; it may also be used after surgery or to control the disease in other circumstances.

Chemotherapy Bile duct cancer does not seem to be sensitive to chemotherapy in most cases, though the use of chemotherapy as adjuvant treatment after surgery, sometimes in conjunction with radiotherapy, is being investigated.

CARCINOID TUMORS

Carcinoid tumors are quite rare, and many have a very low chance of spreading and are considered almost benign. They occur in various parts of the digestive tract and in some areas of the airways in the lungs and are slow growing. They are quite peculiar in that they produce hormones that, when released into the bloodstream, can cause symptoms such as flushing of the face and chest or wheezing. Depending on where they are situated and whether or not they are causing symptoms, they can be removed, or treatment can be given to counteract the hormonal effects (or stop the tumor from producing them), or drugs can be used to try to control their growth.

Cause

The cause of carcinoid tumors is not known. The fact that the cells from which carcinoids are derived are a specialized part of the endocrine (hormonal) system may be significant, as carcinoids are more likely in a few familial conditions in which there are benign tumors of various endocrine glands.

Symptoms

The tumors usually occur in a part of the digestive tract, such as the appendix, the small bowel, or the stomach. Occasionally they occur in the lungs. The tumors themselves may cause no symptoms at all. If there are symptoms, they may include episodes of abdominal cramping pain. Carcinoids may produce two hormones, one called 5-HT (5-hydroxytryptamine, also known as serotonin) and the other known as substance P. If these are produced in large quantities (usually when there are secondary carcinoid tumors in the liver), they may cause episodes of facial flushing, diarrhea, and wheezing.

Diagnosis

Often, because the symptoms may be few or even absent, the diagnosis of a carcinoid is made coincidentally, for example, when an abdominal operation is being done for some other reason. In other circumstances the diagnosis may be made by measuring the products of 5-HT in the urine (the 5-HIAA test). Scans of the liver and even biopsy may be recommended, depending on the circumstances.

Factors That Influence the Treatment and Prognosis

The most important features are, first, whether the tumor has spread, and second, if it has not spread at the time of diagnosis, whether or not it is likely to behave like a malignant tumor and later spread to, say, the liver. The risk of spread seems to be related to size: small tumors (less than a half-inch or so) rarely spread, whereas the risk is higher if the tumor is larger (say, an inch or more).

Treatment

Surgery If a carcinoid has been detected and is removable, it should be removed. In many cases this will already have happened, as the diagnosis is commonly made at the time of operation. Surgical removal of a carcinoid in its entirety cures the patient in the great majority of cases (nearly 100 percent with carcinoids of the appendix, for example).

Radiotherapy Radiotherapy is usually useful only if the tumor has recurred and is causing symptoms.

Chemotherapy There are two basic approaches to using drugs. Some chemotherapy drugs have a direct effect on carcinoids, though unfortunately the success rate is not very high and remissions may not be long in duration. The drugs that may be used include **streptozotocin**, **5-fluorouracil**, **dacarbazine** (**DTIC**), **Adriamycin**, and others. Other drugs such as **somatostatin** and **interferon** can reduce the symptoms associated with the production of hormones by the tumor. There are several different types of the latter, and your specialist will base the selection on the details of your case.

Embolization In certain circumstances it may be possible to control one particular carcinoid tumor if it seems to be producing a lot of 5-HT or causing other symptoms. Sometimes this may be done by injecting into the artery that feeds the tumor (under X-ray imaging) substances that cause the artery to clog up, thus cutting off the tumor's blood supply. This may produce a useful reduction in symptoms.

GALLBLADDER

The gallbladder is the small reservoir or bag in which bile from the liver collects and then passes into the digestive tract, where it helps in digestion. It is very common for crystals of cholesterol to form in the bile inside the gallbladder: these are gallstones. Gallstones make it easy for inflammation and infection of the gallbladder (cholecystitis) to occur. A badly inflamed or chronically inflamed gallbladder may require removal (cholecystectomy). Occasionally a cancer will be found in the gallbladder when it has been removed. If the cancer has been completely removed and has not spread to the lymph nodes, then the prognosis is very good.

Sometimes a cancer may develop in the gallbladder and remain undetected. It can then invade the neighboring tissues (such as the liver) or spread to lymph nodes in the area. In such a situation complete removal is not possible, and the outlook is worse.

Causes

Cancer of the gallbladder is somewhat more likely if there has been a long history of gallstones causing inflammation. Sometimes the gallbladder reacts to repeated episodes of inflammation by making particles containing calcium that accumulate in the wall of the gallbladder. This condition is sometimes called a porcelain gallbladder because of the way it looks in an X ray. People with a calcified porcelain gallbladder have a significantly higher-than-average risk of developing gallbladder cancer. I should stress that having cholecystitis should not cause you undue alarm. Cholecystitis is very common and cancer of the gallbladder is very rare, so clearly the great majority of people with cholecystitis are not at high risk.

Symptoms

Usually there are no particular symptoms of gallbladder tumors. If the tumor blocks bile duct or causes inflammation, it may cause pain in the right-hand side of the upper abdomen, fever, jaundice, or

THE GALLBLADDER

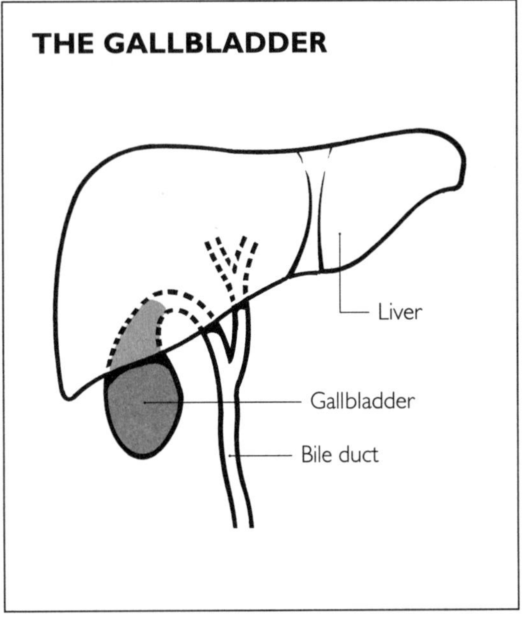

RARER CANCERS IN ADULTHOOD

other symptoms. In general, however, these problems are much more likely to be caused by other conditions (cholecystitis and hepatitis, for example).

Diagnosis

A CT scan of the liver may show up a tumor in the gallbladder. By and large other tests done for other reasons (such as cholecystitis), including ultrasounds, X rays of the biliary system, and so on, are not good at differentiating cancer from inflammation.

Factors That Influence the Treatment and Prognosis

Whether the tumor can be completely removed and whether it has spread to the lymph nodes are the most important factors affecting the outlook. If it can be completely removed, the outlook is good. A good outcome happens most frequently when the discovery of the cancer was incidental, in other words, when the gallbladder was removed for some other reason, such as cholecystitis. If the cancer cannot be removed completely, the prognosis is worse.

Treatment

Surgery Surgery is the mainstay of treatment. If the tumor has not been removed already and if it appears that it can be removed, your surgeon will discuss the full details of the planned surgery with you, as the details will vary considerably from person to person.

Radiotherapy Radiotherapy may provide control of the disease or of symptoms for a time and can be useful in certain circumstances.

Chemotherapy Generally speaking, cancer of the gallbladder does not usually respond to chemotherapy. Chemotherapy is at the investigational stage for this condition. If drug therapies are being investigated at your cancer center, you and your doctor should discuss the potential benefits and hazards in detail.

MESOTHELIOMA

Mesotheliomas are rare forms of cancer that begin either in the linings that cover the lungs (the pleura) or the lining that covers the bowel and lines the inside of the abdomen (the peritoneum).

Cause

Most cases of mesothelioma are related to asbestos exposure. The fibers of asbestos are small and irritating to tissues in a peculiar way. Because the particles of asbestos are so small, they are not coughed up once they have been breathed in. They then appear to make their way through the lung tissue (usually without causing any symptoms) and end up on the outside of the lungs in the pleura. In the majority of cases, the asbestos may cause no damage or some chronic lung damage ranging from very mild to severe. In a small percentage of cases, however, mesothelioma may develop later, sometimes several decades after the exposure. People who work with asbestos are at higher-than-average risk. Their family and household contacts are also at slightly higher-than-average risk, probably because of small particles of asbestos brought home on the worker's clothing or skin. Nowadays the regulations concerning removal of all asbestos-containing material, such as old lagging around pipes, are extremely strict, and it is likely that mesothelioma will become increasingly rare. However, people who were exposed to asbestos in the 1940s and 1950s may still be at risk of developing this cancer.

Symptoms

With mesothelioma in the chest, there may be no symptoms for a long time, and the diagnosis may be suggested when a chest X ray is done for some other reason. Often, however, there will be a cough and shortness of breath, and there may also be chest pain. If it starts in the abdomen, mesothelioma may cause swelling of the abdomen, with pain or discomfort and accumulation of fluid. There may also be weight loss and sometimes some fever.

Diagnosis

Often the diagnosis may be suggested if the person has had exposure to asbestos in the past, although this may be difficult to recall because it may have been the person's parent who had the direct exposure. If a chest X ray or a CT scan show abnormalities that suggest mesothelioma, a biopsy will be required. Sometimes sufficient information can be obtained from taking a specimen of any fluid in the abdomen or the chest. Often, however, a direct biopsy is required, usually done under a short general anesthetic, with an exploratory operation opening the abdomen or the chest cavity as appropriate.

Factors That Influence the Treatment and Prognosis

If the mesothelioma can be removed completely, there is a good chance of cure. Because of the way mesothelioma grows, however, in the majority of cases it will be widespread at the time of diagnosis.

Treatment

Surgery In a few cases, the mesothelioma may be detected at an early stage and may be completely removed by surgery. The exact nature and extent of this surgery will vary depending on the location (for example, whether it is in the abdomen or the chest, what major structures it is near, and so on) and the size of the tumor. You will need to discuss the planned surgery in detail with your surgeon.

Chemotherapy In general, mesotheliomas are not very responsive to chemotherapy. A few combinations of drugs have produced small response rates, however. You should discuss with your specialist what the side effects of any proposed chemotherapy are and what the potential benefits might be. Drugs used in this context may include **Adriamycin**, **cis-platinum**, **cyclophosphamide**, as well as **5-fluorouracil**, **methotrexate**, and others. Sometimes chemotherapy drugs, or other drugs that cause a chemical irritation of the lining, may be put into the chest cavity or the abdominal cavity to try to prevent fluid from reaccumulating after it has been removed.

Radiotherapy In certain circumstances, radiotherapy may control a particular tumor or set of symptoms for a time. The exact role of radiotherapy is difficult to define, however.

VULVA

The vulva is the area around the external opening of the vagina and includes the folds of skin around the vagina (the labia, major and minor), the clitoris, and the tissue around the opening of the urethra. As with cancer of the cervix (see page 81), there are precancerous changes that can occur in the vulva. These can be treated and controlled in most cases. In a few cases there may be cancerous changes within the skin of the vulva, and there may then develop true invasive cancer of the vulva, which are almost always squamous cancers.

In general, the first symptom of cancer of the vulva is itching. (Itching of the vulva is a very common symptom, however, and in the majority of cases is not due to cancer but to an infection or inflammation.) There may be visible changes on the vulva: precancerous changes usually look like white plaques; tumors tend to grow rather like squamous cell cancers of the skin (see page 187) with a heaped-up edge. The diagnosis is usually made by a biopsy, which can be done under local anesthetic.

The most important factor affecting the treatment and prognosis is whether or not the cancer has spread to the lymph nodes. If it has, the chance of long-term control is lower than if it has not. If the tumor has not penetrated deeply into the skin, the chance of spread may be very low. If it has not spread to the nodes, and if the tumor is small and has not invaded deeply into the skin, the chance of cure is high. Hence the treatment depends to a great extent on the individual circumstances. For example, if the tumor is small and has not spread deeply, it may be possible to treat the primary tumor by removing it, and further surgery on the lymph nodes may be unnecessary. In other cases the surgery for the primary tumor may need to be more extensive, and dissection of the lymph nodes in the groin may also be necessary. Radiotherapy may also be used, but the use of radiotherapy, with or without surgery, does vary from center to center. Hence your discussions with the specialists about the treatment options are very important.

The Main Types of Conventional Treatment

5

What's in This Chapter

This part of the book describes the underlying principles of the four main types of conventional cancer therapy, as well as what they do, how they are given, and their most common side effects.

The Four Main Types of Conventional Therapy: A Brief History

Until recently there were three approaches to the treatment of cancer: **surgery**, **radiotherapy**, and **chemotherapy**. In the last few years a new field of investigation and treatment—**biologic therapy**—has opened up. Surgery, radiotherapy, and chemotherapy are in routine use all over the world, and biologic therapy is currently used in certain types of tumors in some situations in a few centers.

Surgery This therapy has been used for cutting out individual tumors for probably two thousand years, and to date it still offers the best chance of cure when the cancer can be totally contained in the area that is removed and has a low tendency to spread elsewhere.

Radiotherapy This form of treatment was invented about a hundred years ago, shortly after the Curies (Pierre and Marie) discovered that a chemical element that they named **radium** gave off a particular type of emission that had certain properties. This type of radiation was later named gamma radiation (gamma rays), and it was first used to treat cancer in France very shortly after the Curies' discovery. Also, in 1895 Wilhelm Conrad Röntgen invented a method of producing what we now know are a similar type of rays. He called these **X rays**, which, because they could penetrate human tissue, began to be used for creating images of the human body. Machines based on the principles discovered by Röntgen now produce X rays in every radiology department in the world. When used in a particular way to make images that can be analyzed by a powerful computing system, they produce CT scans. At much higher doses — say, 10,000 times the dose used for a chest X ray—X rays can kill the cells in their path. This is **radiotherapy**, and the use of radiotherapy to treat cancer is **radiation oncology**.

Chemotherapy Chemotherapy really began in the late 1940s after the Second World War, following a most unexpected spinoff from one of humankind's most inhumane inventions. During the First World War, mustard gas was used as a terrifying and dreadful weapon. It was found that one of the major effects after high doses of mustard gas was destruction of the bone marrow, which ceased to produce red cells, white cells, and platelets — the growing elements in the marrow. Over many years of research, it was found that a derivative of mustard gas called nitrogen mustard or **mustine** had the same properties and would also kill growing cells, including cancer cells. This was the first chemotherapy drug, and others followed. There were occasional dramatic successes in the treatment of what had been previously regarded as hopeless cases. For example, Hodgkin's disease (see page 101), a type of cancer of the lymphocytes, was, in its advanced stages, universally fatal, yet some cases were suddenly being cured by mustine. Another new drug, **methotrexate**, cured some cases of a very rare form of cancer called choriocarcinoma. In the 1960s the modern age of chemotherapy really began when Dr. Vincent De Vita and colleagues combined four drugs (including mustine) and used the resulting combination (called **MOPP** because of the initials of the drugs) to cure a very high proportion of cases with advanced Hodgkin's. From then until today, chemotherapy has produced cures in high numbers for patients with Hodgkin's disease, acute leukemia of childhood, testicular cancer, choriocarcinoma, and some other rare cancers. It has also brought about cures in many cases of adult leukemia and has produced a smaller proportion of cures (and many remissions) in several other cancers. Many new drugs are constantly being tested, and almost all have some advantage over one of their predecessors, although sadly, apart from the tumors just mentioned, the percentage of cures is still low.

At about the same time that chemotherapy drugs were being tried, it was noted that certain hormones—or substances that resemble hormones—could also be used effectively. One of the most significant and important examples is the hormone (or rather antihormone) **tamoxifen**, which is exceedingly effective in many cases of hormone-responsive breast cancer. I am including these modern types of hormone therapy under chemotherapy, although the drugs themselves are very different in their mode of action and their side effects from chemotherapy drugs per se.

Biologic Therapy Over the last ten years, researchers have learned more and more about the complex ways the body responds to cancer and have been trying to modify some of those responses to assist the body (in very specific ways) to deal with cancer cells. Substances that change the response of certain specific elements of the immune system to make it more effective against cancer are therefore called **biologic response modifiers**, or **BRMs**. The most impressive of the BRMs to reach bedside use is **interleukin-2** (IL-2) which has some effect in cases of kidney cancer and melanoma. Another BRM called **interferon** is active in chronic myelocytic leukemia and in a rare form called hairy-cell leukemia (although in this cancer, interferon has now been superseded by a more effective drug).

Other types of biological agents are also being investigated and used. For example, it has been possible to use antibodies (see page 268) to carry toxins or chemotherapy drugs or radioactive isotopes to cancer cells. Although this type of treatment should be enormously effective, there have been major problems in perfecting a system that will deliver very high doses of the toxin or isotope to the cancer.

Note: The biologic therapy described above is a specific and highly technical type of conventional therapy. It is difficult to use and may cause quite severe side effects in some cases. It has no connection with what is called biologic therapy by some complementary practitioners. Such people usually use the phrase to describe, say, a diet that is supposed to strengthen the immune system or remedies that are without effect on any part of the immune system that can be objectively tested.

Combining Types of Treatment: Multidisciplinary Care

In many cases nowadays the best treatment may consist of a combination of some of these four types of therapy. Combining treatments may make a big difference in the effect of the treatment on the cancer and also in the effect of the treatment on you. For example, in many cases of breast cancer it may be possible to preserve the breast using limited surgery (partial mastectomy) followed by radiotherapy and sometimes chemotherapy. In sarcomas, combining types of treatment may make it possible to avoid amputation of a limb, and in colon cancer it may be possible in some circumstances to combine treatments to avoid having to remove or bypass the anal sphincter. In lymphoma, combination of treatment is used in many cases and, again, may achieve better results in terms of both the effect on the disease and of side effects.

So, for all these reasons, many cancer centers nowadays have set up specialized multidisciplinary clinics in which experts in various fields review and discuss the treatment plan (and often see the patient) together. This means that you may meet a surgeon, a radiation oncologist, and a medical oncologist, for example, at the same time (or at separate consultations). Some patients feel a bit anxious about seeing several experts and wonder whether it means that their case is particularly bad or if they are definitely going to need all types of treatment. It's worth emphasizing the point that it may be important for you to be assessed by, let's say, a radiation oncologist, so that it can be clearly established that in your particular case, let's say, radiotherapy will *not* be needed. In other words, the expertise of the expert is just as important and useful in deciding which patients *don't* require that type of treatment as when deciding which patients do require it!

In many centers the multidisciplinary clinic is at the heart of the center's approach to cancer treatment, and it allows specialized services to be adapted to particular clinics (for example, reconstructive surgery and counseling for breast cancer clinics, prostheses and cosmetic services for facial surgery clinics, speech therapy in larynx and throat cancer clinics, and so on). This concentration of specialists and experts might perhaps seem a little daunting or even confusing at your first visit, but do be reassured: it's really worth it in the long run. If you can't remember people's names or who does what (and first time around, most people can't), then don't hesitate to ask them for their card or write down their names, jobs, and phone numbers—you're allowed to do that, and you'll find that health care professionals like it, too. Having a multidisciplinary team working on your behalf and being able to call the right person for your problem will make a big difference to you: it will make you feel much better as well as improving your chances of getting better quickly.

Surgery

The principles of surgery are easy to understand. The objective is to remove the cancer, with some surrounding healthy tissue, in a way that produces the smallest possible change in the normal functioning and appearance of the area and at the same time offers the maximum chance of cure.

The exact nature of the operation—and therefore the effects after it—vary greatly from case to case, even with similar types of tumor in the same area of the body. For that reason the planned surgery, the effects on you, and the plan for care after the operation (such as physiotherapy exercises, remobilization, breast reconstruction, care of a colostomy, limb prosthesis, and many others) are essential parts of the relationship between you and your surgeon and should not be gleaned from a book, even if it were possible to list them all.

Nevertheless, since some aspects of surgery are very common with particular sites, certain topics (such as breast reconstruction, laryngectomy, and so on) are mentioned in outline when the particular cancer is discussed. Also, because care of a colostomy, ileostomy, or urinary stoma (urostomy) is a common and important part of living with the effects of cancer, there is a section of Chapter 10 devoted to this issue.

It needs to be emphasized that in many circumstances, depending on the type of the cancer and where it is, complete removal by surgical means is not feasible. For example, except in very exceptional and unusual circumstances, surgical removal of secondary cancers in the lungs or in the liver or multiple recurrent cancers of the ovary is not feasible. The limitations of surgery are often difficult for patients and relatives to accept, but I hope that the explanations of the different types of tumor biology in Chapter 4 will help you understand some of the things it can and cannot do.

Radiotherapy

Principles

The rays used for radiotherapy are either created artificially (in the same sort of way in which Röntgen created them) by various types of radiotherapy machines (including machines called linear accelerators) or given off by radioactive substances such as cobalt. The radiation given off by the machines is always measured with great accuracy and tested and monitored very closely so that the amount of radiation given out by each machine per treatment is precisely known. The radiation is given to the area where the tumor is, and the skill, expertise, and technology of your radiation oncologist and the radiotherapy department play an important role in the treatment. Two factors are considered in determining the appropriate dose of radiation. First, the dose needs to be high enough to produce the maximum cancer-killing effect. The strength required will depend on the type of the cancer (some cancers are more sensitive to radiation than others) and also on the objective of the therapy (radiation that is given with the objective of curing the cancer may require a higher dose than radiation intended to reduce pain, for example). Second, the dose must not be so high that it damages the normal tissues in the area. Some normal tissues are not easily affected by radiotherapy (bone, for example, is relatively insensitive to radiation, so that higher doses can be given without producing damage). Other tissues, such as the spinal cord, are very sensitive to potential damage, and doses have to be very carefully controlled and given in ways that reduce the dose to the cord. Apart from the spinal cord, there are other tissues and organs that require particular care and attention when radiotherapy is being planned. These include the lining of the digestive tract (esophagus, small intestine, and colon, for example), the lungs, and the kidneys.

Thus, in planning the radiotherapy treatment for any particular situation, the radiation oncologist considers the type and site of the tumor and then carefully works out which normal tissues are likely to be exposed to the radiation given to that area. Rays created by different methods have different

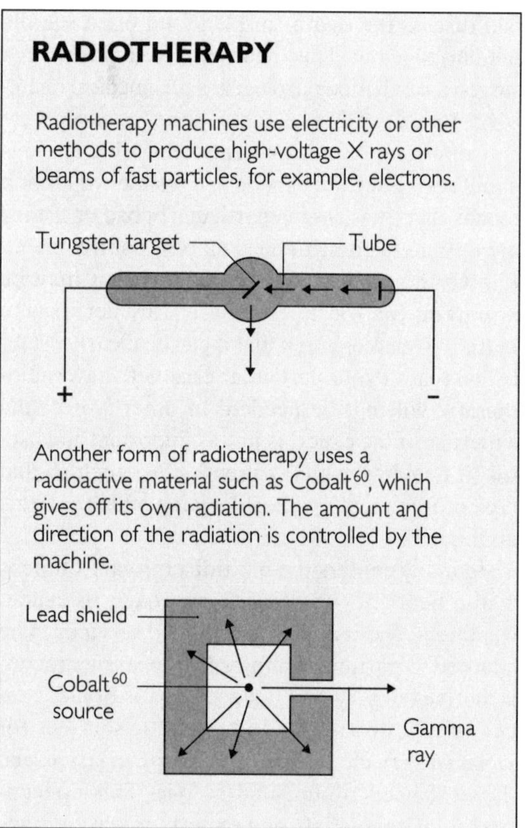

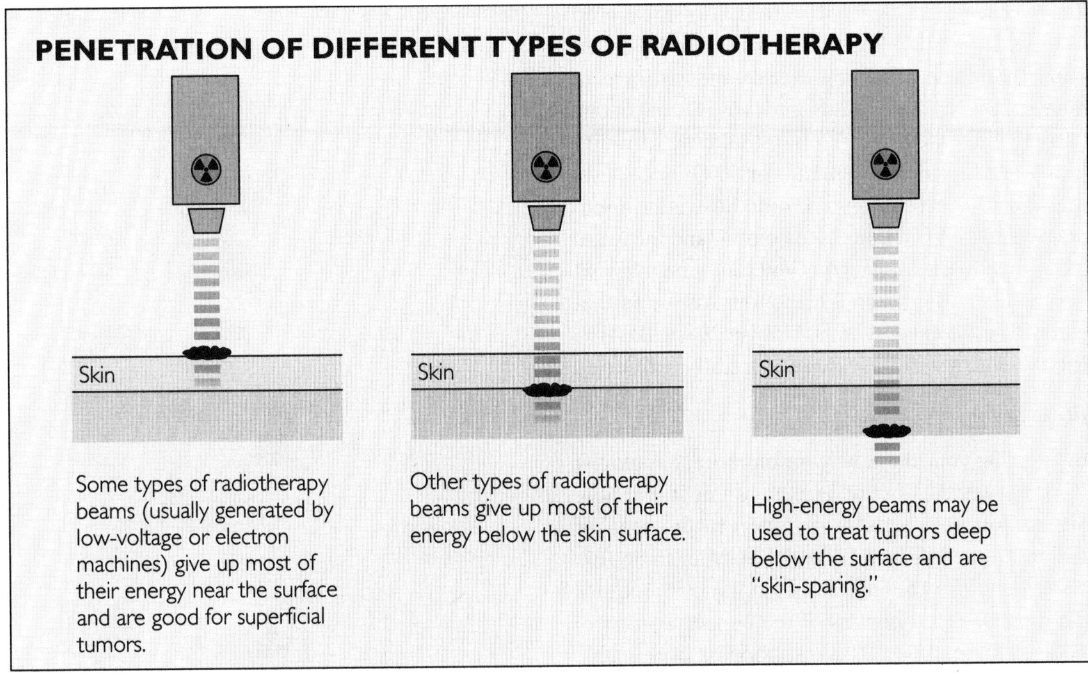

characteristics; in particular, some have a high ability to penetrate through human tissues and therefore to damage the areas around the tumor. This ability varies depending on which machine is producing the rays. For example, if the radiation is being generated by what is called a low-voltage machine, the rays give up most of their energy very near the surface and do not penetrate very far. These rays can therefore be used very effectively for skin tumors. High-voltage radiation penetrates farther and may give the highest dose of radiation deep below the surface. Hence it is extremely important for the radiation oncologist to work out exactly where the tumor is so that the maximum dose of radiation can be delivered close to the tumor while sparing as much as possible of the normal surrounding tissue.

Brachytherapy The radiotherapy that has been described above comes from machines of various types and is often called **external beam therapy**. In addition to external beam therapy, radiotherapy can also be given by placing radioactive isotopes close to the tumor inside the body. This technique may be useful—usually as an adjunct to external beam therapy—in certain cancers such as those of the cervix, endometrium, esophagus, and some others. This type of therapy is called **brachytherapy** (which means "therapy from a short distance"), and it involves placing radioactive isotopes inside thin tubes in the relevant area of the body for a certain amount of time to give the exact dose required. Depending on the area involved, you may need to be in the hospital for a few days.

For example, in treating cancer of the cervix, the tubes that hold the isotope may be placed at the cervix and then the isotope can be moved in and out of the tubes by a machine called the **selectron** without causing you any further disturbance. If brachytherapy is recommended in your case, the full details will be explained by your radiation oncologist.

Terms Used The dose of radiation is measured in units now called **Grays**. They used to be called **rads** (radiation absorbed doses) and still are in many places, so that one hundred rads is equal to one Gray (abbreviated Gy). Thus a total dose of radiation might be called 5,000 rads or 50 Gray (50 Gy) or even 5,000 centiGray. The total dose is split into portions called fractions (see below), and these are often specified as well. Thus you might be told that you will get 50 Gray in 20 fractions, meaning that you will get a total dose of 50 Gray in 20 small doses, each of which will be 250 rads (or 250 centiGray).

Planning the Therapy

In planning your therapy, your radiation oncologist starts by working out where the tumor is and how big an area needs to be included in the area of radiation (the **radiation field**). In order to do this accurately, the radiation oncologist will require the most detailed images of the cancer available. These may include CT scans, bone or liver scans, arteriograms, MRI scans or other methods of showing where the tumor is. The oncologist also has to determine what other structures and tissues are likely to be included in the field, for example, bowel, spinal cord, skin, and so on. In some circumstances, this may require further images of normal structures (produced using barium X rays or other tests, for example). Then the type of radiation can be selected in order to give the maximum dose to the area of the tumor and the minimum to the surrounding normal tissue. The oncologist next works out the best method of giving the dose of radiation, that is, how many doses (fractions) it needs to be divided into. This depends on several factors, mostly on how wide an area is to be included in the field and on the nearby normal tissues and how sensitive they are. For example, if the area is small and in a relatively insensitive tissue such as bone, the radiation may be given all in one fraction. On the other hand, giving a high dose of radiation to, say, a tumor in a breast with the intention of curing it usually requires many fractions (up to twenty or twenty-five) to maximize damage to the tumor while minimizing damage to the skin.

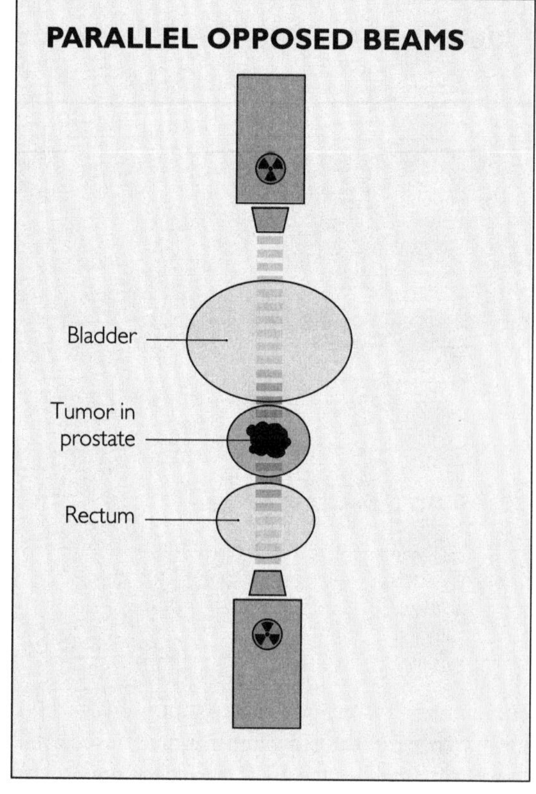

There are also different ways of giving the radiation to spread, as it were, radiation exposure of normal tissues over different areas while the tumor catches the brunt of the radiation each time. Thus radiation may be given from two or more different directions. For example, radiation may be given from the left on one occasion and from the right on another, so that each of the areas of the skin on the left and right of the tumor gets less than half of the radiation (or much less, depending on the penetration of the rays) while the cancer gets the full brunt.

In order to make sure that the radiation is given to exactly the same place each time, the technologists may need to make ink marks on your skin so that the rays can be lined up with perfect accuracy each time. Since ink marks on skin are lost after some days as the skin grows and replaces itself, in some cases it may be necessary to make a small, indelible tattoo on the skin. In certain areas of the body, it may be necessary to make a plastic mold or mask to hold the tissues in exactly the same place each time. If that is necessary, your radiation oncologist will explain the full details.

How Radiotherapy Is Given

Radiation is usually given in small fractions each day.

For each fraction of radiation you will be shown to a room housing the particular radiation machine appropriate for your therapy. Your technologist will help you lie down on a flat table, and the machine will be lined up over the area to be treated, just as if you were having an X ray taken. (An X ray is basically the same thing, but using a much lower dose of radiation.) The technologist will then leave you for a few minutes and will turn on the machine for the exact length of time necessary (usually a couple of minutes). The technologist will monitor the whole process from the control unit. While the machine is on, you must keep still, but you will not feel any effects. There is no pain or heat and no smell or noise. Thus it is very similar to having an X ray taken.

Treatments are usually given on each weekday, and each fraction takes a couple of minutes or so. Usually, taking into account the setting up of the machines and so on, you will probably need to allow up to an hour or an hour and a half for each session from the time you arrive at the radiation center to the time you leave.

Side Effects

By and large, the side effects of radiation therapy depend on three aspects of the treatment. First, the size of the **field** is important: if only a small area is involved, the side effects may be very slight or even absent. If the field is large, the side effects may be more noticeable. Second, the **area** of the body is also important. For example, radiation to the abdomen is likely to cause nausea or diarrhea, whereas radiation to the armpit will not. Third, the size of the total **dose** and the number of **fractions** are important. Generally, higher doses cause more side effects, although I should stress that these effects vary considerably from patient to patient.

It is easiest to discuss the side effects of radiotherapy under two headings: general effects on the whole person (not related to the area receiving the radiotherapy) and local effects (effects that are caused within the area involved).

General Effects

General effects of radiotherapy include **tiredness**, **nausea**, and sometimes **vomiting**. These effects are very uncommon if the radiation field is small (unless it is directed at the abdomen) and also if the total dose is low. Thus general effects like these are very rare if, for example, a few fractions of radiotherapy are given to a painful hip.

In general, the tiredness occurs during the second week of therapy or later, and it may continue for two or three weeks after the therapy is finished. Nausea (if it is going to occur) usually starts within an hour of the therapy and clears up a few hours after the end of therapy.

Unless the therapy is being given to the head or scalp, **hair loss is limited only to the area getting the therapy**. Thus you will not lose the hair on your head if you are having radiotherapy to the chest or abdomen, whereas you may lose armpit hair if you are having radiotherapy to the breast or armpit. Hair lost in this way will often regrow.

Local Effects

The local effects of radiotherapy depend very much on the part of the body involved and the dose of radiation given.

Skin In most cases there will be some effects on the skin included in the radiation field. Sometimes the effects on the skin are virtually negligible. In

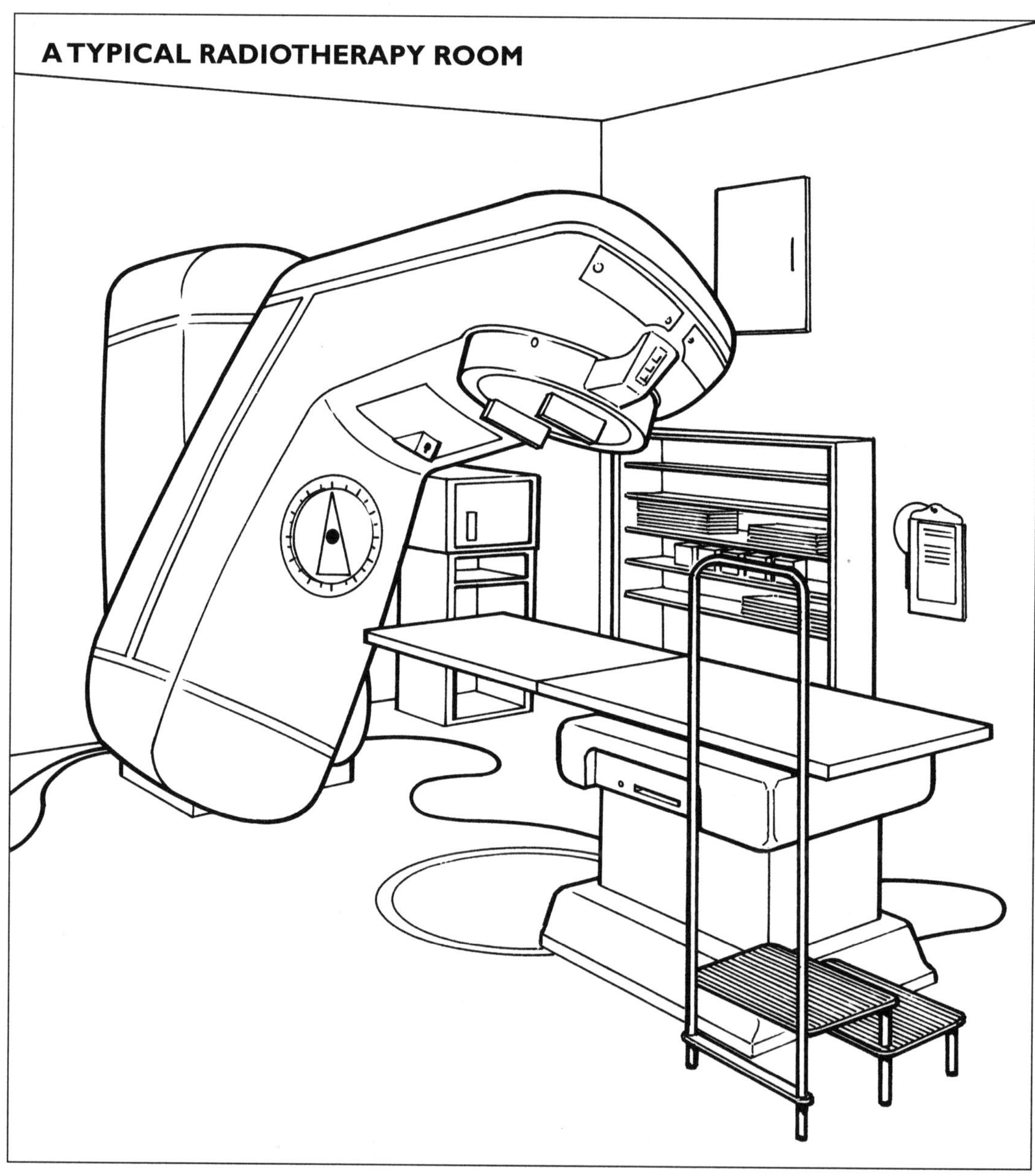

A TYPICAL RADIOTHERAPY ROOM

most cases, they are similar to a mild or moderate sunburn, and in a small number of cases (particularly if the person has been sensitive to the sun in the past) may be like a bad sunburn, occasionally with some blistering and oozing. These effects all heal up within a few weeks, sometimes leaving behind little freckles in the area and, very occasionally, tiny red veins.

Hair Hair that is included in the radiation field is likely to be lost (see above). It may regrow later, but this can vary from person to person.

Digestive Tract If the radiation field includes the abdomen or the liver, there is quite likely to be some nausea (sometimes with vomiting) and also possibly diarrhea, which may continue for several days or a couple of weeks. If the field includes the esophagus, there is likely to be some discomfort or pain on swallowing, again, for several days or a few weeks.

Other effects may occur with radiotherapy given in certain situations. As these may be an important part of your aftercare, it is very important for you to discuss the details of your therapy with your radiation oncology team.

Chemotherapy

How Chemotherapy Works

As we saw in Chapters 2 and 3, cancer cells are unfortunately very similar to our normal cells, and this makes them very difficult to kill with drugs. The treatment needs to be very different from that required to treat, say, an infection caused by bacteria. Bacteria are basically microscopic plants, and their cells are totally different from the cells of all animals, including humans. Thus it has been relatively easy to find substances—antibiotics—that will interfere with the way bacteria grow while not interfering with human cells. That is why most antibiotics have very few side effects and why those side effects are usually quite mild.

Cancer cells, by contrast, are very similar to the normal noncancerous cells from which they develop, and it is extremely difficult to find substances that are selectively toxic to cancer cells and do not affect normal cells (with the exception of some anticancer hormones). In fact, most chemotherapy drugs are effective at damaging any cells that are actively growing and dividing. Fortunately, in many cases there are more cancer cells (in proportion) going through the process of growing and dividing than there are normal cells, so that substances that damage growing cells have a more profound effect on cancer cells than on normal cells. There are, however, several tissues in the human body in which a lot of the cells are going through a growing and dividing phase at any one time. These tissues include the bone marrow (which is perpetually busy manufacturing red cells, white cells, and platelets), the digestive tract (which is constantly renewing the lining of the whole tract from mouth to anus), the hair (which is constantly growing), and some other tissues as well.

Chemotherapy drugs (or most of them) damage anything in the body that is undergoing active growth and division. That is how they produce the effects that they do. If the cancer cells are sensitive to the drugs, the effects will be more beneficial. If the cancer cells are resistant to chemotherapy, the effects will be less beneficial or even absent.

Even with the most sensitive cancers and the best drugs, the margin for error is small. Most chemotherapy drugs will kill the patient if even a relatively small increase in the dose—say, twice the normal dose—is given. (By contrast, in treating bacterial infections with common antibiotics, there would not be lethal or serious side effects at even ten times the normal dose.)

How Chemotherapy Is Given

Chemotherapy drugs are most commonly given by mouth or by injection into a vein. When chemotherapy drugs are given into a vein, they may be given either as a single "shot"—the medical term is bolus—over five to twenty minutes or as a continuous infusion over a few hours or even twenty-four hours or more. Some drugs can be given by either method, whereas some have to be given by injection.

Arterial Route Some chemotherapy drugs can also be administered via an artery (after a special catheter has been placed there). This method of administration is still being investigated in several types of tumors, and it is not yet certain whether it will prove to be more effective than other methods.

Intracavitary Route Some drugs can be given into an area of the body (such as the abdomen or the chest cavity). For example, **bleomycin** can be given in an area where fluid has accumulated to try to control the reaccumulation of the fluid.

Intrathecal Route In some special circumstances, some drugs can be given into the fluid (the CSF) that circulates over the brain and spinal cord. The intrathecal route of administration is used to prevent the spread of malignant cells to the brain and spinal cord in childhood leukemia, some lymphomas, and some other tumors and is also used to treat existing secondaries in certain cancers.

Intravenous Injection Systems (for Injections When Your Own Veins Are Not Easily Accessible)

Some people have big, fat veins in their arms, and some people do not! (Actually, we all have big fat veins somewhere, but in some people they are not near the skin and so cannot be seen easily.) Small veins can make it difficult to get an intravenous injection started. Also, many chemotherapy drugs irritate the walls of veins, so that after several injections the vein becomes clogged (which is no problem in itself) and scarred and cannot be used for taking blood or giving treatment. In those circumstances, your doctor may recommend that a special catheter system with or without a reservoir be put in, which will allow access to veins without any problems. There are several devices like this, and the principle (and practice) actually are quite simple. There are two main kinds.

SUBCUTANEOUS SYSTEM FOR REGULAR INFUSIONS

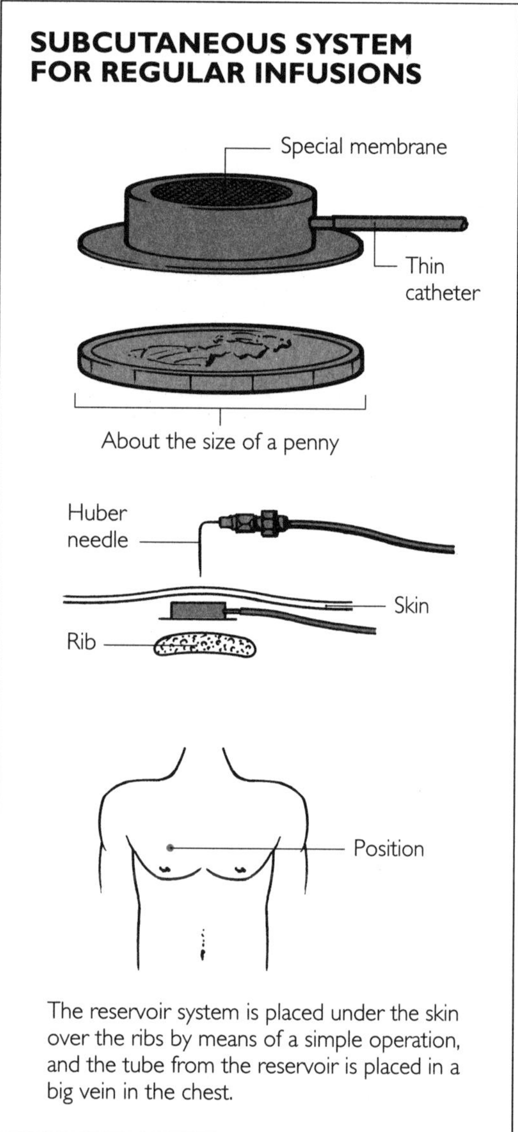

The reservoir system is placed under the skin over the ribs by means of a simple operation, and the tube from the reservoir is placed in a big vein in the chest.

Systems with a Reservoir (Port-a-Cath and Other Types) Putting in a reservoir system is nowadays a simple standard procedure. It is usually done under a general anesthetic, though it can be done with a local anesthetic. The whole system is implanted under your skin so that nothing is actually above the surface or, as one patient put it, *"There's nothing hanging out of me."* A slim, plastic catheter is put into a convenient vein (usually the one deep under your collarbone). It is then connected to a reservoir that is placed under the skin on your chest, usually near the collarbone. This reservoir has a plastic membrane covering it that can be penetrated, without damage, by means of a special needle that can be put into it through the skin. This is called a **Huber needle** (no other type of needle should ever be used with the reservoir because it might damage the membrane). Putting the needle into the reservoir involves firm pressure but causes very little pain. Once the needle is in, fluids, drugs, and anything else you need intravenously (for instance, blood, platelets, or antibiotics) can be given easily. At the end of the injection or infusion, the whole system is flushed with a small amount of saline containing an anticoagulant (heparin) to prevent clotting, and that's all there is to it.

The reservoir system needs to be flushed regularly (usually every few weeks or so) but can stay where it is indefinitely. Most of my patients with reservoir devices have no problems wearing swimsuits or any other clothing—the subcutaneous reservoir cannot be detected easily except by feeling it!

Systems without a Reservoir (Hickman Catheters and Similar Devices) In certain situations, your doctor may recommend that you have a plastic tube (catheter) without a subcutaneous reservoir. In that case, you will have a plastic tube emerging from the skin which needs special care to make sure it does not collect bacteria. The most common type of catheter used is the Hickman, and its advantage over a reservoir system is that it allows larger amounts of fluids or transfusions to be given quickly. Thus your doctor may recommend a Hickman catheter for you if she or he thinks you are likely to need several transfusions or large amounts of fluid at various stages of your treatment. It is installed in much the same way as the reservoir, except that, at the end of the procedure, a short length of plastic tube will be curled up under a dressing on the upper part of your chest. There are quite a lot of "dos and don'ts" about a Hickman, and, if you are willing to participate in its care, your nursing team will show you what to do. Some patients feel very good about participating in the care of their Hickman, while others prefer not to touch the catheter but to let the nursing team do it all. Either approach is acceptable.

Side Effects of Most Chemotherapy Drugs

Almost all chemotherapy drugs (but not hormone treatments) cause some side effects, the most common of which is nausea. A few, such as vincristine, do not; but most of the others may do so.

Fatigue and Exhaustion

Tiredness is a frequent side effect of most chemotherapy treatments. Chapter 10, "Living with Cancer," has a section on tiredness that also deals with the difficult question of when and whether to return to work. By and large, the worst of the tiredness begins to decrease three or four weeks after the end of chemotherapy, but the improvement happens slowly. It is quite usual for people to go for several months feeling noticeably less energetic than they did before the treatment.

Nausea

For reasons that we do not understand, most chemotherapy drugs affect a small center in the brain that is responsible for nausea and vomiting. This area is called the **chemotactic trigger zone**, or **CTZ**. It is not known why almost all chemotherapy drugs stimulate this area, as the drugs are so different in so many other respects. Table 5.1 shows the extent to which different chemotherapy drugs are likely to cause nausea.

In general, nausea caused by chemotherapy depends to a certain extent not just on the drug (see Table 5.1) but also on the dose and how it is given (as a single "push" injection or as a long intravenous infusion, for example). Nausea usually begins a few hours after the drug has been given; three to six hours is typical, though it is less for a few drugs. The most severe nausea usually continues for twenty-four to forty-eight hours or so. Typically it is gone by the second or third day (in many cases, before that), though you may find that your appetite is poor for a day or so after that. It is also helpful to know that very often nausea comes and goes in episodes. You may have no nausea at all in the middle of the second day, let's say, but then have a couple of hours when you feel somewhat nauseated again that evening.

Anticipatory Nausea Many patients find that the nausea begins earlier with each course of chemotherapy. This is often due to "conditioning" (in other words, a conditioned response is created in which your behavior is changed by the strong stimulus of the treatment). Thus, for example, you may come to associate the hospital with nausea and feel nausea when the hospital first comes into view or even when the name of the hospital or something else associated with it crops up. Some of my patients have told me that they experience nausea when they walk past the bus stop they usually use to go to the hospital, and one patient even retched at the sound of my voice when I telephoned her unexpectedly a year after therapy. (I hope you will believe me when I say that most of my patients do not usually retch at the sound of my voice!) This type of conditioning is called **anticipatory nausea** and is quite common: in fact, about one-third of all patients on chemotherapy may experience it. If it does happen to you, remember, first, that it is very common and is not a sign of going mad. Second, you may be able to help control it by taking your antinauseants (such as lorazepam) the night before you go for your chemotherapy.

Scapegoating Another form of conditioning has also been shown to occur with foods eaten in the few hours after the treatment. If, for example, you eat ravioli in the period just after chemotherapy, you may

TABLE 5.1: INCIDENCE OF NAUSEA CAUSED BY THE MOST COMMONLY USED CHEMOTHERAPY DRUGS

ALMOST ALWAYS CAUSE NAUSEA	OFTEN CAUSE NAUSEA	SOMETIMES CAUSE NAUSEA	RARELY CAUSE NAUSEA
cisplatin	dactinomycin	ifosfamide	5-fluorouracil
dacarbazine (DTIC)	cyclophosphamide (moderate doses)	etoposide	6-mercaptopurine
nitrogen mustard	Adriamycin	mitomycin-C	bleomycin
streptozotocin	carboplatinum	mitoxantrone	busulfan
carmustine	daunorubicin	procarbazine	chlorambucil
cyclophosphamide (high doses)	lomustine	epirubicin	melphalan
cytosine arabinoside (high doses)		asparaginase	methotrexate
			cytosine arabinoside
			hydroxyurea
			Taxol
			thioguanine
			thiotepa
			vinblastine
			vincristine
			vindesine
			vinorelbine

find after some weeks that every time you eat ravioli you feel nauseated. It is therefore worthwhile to try to avoid your favorite foods after your chemotherapy. In fact, some research has shown that you can "transfer" this conditioned response onto a scapegoat food by eating it immediately after the chemotherapy. In the research, this was done using halva, a sweet paste made of sesame flour and honey that is available almost everywhere but that few people eat regularly. I recommend this trick to some of my patients. Many of them have found it helpful to eat an unaccustomed food such as halva to deal with hunger after the chemotherapy in order to avoid transferring the conditioned nausea onto their favorite foods.

Treatment of the Nausea Caused by Chemotherapy (see Table 5.2). In the last ten years or so, and particularly in the last two or three years, considerable advances have been made in the treatment and

TABLE 5.2: MEDICATIONS USED FOR NAUSEA

NAME OR TYPE OF DRUG	EXAMPLE OF BRAND NAME	USUALLY GIVEN BY...	NOTES
metoclopramide	Maxeran	tablet or injection	Inhibits the CTZ and empties the stomach.
prochlorperazine	Stemetil	tablet, suppository, or injection	May cause drowsiness or occasionally restlessness.
domperidone	Motilium	tablet or injection	Helps stomach empty.
steroids (for example, dexamethasone)	Decadron	tablet or injection	Mechanism unknown—helpful in combination with other drugs.
lorazepam	Ativan	tablet or injection	Can be used night before. Also decreases memory of nausea.
H3 blockers (for example, ondansetron and granisetron)	Zofran, Kytril	tablet or injection	Very powerful if other medications not working. Effective only in first two or three days—no use later.
nabilone, dronabinol	Cesamet, Marinol	capsule	Synthetic analogue of a cannabis extract—works in some cases.
"anti–side effects" treatment	Benadryl	tablet or injection	Not an antinauseant but may be given to reduce the chance of side effects of some antinauseants that may cause stiffness of jaw or facial muscles.
"over the counter" antinauseants	Gravol	tablet or suppositories	Not meant to work when others don't but occasionally can be wonderfully helpful, particularly the long-acting preparations or the suppositories.

control of nausea. Thus nowadays a very high proportion of patients on even the most nausea-producing chemotherapy drugs have a relatively small number of episodes of vomiting, and many have no vomiting at all.

There are many different drugs that can be used to help you with nausea. They can be given in tablet form, by injections (with or before your chemotherapy), or by suppository. Suppositories are particularly useful if the nausea is bad because they can be used when you are unable to keep tablets down and also because the drug in the suppository is absorbed steadily over a period of hours.

One particularly useful group of drugs has been introduced in the last two or three years. These are the **H3 blockers** (a technical term that refers to the way they work). If the nausea is bad and does not improve with the standard antinauseants, these drugs (of which the most well known are ondansetron and granisetron) can be effective. For reasons that we do not understand, they work against chemotherapy-associated nausea only in the first two or three days, and there is no value in taking them after that time.

Notes (see Table 5.2): The table may give you some idea of the range of drugs available to treat nausea. It is important to be sure that you take the correct doses of the medications. Many people do not take enough of the drug, either taking too few tablets or not taking them often enough or both. Second, if you are having difficulty keeping the tablets down, talk to your doctor about the possibility of using suppositories. Third, chemotherapy-induced nausea is generally slightly worse in the morning so it may be a good idea to keep an antinauseant tablet on the bedside table to take first thing in the morning even before you get up.

Hair Loss

If you are being given chemotherapy that is likely to cause hair loss (see Table 5.3), you will start noticing the loss in about three to four weeks. Usually the hair loss proceeds quite quickly after that, and in some patients it can be complete in a few days. In others, the loss continues steadily over several weeks. If you have not had significant hair loss by about three months, in general that means it will not happen.

TABLE 5.3: HAIR LOSS WITH SOME OF THE MORE COMMONLY USED CHEMOTHERAPY DRUGS

DRUGS THAT ALMOST ALWAYS CAUSE HAIR LOSS	DRUGS THAT MAY CAUSE HAIR LOSS	DRUGS THAT RARELY CAUSE HAIR LOSS
Adriamycin	cyclophosphamide	platinum drugs
epirubicin	fluorouracil	vincristine
etoposide (VP-16)	vinblastine	bleomycin
nitrogen mustard		methotrexate
dactinomycin		mitomycin
Taxol		mitoxantrone
		melphalan
		procarbazine
		lomustine
		vinorelbine

The secret of coping with this is to be prepared. That means going to look at wigs (your nursing team or social services team can usually provide you with information) even before you start the therapy. It may be worth picking out a wig (though not necessarily buying it) so that you know what you will be wearing if it is needed. Many of my patients whose hair was long have bought short wigs. They tell me that not only do they get compliments on changing their hairstyle (most wigs are virtually undetectable as wigs these days), but as their own hair regrows, they can stop wearing the wig after a short time.

By and large, hair regrowth begins before the end of therapy, usually at about three or four months. Regrowth reaches a stage where you can do without a wig by about six to nine months or so. In general, the hair that regrows is softer and curlier and in some cases darker, too.

Scalp Cooling In a few cases it is possible to reduce the amount of hair loss, and sometimes prevent it altogether, by using scalp cooling. This involves putting a cap that has been cooled in a refrigerator onto the head. It needs to be in position for about ten minutes before the chemo and remain in place for about ten minutes afterward. It works only for those drugs that are excreted out of the bloodstream quickly; Adriamycin is one. A cold cap will not prevent hair loss with a drug that stays in the bloodstream for a long time (such as cyclophosphamide).

Infections

Because it affects your bone marrow, chemotherapy can reduce the number of white cells in your blood and lower your ability to fight infections. In general, the time of greatest risk begins about seven to ten days after chemotherapy. If the white cells are very low, they sometimes remain low for three weeks or so after that treatment. During that period you may be particularly prone to getting an infection. The common infections are **chest** infections (with a cough and green sputum) and **throat** infections (with a sore throat and pain on swallowing). A **generalized infection** may also occur, with severe chills, shivering, and fever without any particular problems detectable in the chest. Also possible are skin infections such as **boils**, infections around the **anus**, or **urinary tract** infections (passing urine frequently, pain on passing the urine, sometimes with pain in the loin region [around the lower back near the ribs]).

If you feel ill, and particularly if you feel feverish or have shivers, first **take your temperature**. If your temperature is over 100°F (37.5°C) on two occasions or over 100.4°F (38°C) once, contact your doctor. If you have an infection while your white cells are low, it may be difficult for your body to deal with it. This may mean that you will require antibiotics. These may be given by mouth in some circumstances, but you may also need to be admitted to the hospital for a week or so in order to receive intravenous antibiotics (see also page 125).

Anemia (Insufficient Hemoglobin or Too Few Red Cells)

Chemotherapy can also reduce the number of red cells (hemoglobin) in your blood, so that you become (temporarily) anemic. With anemia, you may look pale and feel tired and perhaps short of breath and weak. If those symptoms are severe, your doctor may decide that you need a blood transfusion.

Bruising and Bleeding

The platelets, which are also manufactured in the marrow, may also be reduced in number when the marrow is suppressed by chemotherapy. If that happens, you may get little pinhead-sized purple spots (like tiny bruises, which is what they are) in the skin. These are called **petechiae**, and you are most likely to see them on the shins. You may also get bleeding from the gums, the nose, or the digestive tract, which may cause you to bring up blood or a coffee groundlike material or to pass jet-black stool. You may also get large bruises within the skin.

If you get any of these problems, let your doctor know so that he or she can check your platelets. If they are very low, a transfusion of platelets may be recommended.

Precautions against Infection

While you are on chemotherapy, you can take several practical steps to decrease the chance of getting an infection. These are given on page 125.

Problems with Appetite and Taste

Both appetite and the sense of taste can be affected by chemotherapy, sometimes to a marked extent. Your appetite may remain poor for weeks or months at a time, and you may find that food tastes peculiar (often patients describe it as a metallic sort of taste). These are difficult symptoms to deal with. In general, it is worth trying out foods that you think might appeal to you and eating in smaller quantities but quite frequently. If you are still eating too little and losing weight, ask to talk to a dietitian about taking high-protein and high-carbohydrate supplements. These are usually liquids or puddings. The instant breakfast mixtures that you can buy at the supermarket may work well, too. If nothing is helping, your doctor may recommend medications such as Provera to increase your appetite.

Does a Special Diet Help?

Many of my patients ask this question. We hear so much about diet and also about the fact that people with major dietary deficiencies (usually in other parts of the world) may become anemic. Although logic suggests that taking extra care over your diet might reduce the side effects of chemotherapy, such is not the case. In fact, provided that your diet was a reasonably normal one before the chemotherapy, there is nothing you should change during therapy. The extent to which the chemotherapy affects the bone marrow is partly dependent on the way your body handles and excretes the drugs and partly on the sensitivity of your bone marrow to the drugs (which in turn depends on things like your age, the amount of chemotherapy you have had previously, and so on). If your bone marrow is greatly affected by the chemotherapy, you need not think that this is your fault or that there is something you should be doing (or eating) to prevent it.

Side Effects That Happen with Particular Chemotherapy Drugs

A few other side effects besides those mentioned above are relatively common. The most common of these are given in Table 5.4, not to alarm you or have you phoning your medical team, but to prepare you for some of the things that may happen and prevent you from panicking at unexpected developments. Most of these side effects go away by themselves.

High-Dose Therapy with Bone Marrow Rescue, Bone Marrow Transplantation, or Stem-Cell Rescue

A problem in treating certain types of cancers is the effect of the drugs on the patient's normal tissues. Very often the amount of a drug that can be given is limited because of the potential for damage to one part of the body or other. The particular tissue or organ that is most easily affected by a chemotherapy drug is called the **dose-limiting organ**, and with most chemotherapy drugs it is the bone marrow. Over the last twenty years it has been possible to devise ways in which higher doses of chemotherapy could be given. Many of these techniques have proved very effective in certain cancers (for instance, the leukemias, some of the lymphomas, and certain cases of Hodgkin's disease), although so far they have not made a major contribution to the treatment of the more common cancers, such as cancers of the lung, breast, ovary, or bowel. There are three basic procedures.

Bone Marrow Transplantation

The medical term for bone marrow transplantation when bone marrow from a donor is used is **allogeneic bone marrow transplantation**, but it is often referred to simply as "bone marrow transplantation"

TABLE 5.4: SIDE EFFECTS OF SOME CHEMOTHERAPY DRUGS		
TOXICITY	**SYMPTOMS YOU MIGHT NOTICE**	**EXAMPLES OF DRUGS THAT MAY CAUSE IT**
Sense of taste	A peculiar or metallic taste to food	Many drugs can do this.
Bowel lining and function	Diarrhea	Large number of drugs can do this, including fluorouracil.
Hearing	Loss of high-tone hearing, buzzing in ears	Platinum drugs
Nerves	Numbness or tingling in toes and fingers (occasionally with weakness)	Vincristine, platinum drugs
Motility of bowel	Bloated abdomen and no bowel action	Vinblastine
Kidney	Usually no symptoms, but blood tests show toxicity	Platinum drugs, several others
Skin pigment	Darkening of skin folds, sometimes mouth	Several, including bleomycin, fluorouracil. Many other drugs also make the skin more sensitive to sunlight, and so sunblocking creams are required. These include fluorouracil, dactinomycin, methotrexate, and others. Please check with your doctor.
Strength of heartbeat	Breathlessness, particularly worse when lying down	Adriamycin and drugs of the same group after many doses.
Fertility	Inability to start a pregnancy	Many drugs (and many tumors) may stop fertility. Ask your doctor.
Fetus	Abnormalities of fetus as it grows	Again, many drugs are potentially capable of this, so if you intend to start a pregnancy (or have started one) make sure your doctor knows.
Veins	Ache or pain over vein where drug injected	Many drugs are irritants to the lining of veins, but the commonest ones are Adriamycin, dactinomycin, nitrogen mustard, vincristine, dacarbazine, and Taxol.

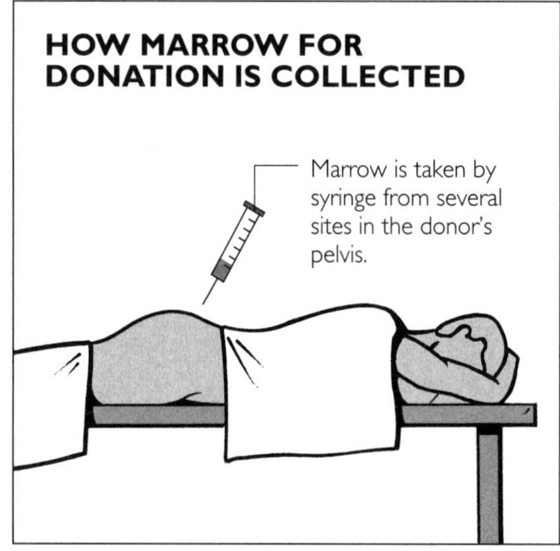

or **BMT**. (When the patient's own bone marrow is used the medical term is **autologous bone marrow transplantation** or **ABMT** [see the next section], although quite often the initials BMT are used to describe both procedures.) Allogeneic bone marrow transplantation is used where there is a primary cancer in the bone marrow; in practice, that means leukemia or other similar conditions. It is necessary to find a relative (or someone on a marrow registry) who has a bone marrow that is genetically very similar to the patient's. A proportion (less than 10 percent) of the marrow is collected from the donor (this involves a general anesthetic and multiple samples of marrow taken from the pelvis). The patient is then given high-dose treatment with chemotherapy with or without radiotherapy. The dose of treatment is very high and is intended to kill all of the cancer cells. Of course, it would also kill the patient if he or she were not "rescued" (the medical term) by the marrow from the donor. When the drug has been excreted by the patient, the marrow from the donor is given as a transfusion into a vein. After several days or a couple of weeks, the new bone marrow establishes itself ("takes" is the medical term) and begins to manufacture red cells, white cells, and platelets for the patient. The patient will usually have to take medications for a long time (perhaps indefinitely) to prevent the new marrow from rejecting the patient (this rejection is called **graft-versus-host** or **GVH** disease). This type of therapy is now the standard therapy for certain types of leukemia (particularly acute myeloid leukemia) and some lymphomas, if there is a suitable donor available.

Autologous Bone Marrow Transplantation (ABMT), Also Called High-Dose Treatment with Bone Marrow Rescue In ABMT the procedure is basically the same as with BMT, except that the patient is his or her own donor. The sample of marrow is collected from the patient first and then carefully preserved in a freezer. The patient then gets high-dose therapy of some description, and when the drugs have been excreted, the marrow is given back (again as a transfusion into a vein). This technique has also been useful in certain kinds of lymphoma and Hodgkin's disease and in one or two other cancers as well. At present, however, the high-dose treatment can only sometimes kill all the cancer cells when the cancer originated in such sites as the breast, lung, ovary, or some other sites. If this is an option, you should discuss with your doctor what chance there is that the treatment will be curative.

Stem-Cell Rescue In the last few years, it has been found that certain types of white cells from the bloodstream will do the job just as well as bone marrow cells. This procedure usually involves collecting the relevant white cells from the bloodstream after the person has been given medications to enhance the number of those cells. The process is called pheresis and is usually done using two intravenous lines. The blood comes out of one line, goes into a centrifuge, a machine that skims off the desired cells, and then is returned to the patient through the other line. This type of treatment is not

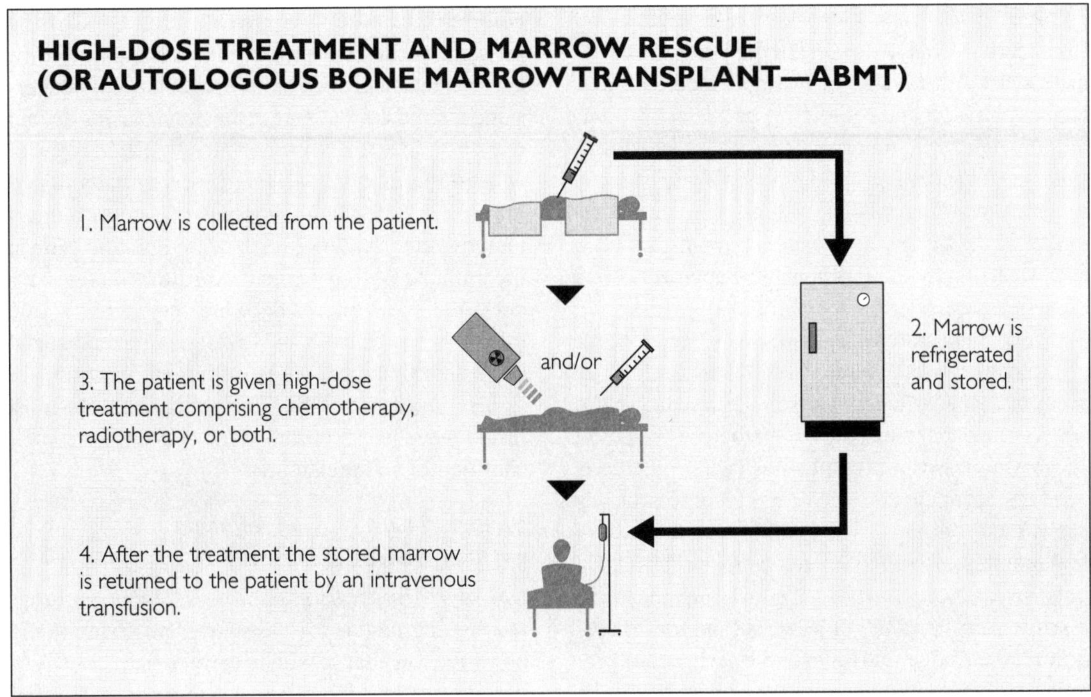

available everywhere but may prove to be useful in the future.

Biologic Therapy

Biologic therapy is in its infancy. It may develop over the next decade into a series of powerful weapons against cancer cells (perhaps to be used in treatment or perhaps to be used in prevention). At the moment, though, it is difficult to know which types of biologic therapy will be genuinely valuable and how and when they should be used. In this section I explain briefly a few of the more important types of biologic agents being investigated and used.

Biologic Therapy as Treatment of Cancer

Monoclonal Antibodies Monoclonal antibodies are explained in more detail in Chapter 9, "Advances in Understanding the Cancer Cell" (page 263). Briefly, they are pure, single antibodies produced in the laboratory to react against a single target. (In "natural" antibody production, when we get ill with, say, the flu, we produce dozens of antibodies against different parts of the flu virus.) When monoclonal antibodies were first invented, it was hoped that they would become the true magic bullets, capable of carrying poisons or radioactive isotopes directly to the targeted cancer cells while avoiding normal cells. There have been enormous problems in realizing these hopes for many reasons, four of which I will outline here. First, cancer cells are very similar to normal cells, and it is difficult to produce a monoclonal antibody that does not confuse the two; second, it is extremely difficult to deliver a sufficient amount of an antibody to the cancer cells for a long enough time to do the intended job; third, in many types of cancer the malignant cells seem to learn quite quickly how to deal with the antibodies; and fourth, the patient's immune system may sometimes produce an "anti-antibody" and dispose of the monoclonal antibody quickly.

Nevertheless, monoclonal antibodies can be useful in certain circumstances. In the laboratory they are used by the dozen in testing blood samples, cancer biopsies, and cells. They give an enormous amount of information about the nature and development of cancer cells and have changed the way in which pathology is done. Although their performance in the treatment of cancer patients has been somewhat disappointing, some of the approaches that have been investigated are of interest.

Monoclonal antibodies can carry small doses of radioactive isotope and can be used to show up areas of cancer when the person has a scan. So far, when used in treatment, they seem to have been most successful in certain lymphomas (where the body does not seem capable of raising an anti-antibody easily) and perhaps in certain selected cases of melanoma and primary liver cancer. They have been used successfully in cleaning up the bone marrow in certain kinds of leukemia and also to condition donor bone marrow so that it does not produce graft-versus-host disease. Unfortunately, monoclonal antibodies have not so far been used successfully in treatment of the more common tumors such as prostate and lung, though they are still being assessed in breast cancer. It is still hoped that a vaccine can be produced that will protect against certain forms of cancer, but that remains a theoretical possibility at the moment.

Interferons Interferons are substances produced by the immune system during acute infections (such as flu). Studies showed that interferons were active against various types of cancer cells. Many years of clinical studies have now shown that interferons are useful but only in certain types of cancer. In general, they are most valuable in the treatment of Kaposi's sarcoma (see pages 106–108). They are often used as the treatment of choice in chronic myelocytic leukemia (CML) and were also found to be useful in the treatment of hairy-cell leukemia, but have now been replaced by something better in the latter disease.

Interleukins and LAK Cells The interleukins, a group of substances produced by cells in the body, act as signals between cells. We do not fully understand all of the many things that interleukins do, but one of them is to activate or "arm" certain types of cells in the immune system. It was initially hoped that if helped by large amounts of a certain interleukin—interleukin-2 (or IL-2)—specific cells in the immune system would be able to obliterate cancer cells. The early results were very exciting. The treatment was difficult and hazardous, but occasional and remarkable responses were seen. With further studies, it seems that the effects of IL-2 may be most pronounced and useful in kidney cancer (renal cell carcinoma) and melanoma.

Biologic Therapy as an Adjunct to Other Cancer Treatments

Colony-Stimulating Factors (CSFs) Colony-stimulating factors are substances produced in the bone marrow that stimulate early precursor cells of the bone marrow to accelerate their production of mature cells (red cells, white cells, or platelets). In other words, CSFs can stimulate the marrow to increase and speed up its production of cells. When the marrow has been seriously affected by chemotherapy—and the patient has life-threatening infections, severe anemia, or bleeding—CSFs can speed recovery. The CSFs have different names, depending on which cells in the marrow they stimulate (G-CSF and GM-CSF are two). The CSF that stimulates red cells is called erythropoietin, usually abbreviated Epo.

Recent advances in techniques have made it possible to produce CSFs in large quantities. Their use with chemotherapy has shown that they do decrease the period of agranulocytosis (very low white cells). In general, however, they are used only when the consequences of marrow suppression are very severe (with life-threatening infections, for example) and where it is clear that proceeding with chemotherapy will make a major difference to the likelihood of achieving a cure or prolonged remission. They are not routinely used in every case in which chemotherapy causes a reduction in white or red cells or platelets.

What Is a "Clinical Trial"?

As one of my patients said, quite gently, to me: *"To put it mildly, Doctor, the treatment of most cancers these days is less than satisfactory."* And she was right. For those patients who are cured, most of the cures will be achieved by surgery, and some will be achieved by radiotherapy or chemotherapy. For most other patients, however, the medical profession is still trying to discover the best method of treatment. And that means that we are constantly looking for ways to improve the treatment.

In cancer treatment that usually means we have to undertake a detailed and careful comparison of any therapy that we believe might be an improvement with the standard treatment. This is usually done by means of what is called a clinical trial. The word "trial" is used to mean that the new treatment is being tried against the old, not that the patient (or the doctor) is on trial. There are different phases of the clinical testing of a new drug to establish the best schedule of giving the drugs and whether there are any important side effects, then in what types of tumors the drug is most active, and finally whether the new treatment is superior or not to the standard therapy. These phases are what are referred to as the "Phase I," "Phase II," and "Phase III" types of clinical trials.

Randomization In order to remove any bias that may come from the doctor (who may believe that he or she already knows the answer) or the patient, the patients are entered into the trial by randomization. That means that whether you get the standard treatment or the newer treatment is decided randomly by a computer in the central office of the trial. Although that sounds impersonal, it is the only way of making sure that the results are truly reliable. Imagine what would happen, for example, if a doctor believed that treatment X was better than treatment Y. He or she might put all the patients whom he or she thought would do well (say, the younger patients with smaller tumors) on treatment X and the older and more ill patients on treatment Y. The trial might then show that the patients on treatment X did fare better than those on treatment Y—not because of the treatment, but because of the way the patients were selected for each treatment. Thus randomization—computer coin-flipping, really—is the only way to make sure that the trial yields results that are reliable.

Closing the Trial If the Result Is Clear If a trial shows that one treatment really is dramatically better than the other, the trial will be stopped and everyone will receive the better treatment. This is not likely to happen unless the results are truly impressive. Nevertheless, it is important for patients to realize that they are not being denied access to any miracle treatment that may be found.

Standards of Care You may be tempted to think: *"If my doctor does not know what the best treatment is, surely he can't be much good."* The answer is that doctors who are actively looking for answers in cancer treatment are generally better at looking after their patients than doctors who are not. Several studies have shown that centers where clinical trials are carried out have a higher standard of overall care than centers where such trials are not being done. Presumably this is because the demands of organizing and running a trial keep standards up to a high level and provide a spinoff effect that benefits all patients whether they are in clinical trials or not.

Ethics All clinical trials have to be reviewed and approved by the hospital's or center's ethics committee. This guards against any chance of dishonest or unethical practices or treatment that is unfair or prejudicial to you. You will be asked to complete a detailed consent form (which will previously have been assessed in detail by the ethics committee) and will be given a copy to keep. If you simply cannot tolerate the treatment any more, or for any other reason wish to stop being in the clinical trial, you have that right. You just have to tell your doctor what you wish. Obviously your doctor hopes that you will not want to do that, but you can if you want to, and the relationship with your doctor—and the care you receive—will not suffer as a result.

Why It's Worth Considering a Clinical Trial

Clinical trials are the only way knowledge advances. It was the way the world learned about the benefits of the adjuvant treatment of breast cancer, the best treatment of childhood leukemia, the fact that bone marrow transplants worked for adult leukemia, and many other aspects of treatment. Trials are awkward things to think about, for the doctor as well as the patient. We have to admit that we do not know the answers, and we are therefore asking for your help in finding out how to improve treatment. Many patients initially feel that they are guinea pigs, and to some extent that is true. Until we know the best and definitive treatment of cancer, every patient will be a guinea pig. A clinical trial is, however, a way of acquiring firm and reliable information. Although clinical trials require a lot of work from the medical team and a certain amount of cooperation from the patient, at present they are our only means of making true and credible progress against cancer.

COMPLEMENTARY, ALTERNATIVE, OR UNCONVENTIONAL TREATMENTS

6

What's in This Chapter

In this section I explain the chief differences between conventional medical practice and the practices of complementary medicine. I then show why it is that complementary medicine is so attractive to many people. As that attraction may depend partly on stories of unexpected or even miraculous cures or benefits, I discuss several of the possible explanations for these.*

By Way of Definition

Complementary (or "alternative," "unconventional," "unproven") treatments for cancer, or for any other condition, are difficult to define. In fact, the only thing that all complementary medicines have in common is what they are not. They are not conventional treatments. That means that we first require some sort of definition of conventional treatments. That is also difficult and itself requires a definition: of what is meant by conventional physicians and conventional medicine. Let's define conventional doctors as doctors who have been trained in medical schools licensed by the governments of their countries, practicing medicine in a way that is approved by the regulatory boards in place. Then we may define conventional treatments as treatments given by those conventional doctors or physicians (and their associated health care professionals, including nurses, physiotherapists, psychotherapists, and so on) that would be regarded as acceptable by the majority of their peers. You will notice these definitions mean that not everything a conventional doctor does is a priori conventional treatment. If one doctor happens to prescribe brown rice as a treatment for tennis elbow, that does not mean that this is by definition the conventional treatment.

The Frontier

These definitions imply that the most important criterion of conventional medicine is general acceptance (of the treatment and the physician) within the medical profession. Naturally we (in the conventional medical profession) hope that nowadays this type of acceptance will be based on objective and valid proof of benefit or (if that proof is not yet available) on a demonstrable method of gathering evidence that will produce proof in time. And this brings us to a partial definition of the frontier between conventional medicine and complementary medicine. In conventional medicine we are

* Some of this section is adapted from *Magic or Medicine?* by R. Buckman and K. Sabbagh (Amherst: Prometheus Books, 1995).

constantly trying to test and prove that what we do *is* genuinely beneficial in dealing with disease or symptoms. It must be said at the outset that this is a task that has been only partially accomplished. In fact, it has been estimated that of all the things that are done or prescribed in clinical medicine, only 15 percent have actually been tested and are objectively proven effective (which means that 85 percent of what we do is the result of habit, fashion, personal belief, or arbitrary decision making). For all new treatments, however—and particularly for all new treatments of cancer—there is now major pressure (backed by law in the case of new drugs) on any doctor or scientist who believes in a treatment to prove the validity of his or her approach. That is why the clinical trials that I mentioned in Chapter 5 are so important. In fact, the clinical trial can be seen as an attempt by conventional medicine to *dis*prove its latest brainchild: if the clinical trial shows that the new treatment is no better than the standard treatment, the new one will be abandoned. That method of proving (by attempting to disprove) the value of a treatment is the hallmark of conventional medicine. Admittedly that hallmark is not (yet) stamped on a high proportion of what we do, but in cancer treatment, and particularly in the last two decades, it has become a genuine and widely respected method of defining and changing clinical practice.

By contrast, in complementary medicine this activity (of testing a treatment and comparing it to another treatment) is absent. There have been a few clinical trials of complementary medicine treatments (for instance, of laetrile), and they were started and organized by conventional physicians and scientists. Such studies can be done and may show impressive results. In fact, some of the studies of complementary medicine remedies in other conditions (that is, not in cancer) have shown astounding and objectively valid proof of the efficacy of the treatment. For example, a flawless study of a Chinese herbal remedy for childhood eczema proved that the remedy was far superior to a "dummy" remedy made from a batch of other Chinese herbs when used in children whose eczema had already shown itself to be unresponsive to conventional steroid treatment. With respect to another condition, two well-conducted studies of chiropractic manipulation for low back pain showed that it was better than conventional treatment.

These studies indicated that it is possible and practical to do research into remedies in complementary medicine and, where the remedy was truly of benefit, to demonstrate and prove its efficacy. In general, however, such cases are the exception rather than the rule. Most practitioners of complementary medicine do not present their accumulated experience with a particular disease in a way that allows comparison with other approaches. They usually (if they present any data at all) offer anecdotal evidence based on one or two cases plus personal testimonials from their patients.

Although the benefits of the majority of treatments used in complementary medicine have not been scientifically verified, practitioners of complementary medicine do often benefit their patients. In fact, testimony from literally thousands of patients shows that people who use complementary medicine almost always feel better. In the rest of this chapter I want to discuss why that is and also why such improvements do not necessarily prove the value of a particular treatment for cancer. First, however, it's important to understand why complementary medicine is so attractive and what it is that people get from practitioners of complementary medicine that they may not be getting from conventional physicians.

Advantages of Complementary Medicine

There are many aspects of complementary medicine that make it attractive to patients. I have listed most of them at length in a previous book, but the main general concepts—the philosophical attractions of complementary medicine—are summarized here in Table 6.1.

TABLE 6.1: PHILOSOPHICAL ATTRACTIONS OF COMPLEMENTARY MEDICINE	
BASIS OF REMEDY	**WHAT THE IDEA IS**
Concept of health	Treatment not only conquers disease but establishes positive health.
Concept of force or energy	Treatment harnesses universal natural forces.
Unifying hypothesis of disease	Treatment corrects an imbalance or counteracts negative force(s).
Concept of self-healing	Forces are accessible within patient that can reverse course of disease.
Concept of the natural	Natural products are inherently better than synthetic products.
Concept of the traditional	Folk wisdom preserves knowledge that ancestors had that was lost.
Concept of the exotic	Different cultures offer knowledge previously unavailable to people of this culture.
Concept of David and Goliath	"Little man" finds answer to major question (for example, cure for cancer) where the might of national or industrial bodies has failed.
Concept of justice	Cure is available to those whose attitudes and beliefs mark them as worthy of it.

What We Want When We Are Ill

It is our individuality or personhood that is most threatened when there is disease. As I said in *Magic or Medicine?*:

> Whatever the cause of disease, the person who suffers from it is threatened with the loss of personal significance unless someone helps him or her rediscover it. Conventional doctors are rarely good at helping the patient with that process: complementary practitioners usually are.

The three major needs that we all have when we are threatened by illness seem to be these: support, participation in control, and hope.

When we are ill we all wish for support, which implies a measure of acceptance by the other person. A rather ugly but probably correct phrase for this is "unconditional positive regard." In conventional medicine we have only just begun to relearn the art of giving support. We are improving rapidly but practitioners of complementary medicine have been good at it for centuries.

Anyone who is ill would like to feel that he or she has some measure of control over the process. The ideal would be to control the disease, but if that is not possible the next best thing is to have at least some control over the treatment. If that is not possible, most people would want some control over the information. In many respects the patient's action in seeking out a practitioner of complementary medicine is a way of taking control of the illness.

The question of hope could be the subject of an entire book on its own. Much of the attraction of complementary medicine stems from the anecdotal evidence it offers of unexpected or miraculous responses, often cures. Because it is important to view stories such as these with some sense of perspective, I discuss some alternative explanations for some of this anecdotal evidence below. It is not my intention to be curmudgeonly and purely negative about these stories. However, in the two and a half years that I spent investigating such stories, I often found that there were alternative explanations that had not been considered.

Possible Explanations of Inexplicable Miracles

No Facts

Of all the explanations of unexpected responses in cancer patients, perhaps the most frequent is that there are no facts available. As an example, here is something that occurred during our research for a television series about complementary medicine.

> A woman in her mid-fifties telephoned our researcher (in response to an advertisement) to say that she had been cured of bowel cancer by herbal treatments recommended to her by an iridologist (an iridologist is a complementary medicine practitioner who diagnoses disease by looking at the iris of the eye) seven years earlier. She said that she had previously been seen at a local hospital by a conventional gastroenterologist who had done a biopsy and told her that she had bowel cancer and needed surgery. The researcher was very impressed by the story, so I asked the researcher to obtain the exact date of the biopsy so that I could get it reevaluated. I suspected that the biopsy would show a premalignant condition, in other words, that the patient had a *risk* of developing cancer, not cancer itself. The woman told our researcher the exact dates, and I contacted the pathology department of that hospital. We searched the pathology records using three different spellings of the woman's name and several variations on her birthdate. We also looked in the previous two years and the two subsequent years. There was no record of any biopsy. At this point I telephoned the woman myself (not having spoken to her directly before that). She confirmed what she had said to the researcher. When I asked her about the biopsy, she then said she had not had a biopsy but that the gastroenterologist had told her that he did not like the look of her colon. In other words, there was no proof that this particular patient had ever had cancer or even a risk of it.

I am not saying that this woman was deliberately misleading our researcher, but I do feel that she gave in to wishful thinking. She very much appreciated the attention of her iridologist and was, in her view, simply trying to amplify the benefit of what she thought the iridologist had done for her. Yet three other members of the office staff who heard this story firmly believed, when they first heard it, that it was proof that cancer could be cured by herbal remedies. It was only because I was able to track down the essential evidence that it was possible to see that there was none. Had I been unable to search the records of that hospital, this story might have gone unchallenged as a proof of a complementary medicine treatment of bowel cancer. We found many such examples during our research.

> A similar exchange occurred during a television phone-in program in which I was involved. A woman telephoned and said that she had founded a complementary health center where complementary medicine practitioners and conventional doctors worked side by side. She said that they used methods of treatment that helped patients with diseases such as multiple sclerosis, and that by doing some diagnostic tests before and after treatment, they had proven the effectiveness of their therapy in up to 60 percent of cases.
>
> I was somewhat dubious about this claim, as I was not aware of any diagnostic tests that could give objective measurements in this way in multiple sclerosis. The woman and I wrote

> to each other over the course of the following eighteen months, during which correspondence I pressed her to let me see the results of those tests that could substantiate her claim. At last she admitted that there were no such results and that because hers was not a research center, there never would be any such results.

I don't doubt that her patients felt better after attending her clinic, but in my opinion it was untruthful of her to make an unsubstantiated claim like that on public television, and it was unfair to any patients with multiple sclerosis who might have been watching the program.

Premature Reporting

Another reason why anecdotes of individual cases may be misleading is that results may be reported prematurely. In other words, the patient may sincerely believe that he or she is cured and that an unexpected or miraculous remission has occurred, but it may not be so. This will not intrinsically harm the patient him- or herself—after all, it may be very beneficial to believe that you are doing well and to have a genuinely positive attitude. Unfortunately, the story may mislead people into believing that treatment has a genuine effect when it does not. Perhaps the most widely known story is that of the much-loved movie actor Steve McQueen.

> Steve McQueen had a mesothelioma, a rare and extremely aggressive form of cancer, which in his case occurred in the abdomen. His conventional physicians told him that there was nothing further they could do, and so he went to a private clinic in Mexico. There he was given a variety of treatments including herbal remedies, colonic irrigation, diet supplements, and meditation. Steve McQueen was so impressed by the way he felt that he made a public broadcast on Mexican radio thanking the president and people of Mexico for allowing the clinic to exist and allowing him to be cured of his disease. On the recording, he sounded extremely ill, and in fact he died a few weeks later after a hazardous part of his treatment at the clinic that involved surgery.

At the time that broadcast went out, most listeners—particularly because they so revered Steve McQueen and wanted him to recover—believed that he had been cured. In fact, many people still believe that today. When a person announces, *"I have been cured,"* it is very difficult to say, *"Perhaps things are going well now, but to call it a cure may be overoptimistic."* Another example occurred a few months ago when I was giving a talk.

> After my talk, I invited questions and comments from the audience. One man asked me why it was that he had not been told about the long-term risks of treatment, adding that he had beaten cancer against all the odds. The audience applauded. He and I happened to talk after the lecture, and I asked him (guessing from what he had said) whether his cancer was actually a low-grade lymphoma. He said that it was. I asked him how long ago it had been diagnosed, and he told me just over a year.

Low-grade lymphoma is one of the rare cancers that fluctuates (with or without treatment), and many patients have long periods of time when they are completely free of disease. In fact, the average survival with this condition is many years (more than seven, probably), so that any statement about having beaten the disease against all the odds at one year after diagnosis is premature. Similar stories are very common. I met several women who were taking complementary medicine remedies after recent surgery for breast cancer (which is very unlikely to recur in the first year), people who had had lymphomas or bowel cancer diagnosed in the last year or so and who also did not yet know whether or not they had truly been cured. Thus prematurity is one possible explanation of a personal history of recovery.

Variations in Natural History

Another possible explanation is the variability of many forms of cancer. Cancer does not behave "by the book" in every case. For example, if there is a particularly aggressive form of cancer that, let's say, usually results in the patient's death within two years in 95 percent of cases, that still means that one out of every twenty patients will be alive beyond that time. I have seen many such cases myself. When I was a junior doctor, one of the first patients I looked after was Brian, a man with acute myeloid leukemia. At that time there was virtually no treatment for it, and yet Brian was alive and completely well nearly three years after diagnosis. He was an immensely likable man, and we were all very glad for him, but the disease did eventually progress. Similarly, I remember Phyllis, a woman with malignant melanoma that had spread to her liver (many years after the initial diagnosis), who remained alive and functioning for more than four years with those metastases in the liver—something that happens very rarely. Another patient of mine at present has breast cancer with metastases in the lungs that have remained basically the same size for more than three years despite her refusal to take any treatment. These are all examples of how impressive and memorable individual stories can be if they concern something that is very different from the average course of events.

Simultaneous Conventional Therapy

Another possible explanation for an apparently unexpected or miraculous remission may be that the patient was receiving conventional treatment at the same time as the complementary medicine remedy. This can happen even without the patient's consciously realizing it.

> A couple of years ago I interviewed a woman who was a co-founder of a very well-known complementary cancer help center in Britain. She herself had had breast cancer and had written a book in which she outlined the various complementary medicine remedies she had used. At one point the breast cancer recurred on the chest wall, and it was recommended she take tamoxifen. She then went on to write about various herbs and other treatments and said that her conventional doctor was later very surprised to find the cancer was not behaving as he expected. When I interviewed her, it turned out that she had in fact been taking tamoxifen for several years during this whole period. I do not know whether she realized that tamoxifen causes regression of breast cancer (if it is receptor-positive, as hers was) in about 60 percent of cases. In other words, the course of her disease was exactly as one would have expected in those circumstances. Another woman I interviewed in Mexico told me, point-blank, that she was not taking any medication for her cancer (breast cancer with positive lymph nodes) except the complementary medicine remedies given to her by the clinic. After our filmed interview, I asked her again, and it was only at this stage that she remembered that she had indeed been taking tamoxifen every day since her surgery two years ago. Had we shown the filmed interview as she gave it, the viewer would have believed that the complementary medicine remedies were controlling her breast cancer.
>
> Another patient of mine received what she had been told were alternative remedies. She showed me the bill for these remedies, and I was surprised to see that among the nonconventional substances that she had been given were some standard chemotherapy drugs. She and her husband were extremely upset that she had been given chemotherapy without knowing it. Had her disease responded to them, she also might have believed that alternative remedies can control cancer.
>
> More recently, a man with Kaposi's sarcoma (a tumor that occurs frequently in AIDS) wrote an article about his treatment. He had Kaposi's sarcoma in both lungs and had been taking an

extract of shark cartilage. The tumors got worse, and his doctors gave radiotherapy to one lung (Kaposi's sarcoma quite often responds to radiotherapy). The tumors in the lung that got the radiotherapy began to shrink, whereas those in the other lung did not. The patient's interpretation was that the shark cartilage must have had something to do with it (despite the fact that the shark cartilage was taken by mouth and therefore reached the tumors in both lungs) and that the radiotherapy could not have been the cause of the improvement (despite the fact that only the irradiated lung showed improvement, as one would expect with Kaposi's sarcoma). Here again it requires some understanding of cancer and its treatment to put the patient's interpretation in perspective.

There are many such examples. One complementary medicine clinic in Mexico is quite open about its use of conventional medicine, and the patients there regularly—routinely, in fact—receive chemotherapy and radiotherapy in addition to their complementary medicine remedies such as laetrile. Hence any statements about the efficacy of a complementary medicine remedy (as opposed to a conventional treatment) need to be evaluated very carefully, because many patients receive (knowingly or unknowingly) conventional treatment at the same time.

Misinterpretation

There are several ways in which it is possible to misinterpret what a doctor says, and this may lead to an apparently unexpected outcome. Selective recall is one of these. Discussion of the prognosis is one of the most emotionally charged conversations imaginable. As a result, what is recalled and recounted may not be necessarily what the doctor said. Many patients ask directly, *"How long have I got?"* And many doctors, myself included, feel that we have to give an honest answer and not simply avoid the discussion altogether. In almost every situation, no one can say exactly what is going to happen, but it is usually possible to give the most likely range of possibilities. For example, there might be a type of cancer in which, in an advanced stage, half of the patients will be alive at two years, and 5 percent will be alive at five years. It would be fair to say that probably the prognosis is measured in a small number of years for most people, but a few will do better than that. The patient may then ask whether that means the prognosis could be less than a year or two years. As a few people in this situation will die of the disease in a short time—say, less than six months—the doctor might say. *"Yes, this could happen, but it is not very likely."* The patient might then ask, and many people do, *"Do you mean I might not be around in three months?"* The doctor might reply, *"Well, that is not very likely, but it could happen."* The patient might then say to a friend or relative, *"That doctor gave me three months."* If the patient then uses a complementary medicine remedy and is alive at two years (as half of all such patients would be anyway), often the credit for that extension of prognosis is given to the complementary remedy.

On another occasion, during the making of our television series, I received a letter from a man who said that three years earlier he had had a sarcoma on his left thigh. CT scans of his lungs had shown secondary tumors, which would usually mean that his chance of surviving would be very small. His doctors had treated the tumor on his thigh (with surgery and radiotherapy to the leg) but had given him no treatment for the secondaries. He then embarked on a major lifestyle change, taking up intensive prayer, meditation, psychotherapy, dietary change, and exercise. Now he was completely well. Once again, several members of the production staff took this as clear evidence that lifestyle change, including prayer and meditation, could of itself control the growth of cancer. We visited the hospitals where he had been treated and had had the lung CT scans. In fact, his first CT scan had shown two shadows that his doctors thought might be secondaries but could be other things, including little pieces of scar tissue. They had told him that and had also said that they would repeat the scans every three months. If the shadows got bigger, that would prove they were secondaries; if they stayed the same, that would suggest they were scars. In fact, the shadows stayed the same size, which meant that they were scars after all. It turned out that the man had had some exposure to asbestos when he was younger, asbestos being one of the substances that often leaves tiny scars in the lungs. When we interviewed the patient a little later, he said that he did remember being told that the shadows had remained the same size and therefore were not secondaries. However, as the reaction of our production team showed, it would have been very easy to accept this patient's version of events at face value and therefore believe that there was evidence that cancer was controllable by lifestyle changes.

Wrong Diagnosis

In some cases the diagnosis is wrong. Such errors are not very common, but they do happen. A recent article in a medical journal identified six such cases in a hospice. All of these people had been admitted for care at the end of life, having been told that they had a terminal illness. In review, it turned out that the diagnosis had been wrong. Occasional misdiagnoses do happen, particularly with certain cancers where distinguishing a true cancer from a benign or less aggressive condition may be difficult. (For example, once in a while a small-cell lung cancer might be indistinguishable from a much more slow-growing tumor called a well-differentiated neuroendocrine carcinoma.)

> A patient of mine who is very much alive and well had breast cancer diagnosed fourteen years ago. (That in itself is not remarkable—many patients may be cured after primary surgery.) Nine years ago she developed an enlarged lymph node in the neck, and a biopsy was done, which showed recurrent cancer. This condition (recurrence in the neck) is not usually curable. At that time it was the standard treatment to remove the ovaries to change the hormonal environment. However, shortly afterward she developed another lump in the neck, which was monitored for several years and did not change in size. It was believed by the doctors looking after her that she had recurrent breast cancer that was, for some unknown reason, stable. She then moved away and was referred to see me because I was geographically the nearest. With the benefit of not having assessed her before, I was puzzled by the lump in her neck and ordered a CT scan. The lump turned out to be not cancer but a malformation of the vertebral body called a cervical rib. Having had biopsy-proven cancer in the neck nearly ten years previously, this woman had (probably) been cured by the removal of her ovaries and now was free of cancer, although she had a cervical rib. Had she been taking any complementary medicine remedies, her case might have been widely publicized as a case of incurable cancer held in check for a decade by the remedy. As it was, she had probably been cured (although such cases are very unusual) by the second operation.

Spontaneous Remissions

Spontaneous remission (or spontaneous regression) means that the cancer gets smaller or disappears completely (and with no new tumors developing) without any conventional treatment. A pathologist called William Boyd collected a large series of such instances, all documented in great detail, in a book he published in 1961. He estimated that approximately one in every 100,000 cases of cancer will show spontaneous regression. In his series, collected from data extending over a hundred years, more than half of the proven cases of spontaneous regression came from four types of tumor. Those types were: renal-cell cancer, melanoma (the pigmented cancer of the skin), neuroblastoma (a rare cancer of childhood), and choriocarcinoma (a rare cancer of the placenta). In the other half of the cases, there were one or two examples of almost every type of cancer. These facts are very important. First, they prove that almost any type of cancer can regress without apparent cause. Second, they show that spontaneous regression is much more common among those four rare types of cancer than it is among all the others. It has to be said that, in melanoma, skin lesions frequently regress. In fact, the chance that any particular skin lesion will shrink at some stage is about 10 percent, but this usually happens while other skin lesions are growing, and this type of regression would not be included in a definition of true spontaneous regressions.

Feeling Better versus Getting Better

Do the explanations listed above explain the very widespread, almost universal, feelings of satisfaction and benefit that most patients experience when they go to a complementary medicine practitioner? Of course not. Most patients who try complementary medicine come out of the experience *feeling* better, whether or not they are *getting* better. Many of my patients who see complementary medicine practitioners state, honestly and genuinely, that they feel better. And they may feel better even while tests (say blood tests of liver function or measurements of the tumor) show that the cancer is progressing. Feelings of improvement are an end in themselves (as one patient said, *"Feeling good is good in itself"*), even though they should not be confused with a true regression of the cancer.

Sometimes there are additional reasons why the patient may feel better. For example, at a recent faith healing demonstration in Britain, the healer brought on a nine-year-old girl who had a rare cancer in the bones. (It was, I later found out, a neuroblastoma.) She was on very high doses of morphine but could walk only with difficulty. In the presence of more than ten thousand people, the healer encouraged her to get out of her wheelchair, which she did. She walked across the stage, and the healer told her that the next time she saw her doctor, she would be told she had no cancer in her bones. Sadly he was wrong, and the poor girl died a few weeks later. Why had she been able to walk? Partly because the healer and the entire audience so wanted her to get well that she overcame (probably subconsciously) her feelings of pain and was able for a moment to stand and walk.

A few months after this, I experienced the value of that kind of support for myself.

> I went to a healing ceremony in Mexico at which, each year, it is thought that a charismatic healer called El Niño is reincarnated inside the body of one of his followers. I was there to observe the ceremony, but (without my knowledge) the film producer told the healer that I was ill and partially crippled (both of which are quite true). Suddenly, in the middle of the ceremony, the healer turned to me, and all the audience also focused on me. Without warning I was suddenly the center of more than a hundred people's attention and wishes—and prayers—for my recovery. Although I did not believe in the reincarnation or the healing powers of El Niño, the feeling that I experienced in that instant was tremendous. It was like being warmed and wrapped up in a cozy blanket of affection and regard. I felt, as I have never felt at any other time, that here were dozens of people sincerely wanting me to get well. It was a truly remarkable and pleasant moment. It did not make any difference to my physical disability, but it certainly made me feel wonderful and taught me the value of knowing that other people want you to get well.

Should You Try a Complementary Medicine Anyway?

For all these reasons, then, remedies touted as being effective against cancer may not be so. Knowing that that might be the case, then, should you go to Mexico or Switzerland or Zaire or Berlin and try the herbal remedy or the ozone therapy or the laetrile or the shark cartilage? Like so many things in life, it matters more *why* you do something than *whether* you do it.

If you go to try a complementary medicine remedy with the attitude that it would be nice if it worked, and would not be a disaster if it didn't, and if you can afford it (in terms of money and time), then you will lose nothing by going and may feel a fair bit better in yourself for doing it. If, on the other hand, you feel desperate and want more than anything else to be cured, and are prepared to sell anything and go anywhere to get a cure, then you are setting yourself up for serious disappointment and may find that you have lost both time and money when both are scarce. So in some respects the most important question to ask yourself is not *"Shall I go?"* but *"What are my feelings about going and what am I expecting?"*

Summary: Hopes and Facts

In conventional medicine, treatments appear that are at first greeted with tremendous enthusiasm (often overenthusiasm) and may earn headline phrases such as "major breakthrough." Over the next few years, these new treatments are usually evaluated and found to be less astounding than was first thought, and the situations in which they are most useful are more carefully and accurately defined. Thus interleukin-2 was at first, not inappropriately, hailed as the dawn of a new age. Now it is seen as a very important therapy for renal-cell cancer and melanoma. Similarly, Taxol was first thought to be a quantum leap ahead of the current treatment of ovarian cancer. Now it is seen as an active agent in ovarian cancer therapy, perhaps deserving to be used in the first-line therapy of that cancer, and perhaps having something to offer in the treatment of drug-resistant breast cancer as well, but not a miracle drug. If we go back twenty-five years, the same pattern emerged for L-asparaginase (at first heralded as the major breakthrough for childhood leukemia, now used as part of the therapy), for interferon (now used in the treatment of Kaposi's sarcoma), for bone marrow transplants (now part of the standard therapy for certain leukemias and lymphomas), and for many others. In conventional medicine, reevaluation usually leads eventually to finding a well-defined place for a drug or a treatment.

In complementary medicine, that process does not usually happen. Laetrile was thought to be a major advance in treatment. It is still used by a few practitioners, but none of them can say which cancers it is useful for and which it is not. Similarly, nobody can demonstrate under which circumstances iscadore is most effective or essiac or shark cartilage. Although there are tides of fashion and usage in both conventional medicine and complementary medicine, those tides leave a firm and well-established pattern in conventional medicine but not (usually) in complementary medicine. In complementary medicine, almost all remedies will have a phase of high popularity that lasts five to ten years, and then the remedy fades from view. Few people nowadays use Hoxey's remedies or Colley's toxin or the apple cider vinegar-and-honey diet.

It is so difficult to keep a cool head when you are a patient with cancer and you feel that your clock is ticking and that your conventional doctors have told you the situation is not curable. Yet I hope that the information I have given you in this section will at least give you a sense of perspective and perhaps allow you a bit of intellectual breathing space to evaluate what you are being told (by anyone) and to decide whether it is what you really want.

CANCER, ATTITUDES, AND THE MIND

7

What's in This Chapter

This section deals with the most controversial aspect of cancer, the role of the mind. There are two important questions here, and each is a center of great debate and argument. First, there is the question whether a person's attitudes or the psychological events in his or her life or personality may contribute to *causing* cancer (or protecting against it). Second, there is the question whether the mind can affect the outcome of cancer: if a person has cancer, will a change in attitude or personality, of itself, alter the *progress* of the cancer? The arguments on both sides of these two issues are exceedingly complex.

A related issue, one that has been pushed into the background of this debate, concerns the value of changing one's attitudes and coping skills not with the sole objective of prolonging life but for the sake of enhancing the *quality* of life. In the debate about whether attitudes can cause or help in fighting cancer, we seem to have largely overlooked the value of trying to change one's responses to what is happening purely for the sake of coping with the situation better. As one of my patients put it: *"Even if feeling better is not the same as getting better, isn't feeling better a whole lot better than feeling worse?"*

Humankind's Attitude to Cancer

In order to place this discussion in the right context, we need to look briefly at the origins of our current attitudes to cancer. As we shall see, several different diseases have, in past centuries, filled the bogeyman role that cancer does now.

Of course, we have had cancer in the human species almost since its origin. But at earlier times in our history, other diseases were more terrible and more dreaded. Cancer was not, until recently, one of the Four Horsemen of the Apocalypse. In our past it was no less serious a disease than it is today, but there were other diseases that were far more threatening and catastrophic. So although cancer was known and recognized, it was way behind bubonic plague, smallpox, tuberculosis, syphilis, cholera, and many others.

It is only recently, in fact only during the last few decades, that many of the infectious diseases that used to be the true scourges of civilization have been brought under control, and even then only in the developed countries. It was when the impact of those diseases was reduced that cancer rose to its current prominence in our consciousness.

Historical Attitudes to Illness

That prominence is not really a matter of statistics; it is a matter of perception. Diseases have always been part of humankind's mythology as well as the environment. Diseases traditionally have been regarded as more than simple physical afflictions. They have always been laden with symbolism and in the past were often seen as part of the divine machinery by which the world is regulated. Hence the designation of Plague or Pestilence as one of the Four Horsemen. Many diseases—even non-infectious ones such as epilepsy, Down's syndrome, hypothyroidism, and others—were commonly regarded as visitations from God or the Furies. Sometimes they were thought of as instruments of divine justice and the ultimate and equitable punishment for wickedness. Many people in the Middle Ages thought that the Black Death was God's second Flood, a way of ridding the world of evil. Sometimes diseases were regarded as random shafts of unpredictable arbitrary death, and sometimes as reminders that we are a puny and humble species and deserve to be shown our place from time to time.

The interpretation of illness—the meaning that we apply to an illness and then appear to take from it—is part of our way of coping with what we do not understand. For a brilliant analysis of the role of illness in our social consciousness, it is worth reading Susan Sontag's book *Illness as Metaphor*.

Cancer, then, is the contemporary bearer of the symbolic baggage that mysterious illnesses have borne through the centuries. In fact, the process seems to begin quickly and effortlessly anew with any new illness. In the case of AIDS, for example, even nowadays there are people who regard AIDS as an instrument of divine retribution and an inevitable consequence not of our physical habits but of our moral laxity.

Thus a major source of our current dread of cancer is the attitude that we have always had about mysterious illness, of which cancer is now the foremost example.

Diseases and Longevity

Another factor that may contribute to the magnitude of the threat is the apparent epidemic of cancer we are experiencing.

Cancer is predominantly a disease of the older age group—the late fifties, the sixties, and beyond. A century ago, because not many people reached that age, cancer appeared to be rarer. Nowadays, partly because we can control many of the major infectious diseases, and partly because of measures to improve the general health of the population, the proportion of people in our society who are in their seventies and older is higher than it has ever been. Thus cancer, among other problems of advancing years, is more common than it has ever been because there are more people of the right age to get it. In short, it is not an epidemic.

Can the Mind Cause Cancer?

Because cancer inspires such a feeling of dread, we tend to search for understanding of the cause of the disease and of its course wherever we can. In their hunger for explanations, many people turn to the idea that cancer may be the consequence of an unhealthy mental attitude or of major stressful incidents in a person's life. Healers, doctors, writers, patients, and people from many different disciplines and parts of our society suggest—or even state as a proven fact—that by some means cancer is the outward expression of unresolved emotional processes involving either moods or life events or both. Although there are many variations on this theme, in general, they all suggest that in some way the person who later develops cancer has partly contributed to causing it by bottling up emotions, by not expressing anger, by allowing external stresses to build up internally, or by some other psychological "error."

Clearly, if this were proven to be true, the world would be a more understandable place and perhaps more fair and just. It would, in some respects, be a form of justice if the people who held unhealthy attitudes had a high risk of developing cancer, and if the people who had the correct attitudes or beliefs could thereby reduce the chances of getting the disease.

By and large, the evidence that supports the idea that attitudes play a part in causing cancer comes from individual stories or case histories, but some research on larger groups of people has been done as well.

Individual Stories and Case Histories

Almost everybody knows someone or knows *of* someone who was diagnosed with cancer shortly after a time of great stress. A man's wife dies, and three months later he is found to have cancer of the bowel. A woman nurses her dying mother through the last year of her life and shortly afterward finds a lump in her breast that turns out to be malignant. Another woman, looking after her daughter on her own, spends three years of high stress and anxiety while her daughter deals with her drug addiction; then, shortly after things begin to settle down, the mother is found to have cancer. An important lawyer in a law firm is suddenly "let go" after fifteen years. Following six months of deep depression and feelings of uselessness, he is diagnosed with cancer of the lung.

There is no lack of stories such as these, and they all make intuitive sense. It seems logical that a catastrophic stress—a divorce, a bereavement, a dismissal—should be followed by a catastrophic illness such as cancer. Yet, although it seems logical and makes intuitive sense, it may not necessarily be true. Several factors may contribute to make the idea seem intuitively "right."

"Set" Thinking

The phrase "set thinking" describes the habit we all have of putting things we see into groups—filing our experience as sets of data. (I do *not* use the phrase to mean fixed or unalterable thinking, as in *"set in his ways."*) For example, if you have just bought a blue Volkswagen, every time you see another blue Volkswagen, you are likely to notice it. Suddenly blue Volkswagens have special significance for you. As a result, after you have bought your blue Volkswagen, it may seem to you that there is a sudden surge in the popularity of blue Volkswagens. Although it is possible that there actually are more blue Volkswagens—you may have started (or be part of) a fashion trend!—it is much more likely that the number of blue Volkswagens on the road has not altered; it is just that you are now noticing the ones that are there.

The same is true of individual case histories. We see links that make sense to us between, for example, cancer and divorce, bereavement, and so on. But we do not measure them against stories of people who have divorces, bereavement, or job loss but who have not developed cancer. Nor do we include in the equation people who have been diagnosed with cancer who have not had a trauma. In other words, there is a particular set of stories (where cancer follows trauma) that we remember and take note of. We do not know, however, whether people who have divorces are more likely to have cancer than people who do not, or whether people who have cancer are more likely to have been recently divorced.

Are There Other Factors That May Be Important?

Often when we hear stories such as the ones above, we are not given other facts that may be important in the causing of a cancer. For example, the lawyer who lost his job might have been a heavy smoker for many years (although he might have given up smoking five years ago, let's say). If that were the case, his lung cancer might be explained more easily by the cigarettes than by the job loss. Similarly, the woman whose mother died might now be in her sixties, an age when cancer is generally more common anyway.

In order to answer these questions definitively, we need to know whether a group of people who have, let's say, gone through major stress in the last two years have an increased chance of getting cancer compared to another group of the same age who have not had significant life events.

As we have seen, cancer is not a rare disease—1,250,000 cases per year make it a common disease—so it is very important to know whether it is more common among people who have experienced recent trauma or stress or not.

Is the Time Interval Appropriate?

We do have some idea of how long it takes for a cancer to develop. For example, we now have very clear evidence that people who have been exposed to large doses of radiation (such as survivors of Hiroshima and Nagasaki and those involved in accidents at nuclear reactors) did develop more cancers than the general population. Those cancers were mostly leukemias and lymphomas. Most of these cancers developed ten to twenty years after the incident, however, as did the other types of cancer such as breast cancer or sarcomas. This suggests that there is a latent period—a lag—between something that causes a cancer and the development of the cancer.

Exactly the same is true of cigarette smoking and lung cancer. In parts of the world where cigarette smoking is on the increase, there is always a demonstrable increase in lung cancer, but twenty years later rather than two years later or five years later. As smoking decreases in a group of the population (among males, for example), the incidence of lung cancer goes down, but again, twenty years later. It therefore seems that whether the factor is a single major insult (nuclear exposure) or a chronic continuing factor (cigarette smoke), the gap between the incident and the cancer is at least ten and usually twenty years. Hence it is legitimate to doubt that recent life stresses could be a major factor in causing a cancer. Of course, it is possible, in theory, that a stressful life event might be more powerful than a nuclear explosion or twenty years of smoking and might trigger a cancer in a way that is very different from anything we know of; it is not likely, however, and there is no evidence to support this.

Is the Story Truly Unexpected?

Often the way a story unfolds as it is told suggests a causal relationship. Yet sometimes the details provide a more logical and less unexpected explanation. Here is an example known to me.

> A woman in her late sixties developed swelling of the abdomen. An ultrasound showed a mass in her pelvis. Her surgeon did an exploratory operation, and a biopsy showed that it was caused by cancer of the ovary. Normally this exploratory operation would have been followed by a more extensive abdominal operation to see if there were any microscopic traces of cancer around, as there often are with cancer of the ovary, and it would have been followed by chemotherapy. For reasons that are unclear, her doctor did not do this but simply removed one ovary and told the patient she was clear of cancer. A year later she was involved in a car accident and spent three weeks in the hospital with chest injuries, including several broken ribs. Shortly after recovering from that, she developed a recurrence of her ovarian cancer. In a letter the woman's family practitioner stated that the recurrence of the ovarian cancer was clearly due to the anxiety and trauma caused by the car accident.

In fact, this woman's cancer was, unfortunately, treated wrongly in the first place. After her operation she was almost certainly not clear of disease, and, sadly, a recurrence within two or three years is quite typical of such a case. The chance of recurrence was already very high because she had not been treated adequately.

These perspectives should lead us to wonder whether any individual stories can truly prove that a cancer (or a recurrence of a cancer) is the result of stressful life events or of personality traits.

Data from Large Studies

Many studies of large groups of people have now been done in an attempt to prove or disprove the idea that either the mood of the person or the events that happen in a person's life may contribute to the cause of cancer. At present these do not show that there is a causal relationship.

Depression There is no confirmed evidence that depression contributes to the cause of cancer. For example, one major study evaluated communities in five cities and compared the incidence of cancer after a period of ten years. If depression were even a minor contributory cause to cancer, the study had a very high chance of showing that connection. In fact, there was no such link. The people with depression had the same chance of developing cancer as the general population.

Bereavement It has long been known that bereavement is one of life's most stressful events. A study in Israel looked for an increase in cancer among parents who had lost a child. No increase in cancer was found.

Thus the lack of evidence from larger systematic studies suggests that, as far as we can tell at present, neither the person's mood nor events in the person's life increase the chance of developing cancer.

Can the Mind Change the Outcome?

The idea that the mind can change the *outcome* of cancer is as important and as popular as the idea that the mind can cause cancer in the first place. The hypothesis is also intellectually appealing: if you have cancer, then your attitude or personality can change the progress of the cancer. In other words, you—and how you choose to think and feel—can make a difference. There are many publications in this area, and some of them are quoted often and widely. Because of the importance of this issue, I have selected some of the most widely known workers and studies and discuss them individually.

Attitudes and Breast Cancer (United Kingdom, 1979)

A British study by Dr. Stephen Greer and Dr. Tina Morris, published in 1979, showed some very remarkable findings. The study involved a group of patients with diagnosed breast cancer. With semi-structured interviews the doctors assessed the attitudes that the patients had to their illness before the diagnosis was made. They then correlated those attitudes to their survival. They found that patients who were extremely angry and patients who went into denial did very well. By contrast, patients who simply coped with the disease and carried on as best they could, and patients who went into a helpless/hopeless state, did less well. This paper was very significant, and the methodology (of classifying patients' reaction in this particular way) has been used in many centers since. However, the results have never been successfully repeated in another study. This is somewhat unexpected, as the original study was on a small group of patients and should not have been difficult to repeat. This 1979 study, therefore, offers interesting but isolated data.

The Bristol Example

Bristol Cancer Help Centre is one of Britain's most well known complementary medicine centers for cancer patients. The treatment offered there includes a wide range of psychological and spiritual techniques as well as a stringent diet. In its early publications the center had claimed that its treatments could and would prolong life. After several years the center collaborated with conventional physicians in a study of people with advanced breast cancer. Patients at the Bristol center were matched with approximately twice the number of patients at conventional centers. Preliminary results were published in 1991, carefully excluding from the survey any patients who died within three months of arrival at the Bristol center in order to prevent any unwitting bias against the center. These results showed that the chance of dying was actually higher at the Bristol center than at the conventional centers. The publication of this paper caused immense political furor. Undoubtedly the contractual agreements between all the participants about how and when the results were to be published had not all been honored, and there was no attention paid in the publication to the quality of life of the patients. Eventually, after major political activity, the sponsoring charity apologized to the women in the trial whose first knowledge of the results reached them by the press and television. Nevertheless, the data did not show that patients lived longer at the Bristol center, and the conclusions in the paper reflect those in a similar study that compared patients at a complementary medicine clinic in the United States with patients in a conventional center. The same conclusion is supported by the two Siegel studies below.

Life Events and Breast Cancer

In addition to studies on patients' reactions to illness and to the use of complementary approaches, there have been several studies on the impact of life events on the survival of patients after the diagnosis of breast cancer. Two studies at one hospital in the United Kingdom showed a possible influence but were based on recall of life events by patients after the time of relapse. Clearly the timing had the potential for introducing a bias, as people's ability to recall stresses might increase if they thought that the stresses had played a causative role in their medical problems. By contrast, a larger study in the United Kingdom (designed to exclude this recall bias) showed that there was no connection between life events and survival. The researchers reexamined their data at ten years of follow-up and again found no connection between life events and survival.

Dr. Bernie Siegel

Dr. Bernie Siegel is a Yale-trained surgeon specializing in cancer who in recent years has concentrated on the psychological aspects of serious illness, particularly cancer. Specifically, he noticed that certain psychological characteristics and behavior patterns seemed to be associated with a longer survival. He called these patients "exceptional cancer patients" or ECaPs and started therapy groups and meetings of ECaPs and of those who wanted to be ECaPs. He has published several books about the influence of the mind on serious diseases, particularly cancer. The first of these, *Love, Medicine and Miracles,* was enormously popular. There seemed to be two main reasons for this. First, the book contains a great deal of good and sound advice about how to cope with illness, how to organize one's life, and so on. Second—and perhaps even more important—through the stories and examples in the book, Bernie (he prefers to be called by his first name) implied that psychological attitudes were a determinant of survival, in other words, that the state of mind of the patient affected the progress of the cancer.

"HOPE versus EPHO" Bernie gave—and gives—many lectures all over the world on this subject, and I attended one of them. At that lecture he talked about caring and coping and gave what were clearly sensible and useful guidelines and anecdotes. However, he mentioned only two pieces of medical research, what one might call "hard data." The first was a study done by Dr. David Spiegel (see below). Immediately following that, Bernie mentioned another piece of data that I found most surprising. Here is the transcript of the tape of that part of the lecture:

> When I just think of the word "hope," there were two oncologists who wrote something about the work they were doing, because each one started a new protocol with four drugs, and the first letter of the drugs were E-P-H-O. And what one noticed was that approximately three-quarters of the patients who he was treating had their cancer respond. And the other noticed that only one-fourth of the patients he was treating

> responded. All doing the same thing with the same drugs. When they met and started talking they discovered one significant difference in what they were doing. One took the E, P, H and O and called his protocol HOPE—and the other called it EPHO. And HOPE was significant and symbolic. And what I also know is that people are what I call possibilities not probabilities.

The audience was profoundly impressed by the idea that an attitude—hope—could make such a difference to the way cancer responds to treatment. Personally I found that story unbelievable, for four reasons. First, I guessed from the initials of the drugs that the cancer mentioned was non–small-cell cancer of the lung (it could hardly have been any other). Second, I had never heard of any research involving the use of a combination of chemotherapy drugs called EPHO (or HOPE for that matter). Third, in any cancer treatment nowadays a response rate of 75 percent would be banner headlines. Fourth, I had never heard of any study of any chemotherapy in any tumor that showed a difference as large as a threefold divergence between responses to drug regimens (25 percent versus 75 percent). In short, I thought that if the results quoted were correct and provable, they indicated a discovery as major as splitting the atom or landing on the moon.

I interviewed Bernie Siegel for a television series the following year and asked him about the data he had mentioned. He told me that he no longer used that illustration, but he did manage to locate the source of the story for me. It turned out that the story had been quoted in a book by Norman Cousins. That quotation referred to an article in a little-known medical journal in which the author describes overhearing two oncologists talking at breakfast during an international cancer conference. The author of this article was a medical oncologist practicing in La Jolla, California.

Being curious about such important and unusual data, I telephoned the author of the article and asked him about the two doctors and their extraordinary findings. The author told me that he wrote the story as an example or illustration, not as fact. The article was really a parable (and a rather witty tongue-in-cheek one at that): the moral of the story was to tell physicians that there is more to treating cancer patients than giving the drugs.

Specifically, the author told me that (a) there never was a drug combination called EPHO (or HOPE); (b) he had not had a breakfast at which he had overheard two oncologists describing their papers to be presented at a major cancer conference; (c) a response rate of 75 percent in non–small-cell lung cancer would indeed be extraordinary; and (d) he had invented the anecdote in its entirety to illustrate the point he wanted to make. He referred me to another very witty article on hope (the emotion, not the drug regimen) he had later written for a major medical journal in which he specifically did *not* mention his previous anecdote.

So as it turned out, the EPHO versus HOPE anecdote was a witty parable that had been taken as scientific truth and had grown and acquired an aura of fact through being quoted by both Norman Cousins and Bernie Siegel.

The point of this story is to illustrate the power of an anecdote if it reflects what we all want to believe. Had that piece of data been a genuine and verified fact, it would have changed everything we know about cancer and its treatment: for if drugs work three times better when they are given by an optimistic physician, then optimism is the most powerful anticancer agent yet discovered. Unfortunately the real point of the story—that optimism and attitude *are* important parts of the treatment—was lost when the parable was retold as fact.

The Connecticut Study When I interviewed Bernie Siegel, he told me that he was engaged in a research project that would scientifically test the hypothesis that attitudes could make a difference to survival. He had already participated in one study that had not shown any improvement in survival and was now engaged in another and larger study. The second study involved two groups of patients with advanced breast cancer. One group (thirty-four patients) attended Bernie's ECaP sessions, and the other group (102 patients, matched for all the major factors that might make a difference to survival) were treated by medical oncologists in the same area of Connecticut but without ECaP sessions. The design of the research was very good: if the process of attending an ECaP group does prolong survival, then the ECaP group of patients should have done better and should have lived for a longer time than the non-ECaP patients. In fact, the study, published in early 1993, showed no benefit in terms of prolonging life. There was no difference in survival between the ECaP groups and the non-ECaP patients. Now, along with many observers, I feel it is very likely that attending the ECaP groups made the participants feel better, and that if the study had looked at their quality of life, it would have found a psychological benefit. Nevertheless, it did not support the idea that this type of positive attitude actually changed the outcome.

As I said to Bernie at the time, his participation in this kind of research is very admirable. That sort of intellectual honesty and curiosity sets him apart from the majority of other popular figures in this field. It is to his lasting credit that he carefully and deliberately set out to test the idea that ECaPs do better than other cancer patients. The fact that there was no demonstrable benefit *in terms of longer life* does not diminish the value that the groups have for the people who attend, but it does support the conclusion that ECaP groups do not extend life.

Dr. David Spiegel

Dr. David Spiegel is a psychiatrist practicing at Stanford University in California. In 1989 he published a fascinating and important study. In the late 1970s and early 1980s, Dr. Spiegel had set up some psychotherapy support groups for women with breast cancer. These group sessions were carefully designed and did not simply encourage the participants to take a positive attitude or hope that things would turn out better if they did. In fact, the groups did several things that were unusual. First, the participants in the groups were actively encouraged to face the facts of their situation and to confront—and cope with—the possibility, for example, of dying of breast cancer. Second, the groups actively encouraged networking and social contacts between the participants outside the group sessions. Thus, although the groups met only weekly, the women who took part met more frequently and often became close friends. They visited each other's homes, supported each other when things went badly (for example, they visited each other in the hospital), and so on. Third, the group were also offered additional benefits such as support for the husbands and new techniques for pain control. The patients were never told, or encouraged to believe, that any of these techniques could improve their survival.

The original research study, published in 1981, was designed to see if sessions like this could improve the quality of life, and the results clearly showed that these techniques did so. After several years had elapsed, and Bernie Siegel's concept of hope as a therapeutic agent became popular, Dr. Spiegel decided to see if the group sessions had made any difference to survival, fully expecting that there would be no effect. To his surprise, the long-term follow-up of the women who had attended these groups showed that they lived longer than the people who did not. This was a very important finding because it was the first—and the only—evidence derived from a prospective study (see page 30) that shows that survival might be affected by psychological and social factors.

I met and interviewed Dr. Spiegel as part of the same television series for which I had interviewed Bernie Siegel. I found David Spiegel to be a serious, thoughtful, and original researcher. Perhaps the most important aspect of his work is that his immediate response to his 1989 findings was to insist that the work be repeated in several different cities to see if his results are valid and reproducible. In fact, studies are going on at the moment in several different places (our own clinic in Toronto is one of the participating research centers). When those studies are complete, there will be a definitive answer. If those studies produce the same results as Dr. Spiegel's, there will be very strong evidence that group support can prolong life in advanced breast cancer. If they do not show the same results as the 1989 findings, then it could mean one of two things. Either the 1989 results were a chance finding or there was some factor at work in Stanford in 1989 that cannot be reproduced or translated to other centers.

David Spiegel also had many interesting views on the meaning of his research. As he said, if the findings are confirmed, there could be several different mechanisms at work. There might be simple, observable differences in, for example, getting and persevering with treatment. If you are part of a group, you might get to your doctor's office more quickly if there is a problem, and you might be more likely to persevere with the treatment when you have friends and support than when you do not. Or it might be that when you are in a group your ability to handle stress is increased, and, in particular, your anxiety level is lower. As he said, think of the difference between a single person walking through Central Park at 2:00 A.M. alone and the same person doing the same thing in a group of twenty people. Or it might be that our grandmothers were right after all, and if you simply look after yourself well, things will go better. Thus, if the findings are confirmed, there may be several different explanations. At present we are still awaiting the results of that confirmatory research. There will probably be important news about this topic in the next year or two.

Psychoneuroimmunology

If it were established as a proven and reproducible fact that the mind can influence either the cause or the course of cancer, we could suggest a number of possible mechanisms that would cause this to happen. In fact, a large amount of work is currently being done into the ways that psychological factors influence various systems in the body, particularly the immune system. This broad area of investigation is called psychoneuroimmunology.

Much of the work related to psychoneuroimmunology concerns the effects of mood, stress, or personality on some measurable aspect of a body system. So, for example, some researchers have measured the level of certain lymphocytes in the blood and compared these levels with various aspects of the person's life (mood, stresses, life events, and so on). Other researchers have done the same sort of thing with levels of stress hormones in the bloodstream or with the ability of certain immune cells to do certain things in the laboratory or with allergy skin tests or other aspects of body function. Some of these studies have shown some relationship between psychological states and the results of the tests. At present, however, nobody knows what bearing such a relationship can have on the progress of serious or chronic diseases, particularly cancer. It might well be that changes in, say, lymphocyte levels or other immune function tests can alter some things. For example, there is some evidence that major stress can increase one's chance of getting a cold. However, there is a considerable difference between getting a cold and developing (or altering the course of) cancer. At present the term "psychoneuroimmunology" is a reasonable and valid description of an active area of research. It also suggests a possible explanation of the way in which the mind may affect cancer, *if* it is proven in the future that it does. At present, however, psychoneuroimmunology cannot be used to prove that there is an effect of the mind on cancer—that proof is still awaited.

Blaming the Patient

Humankind has a long history of blaming the patient, and some contemporary attitudes about the connection between the mind and cancer may stem from that long tradition.

Blaming the patient helps people who do not have the disease to feel safe and perhaps superior. If we, the healthy, can identify something the patient has done—and has *chosen* to do—that has caused the cancer, then maybe (according to that line of reasoning) we will not get that cancer if we are careful (the implication being that we can *choose* not to get cancer). Hence our desire to find things in patients' lives that set them apart from healthy people. Many examples from history illustrate this tendency in human nature. We used to think that tuberculosis selectively struck artists and sensitive people: the "TB personality" was actually called the phthisic personality because another word for TB was phthisis. We used to believe that people with obsessional personalities were more prone to the diarrheal illness ulcerative colitis. In Victorian times, Down's syndrome was thought to occur in children because the parents were drunk at the time of conception! We used to believe that stomach ulcers were caused by stress coupled with a goal-seeking personality (before we discovered that the bacterium *Helicobacter pylorii* was a major factor and if you did not have the bacterium, you would not get an ulcer).

In my opinion, cancer and our attitudes to it are in the same tradition. Of course, in some cancers, a patient's actions are a known contributing factor (smoking in cancers of the lung, mouth, bladder, pancreas, kidney, and others; sunlight in skin cancers, and so on). Most cancers, however, arrive mysteriously and apparently randomly. As human beings, we do not like that randomness, so we impose a (spurious) order on the events: we blame the patient. Although it is possible that the mind does play an important role and the patient is in part to blame, the evidence so far suggests otherwise. Some—or much—of this feeling that cancer is caused by the patient in some way may simply be our time-honored way of dealing with fear of the unknown.

Summary: The Importance of Mind-Body Interactions

There is, of course, no doubt that "the mind" interacts in a multitude of ways with "the body." Most of these interactions are so commonplace and everyday that we do not think of them as mind-body interactions but regard them as a perfectly normal part of our existence.

Like everyone else, when I am anxious I can feel my pulse rate rise: my mouth feels dry and my stomach does that peculiar thing that I have learned to call "butterflies." When I am angry, I can feel my jaw muscles tighten, my voice become louder and (if I am very angry) the tips of my ears get hot. When I laugh, I feel good and I notice that my awareness of pain is reduced. And, of course, most of the human species are not surprised that sexual arousal can be achieved by erotic photographs, drawings, poems, stories, or even phone calls! There is no real dispute about the fact that many aspects of the human body and its internal environment can be changed simply by sensory data received through the eyes, ears, nose, mouth, and so on. Nor are we surprised to find that these changes may have unhealthy effects as well as healthy ones. For example, there is a small (smaller than previously estimated) correlation between heart disease and a person's general level of competitiveness and stress. However, whether there is any such mind-body connection operating with the causes or the course of cancer is still unresolved.

Although the debate and the research around this issue continue, we should not underestimate the importance of mental attitudes and coping skills. Viktor Frankl, a survivor of the Holocaust and concentration camps, wrote a brilliant and thoughtful book about his experiences and what he had learned from them. The message of his book, *Man's Search for Meaning,* was clear: they can take everything from you, except the choice of how you will react to what happens. What was true of an enemy is no less true of an illness. Altering your attitudes to diminish the stress and the distress caused by the cancer can only help you. Whether that effort prolongs survival or not, it is undeniable that, to repeat the words of the patient quoted at the beginning of this section, *"Feeling better is a whole lot better than feeling worse."*

SCREENING, EARLY DIAGNOSIS, AND PREVENTION

8

What's in This Chapter

This chapter looks at how our society could decrease the number of cancers that occur every year and help diagnose the ones that do occur at an earlier and perhaps more treatable stage. Although this sounds simple, in practice it is extremely difficult, and I explain why that is. I also discuss what is known about screening and prevention and summarize the things we can all do to decrease our risk of developing a cancer or to identify and deal with a cancer at as early a stage as possible.

Definitions

Screening means doing a test on people who have no symptoms. It may be that a test can or should be done on absolutely everybody or only on people who have an increased risk of developing a particular type of cancer (for example, the Pap test should be done on all females who are or have been sexually active; a rectal examination might be done routinely on all males over the age of forty). In some circumstances a screening test might be used only on those people who are at very high risk indeed (for example, it might become routine to test women who have two or more relatives with breast cancer for the presence of certain genes). Screening for a particular disease means using a test on people who have no signs of trouble and have not noticed any problems suggestive of that disease. The ideal screening test is one that can detect a cancer at an early stage in its progress or, better still, before the cancer has developed, while it is still in the precancerous stage.

Early diagnosis means detecting a cancer at an early stage. Early detection may occur as a result of a screening test or through educating the general public (so that, for instance, anyone who notices a mole that is growing or becoming irregular knows it is important to seek medical advice because the mole might be a malignant melanoma). Early diagnosis, like screening, is especially important if the treatment of the early stages of a disease produces better survival than treatment at a later stage.

Prevention of a cancer means removing the cause or causes so that the risk of developing that cancer is reduced. For many cancers this could involve changing your lifestyle, so by definition, then, prevention means avoiding behavior that is known to increase a person's risk of developing cancer. The classic example is stopping smoking. At present, in the United States, about 160,000 people die each year of lung cancer. If everybody in the United States could be enrolled in prevention—that is, if everybody gave up smoking cigarettes—in about twenty to thirty years' time more than 90 percent of lung cancer would be prevented and the number of people dying from it each year would be less than 10,000.

Why Is Cancer Detected So Late?

As I mentioned in Chapter 2, cancer cells, like all human cells, are very small, so they are usually not detectable until there are several million of them. Unfortunately, by the time a cancer is detectable, it is usually more than halfway along the road to becoming a lethal condition (see page 13). That is the case with most of the common types of cancer. There are a few exceptions. For example, the Pap test is a method of detecting cells before they are cancerous but when they are in a state that carries a high risk of progression to cancer. Such exceptions apart, at present there are no methods of detecting cancer cells when they number hundreds or thousands rather than many millions or billions. That is why research into methods of prevention and following whatever guidelines emerge may be so important for the future.

Screening

For a screening test to be useful it must do two things. First, it must give an abnormal reading when there is a cancer there; in other words, the test must be able to detect all (or nearly all) of the cancers it is designed for. Second, it must not give abnormal readings when there is no cancer; in other words, it must not create a large number of false alarms.

1. Sensitivity Technically the ability to detect cancer is called the **sensitivity**, and it is best explained in this way: *If there are a certain number of cancers in a population, how many of those cancers will yield an abnormal result in the test?* Let's imagine a population of 1,000 people, of which 100 have developed Cancer X. If we test the whole group of 1,000, and if our test gives abnormal results in 90 out of

TABLE 8.1: SCREENING TESTS

TEST	CANCER	CONSEQUENCES OF TEST	NOTES
Pap test	Cervix	Repeat Pap test or colposcopy	Should be done (with pelvic examination) at age eighteen or when sexually active and annually thereafter. After three negative Pap tests, should be repeated when suggested by health care provider.
Bowel screening tests	Bowel	Biopsy	People with average risk should have an annual digital rectal exam from age forty, and annual fecal occult blood test from age fifty. If risk is high, flexible sigmoidoscopy every three to five years as well. If previous diagnosis of polyps or cancer, colonoscopy six to twelve months after diagnosis and every three years thereafter.
Breast screening	Breast	Repeat mammogram, ultrasound, or biopsy.	Physical examination every three years to age forty; annually thereafter. Mammograms every one to two from age forty to forty-nine; annually thereafter.

those 100 cases of Cancer X in that population, we would say that the sensitivity of that test is 90 percent. (In this group of 100 people, there are 10 who have Cancer X but whose test results are normal. Those results are termed false negatives.)

2. Specificity The specificity of a test is a way of expressing how reliable a normal (negative) test result is. That is, if there is a normal (or negative) result, how confident can one be that the cancer is *not* present? Let's go back to that population of 1,000 people. Of that 1,000, there are, as before, 100 people who have developed Cancer X. As before, the test gave an abnormal reading in 90 of those 100 cases of Cancer X and therefore has a sensitivity of 90 percent. But of those 1,000 people, 900 do not have Cancer X. Now let's imagine that of those 900, there are 10 in whom the test gave an *ab*normal result. In other words, an abnormal test result (presumably caused by something other than Cancer X) was produced in 10 out of the 900 people who did not have cancer, and these results are called false positives. The specificity of the test is defined as the number of times a negative result occurs in people who do *not* have the disease—in this case, 890 out of 900, or 98.9 percent.

Thus the usefulness of a screening test is related to how often (or how seldom) it misses a case of cancer and how often (or how seldom) it gives an abnormal reading when there is no cancer there. Research into potential screening tests looks particularly at these two issues and also at the consequences of (a) having an abnormal test and (b) missing a case of that cancer. For example, if a woman has an abnormal mammogram result that looks like cancer, it might be recommended that an ultrasound be performed and then a biopsy if there is still some possibility of cancer. Thus, in assessing the usefulness of mammograms, we must ask how many unnecessary biopsies result compared to the number of times cancer of the breast is missed. Similarly, with the Pap test: if the Pap test is abnormal, it can be repeated without too much inconvenience to the patient. If a cancer of the cervix develops and is not detected, however, the consequences may be very great.

Studies along these lines go on with every potential screening test. As you can see, a lot depends on how common the cancer is among the population studied, and often the results in one city or area may not be quite the same as those in another. The details of the way the test is used may also vary. For these reasons, results sometimes seem to be contradictory, making research in this area difficult.

Certain screening tests are of proven value, however. These are summarized in Table 8.1.

Tests That Are of No Value Some tests have been tried to detect cancers at an early stage and have proved to be of no use. For example, chest X rays

TABLE 8.2: PROCEDURES THAT HELP IN EARLY DIAGNOSIS

METHOD	CANCER	CONSEQUENCES OF AN ABNORMAL TEST RESULT	NOTES
Breast self-examination	Breast	Medical checkup	Is of some value.
Reporting any change in skin moles	Melanoma	Medical checkup and perhaps biopsy	Is very useful.

were done (for cancer and for TB) and were found to have no impact on survival; in other words, the X rays did not save lives.

Tests Whose Value Is Not Proven at Present Some tests are going through the process of evaluation; for example, the use of the PSA blood test to try to detect prostate cancer. At present it is not yet known whether taking action on the results of the PSA test does influence the treatment of early cancer of the prostate. In other words, we do not yet know whether the results of the PSA test can influence the outcome of the disease.

Early Diagnosis

Early diagnosis—detecting the cancer as early as possible—may be achieved by a screening test or some other means. Of the screening tests discussed above, only the Pap test can detect the potential for developing a cancer. All the others detect the cancer after it has developed. Apart from screening tests, early diagnosis may be assisted by the means outlined in Table 8.2.

Prevention

Prevention may be the only way of changing the impact of cancer on our society in the next ten or

TABLE 8.3: USEFUL PREVENTIVE ACTIONS

PREVENTIVE ACTION	CANCERS PREVENTED	NOTES
Stop smoking.	Lung Bladder Pancreas Larynx Mouth, esophagus, pharynx Kidney	Number of lives saved each year (including deaths from heart and lung diseases) could be more than a million by the year 2015.
Avoid any sunburn and reduce exposure to sun.	All skin cancers	
Eat a high-fiber (more than 20 gm a day) and low-fat (about 25% of calorie intake) diet.	Probably cancer of the bowel, breast, prostate, ovary, endometrium, mouth, lung, bladder, pancreas	
Defer the start of sexual activity until at least late teens or early twenties, small number of partners, *and* use barrier methods of contraception.	Cancer of the cervix, AIDS and AIDS-related cancers such as Kaposi's and lymphomas	
Have a vaccination against hepatitis B.	Liver (hepatocellular) cancer	Worldwide would prevent one million deaths per year.

TABLE 8.4: HOW TO INCREASE YOUR CHANCE OF GIVING UP CIGARETTES

1. Cigarette smoking is an addiction and, by and large, extremely enjoyable. Unfortunately it is also extremely dangerous and causes death by heart disease, chronic bronchitis, emphysema, and strokes as well as cancers of the lung, larynx, mouth, esophagus, bladder, pancreas, and kidney.
2. As with all addictions, you can't quit simply by being scared.
3. You have to progress from *"I should quit smoking for my health's sake,"* through *"I want to quit smoking,"* to *"I want to be a nonsmoker."*
4. If you do want to become a nonsmoker, it is a good idea to write a brief list of the reasons why you want to quit. Then make a list of the things you enjoy most about smoking. Tape both lists to a place where you can see them every day—the bathroom mirror or a cupboard door.
5. Nicotine chewing gum or skin patches may help, particularly if your smoking is of the "nicotine-addiction" type (and you get edgy without a cigarette after an hour or two).
6. Counselling may be very helpful indeed. Self-help groups may be very good (if you are the kind of person who handles stress better in company).
7. Pick the right time to try quitting, and do it seriously. Plan it a few weeks in advance.
8. Get all the brochures and pamphlets you can to give you extra help and advice.
9. If you find yourself smoking one cigarette or so after you've said you were quitting, don't give up the whole thing and start smoking all over again. Step back, regroup, and quit again.
10. Being a nonsmoker has many advantages, but you will miss cigarettes every day. Be prepared for that and don't relax after six months.
11. Each cigarette you ever smoked was the result of a decision at that moment to smoke that cigarette. You can make the decision not to smoke, but you need to make that decision every day, many times a day. The good feeling and confidence you will gain from that process is absolutely wonderful. You will like yourself much more if you have control over your actions.

twenty years. The problem is that prevention is not a particularly easy idea to sell. Prevention is not, as they say in advertising, sexy. One of the clearest examples was the famous case of President Reagan's bowel. When President Reagan had surgery for what the media were told was an early cancer of the bowel, the repercussions were felt around the world. Medical reports were issued frequently and studied and analyzed in detail, and in Japan the Nikkei stock index plunged. That was the impact of treatment of an established cancer. Prevention of that cancer would have had no impact. A daily announcement from the White House that *"Today the President of the United States passed a large soft stool with no effort at all"* would be of no interest to anyone. The example is flippant, but the moral is serious: the world is not generally interested in prevention, even though it may be our only chance of changing the course of cancer in the immediate future. As a society we find the idea of high-tech cures and treatments exciting and the idea of prevention relatively dull. Nevertheless, there are some encouraging signs that we are in the process of changing our attitudes. In the United States, smoking is decreasing among some groups of society, and slowly the idea of a low-fat, high-fiber diet is beginning to be taken more seriously. Table 8.3 lists the things we are certain or relatively confident about that, if practiced on a wide scale, would reduce the number of cases of cancer seen every year.

You Can Quit Smoking

Finally—and I don't want to seem to be repetitive about this—cigarette smoking is the greatest preventable cause of chronic disease including cancer in the Western world. Giving up smoking is extremely difficult (I have done it, so I know how really difficult it is).

Basically, there are three main approaches that do work, and if you have decided you want to quit, you'll probably do best if you use the three methods together:

1. use the nicotine patch or gum;
2. get support and encouragement; and
3. learn how to handle urges to smoke and how to handle stress.

Nicotine patches or nicotine gum do lessen the urge to smoke. When you buy either of these, it's important to follow the directions carefully, so get help from your doctor or medical team if you have any questions. Counseling, even brief counseling sessions from your health care provider, can help a lot. You may also want to join a "quit smoking" program. Ideally, look for one that offers sessions about twenty to thirty minutes long, for at least four to seven sessions over at least two weeks. Another point about support is to use it when you get the urge to smoke a cigarette—phone someone you know to help talk you out of it (preferably an ex-smoker). Third, try to be aware of the things in your life that make you want to smoke and change them a bit where you can. (For example, if you smoke a cigarette with coffee after a meal, try to drink your coffee in a no-smoking area or have it at a separate time from your meal. If you smoke when you're on the phone, make sure you have no cigarettes or ashtrays near the phone.)

Above all, it's really important to plan to quit in advance and get everything on your side to help you. There's lots of good information and help available from the Agency for Health Care Policy, and they have a very useful (and short) booklet called *How to Quit Smoking*. You can phone them at **1-800-358-9295** for copies of the booklet and other information (fax number: **301-594-2800**; web site: **http://www.ahcpr.gov/**).

In Table 8.4, I summarize some hints that may help you if you really want to become a nonsmoker. As the saying goes, *"quit for life—your life,"* and even more important, ***"no matter how hard giving up is, don't give up on giving up."***

With So Many Breakthroughs, Why's There No Progress?

9

What's in This Chapter

This chapter examines the world of cancer research, but not merely from the point of view of exciting scientific discoveries in the past, present, or future. This chapter attempts to explain why, with all these promising approaches, the situation from the cancer patient's point of view does not seem to have changed as dramatically as we've all been hoping over the last few years. I also try to explain why the gap between laboratory and bedside is often so wide and so long. As you will see, this part of the book explains what is actually going on: the work, the progress, and a few of the difficulties. Certainly some of those difficulties have been created by the public relations aspects of cancer research—the way in which complicated scientific information is given to the general public. Sometimes positive results have been almost hyped into overoptimistic claims that are not later substantiated. This chapter explains how, for the best of reasons, that happened (and sometimes still does), how research actually takes place, and what is needed to help it continue being productive and useful.

A Near-Crisis of Confidence: Public Perception of Cancer Research

One of my patients once said to me something that many people may have felt at one time or another: *"If there are so many major breakthroughs every week, how come there's no progress?"* And she neatly expressed a very common question: if so many major discoveries are apparently being made every week, when are their benefits going to reach the patients? Why the delay? Is somebody not telling the truth? How can there be major breakthroughs if the treatment of cancer doesn't seem to be changing very much? It's true to say that, at times, the public's confidence in the orderly advance of science against cancer has become strained; in fact, sometimes it has almost been on the verge of a crisis of confidence. While many people are genuinely gladdened to hear or read of a new major breakthrough in cancer research, a proportion of the public is asking what happened to the last major breakthrough, and the one before that, and the one before that. The explanation of this apparent discrepancy between promise and fulfillment involves two issues. First, there is a wide gap between research findings in the laboratory and any advances in treatment that may result from them. This means that the scientific community may experience major breakthroughs and quantum leaps in its *understanding* of cancer. Sometimes researchers may feel as if the very foundations of tumor biology have been shaken to the core. But there may be little or slow progress from the *patient's* point of view because, unfortunately, advances in knowledge are not necessarily the same as advances in *treatment.*

The second problem is a fundamental trait of human behavior. It may be called herd behavior, trend-following, or peer pressure, but it is a fact of human behavior and it applies to all of us, in the medical profession, in the media, and everywhere else. We all have a yearning to be part of a story that makes front-page news. This tendency is made a bit worse by the fact that it's the job of the news media to catch and hold people's attention—we really do live in the age of the sound bite and the headline. This means that slow, steady, plodding progress is not usually regarded as very newsworthy. For all these reasons, then, it is relatively easy for a new piece of information or work to become front-page news, even at an early or premature stage of its development.

The Gap between Lab and Bedside

In the late 1940s and early 1950s, some advances in cancer research and treatment actually happened as if in a movie. While surgery and radiotherapy continued to advance and progress in many ways, steadily increasing the number of cured patients, the new field of drug therapy for cancer emerged suddenly, as dramatically as if the script had been written in Hollywood.

Early Victories

Some of the early discoveries, or rather inventions, of anticancer drugs did happen as if by magic. A scientist might be working in a lab (and I have personally spoken with some of those pioneers) and, with a combination of knowledge, diligence, persistence, inspiration, and serendipity, would produce a substance that happened to be extremely active in killing, for example, breast cancer cells growing in a glass dish or cells of a mouse leukemia. The researchers, often working in a corner of some damp, rundown, old building, would quickly manufacture a bit more of the substance, purify it, test it to make sure it contained no impurities or toxins, and (this happened in the 1940s, remember) it might be given to a patient with advanced incurable cancer within weeks. Sometimes the gap (particularly in Britain) between laboratory and bedside was, as one of those pioneers phrased it, *"two months and a hundred yards."*

But *"that was then, this is now."* The fortuitous findings that marked the early successes of chemotherapy set very high expectations, and we have been trying to live up to those expectations ever since. Among the many types of advanced—and hitherto incurable—cancers on which these new drugs were tested, some responded dramatically, and some patients were cured or had wonderful remissions. This happened, for example, in some cases of Hodgkin's disease, choriocarcinoma, childhood leukemia, non-Hodgkin's lymphoma, and later in testicular cancer and a few others. We still do not know exactly why tumors of these types are so responsive to chemotherapy and can sometimes be cured (although we now have some clues), but of course everyone who heard about these cures was elated.

The problem was, and still is, that the cancers that respond in this way make up only about 5 percent of all cases of cancer. The feeling was that after these early victories, the rest of the cancers would eventually respond to drug therapy in due course. The first 5 percent was just an example of what chemotherapy could do—the remaining 95 percent would follow.

At the time, and for many years afterward, this explanation was entirely reasonable and justifiable. Thus cancer research inched forward, pressed from behind, as it were, by the expectation that somewhere there was a drug or a combination of drugs waiting to be discovered. Some research was directly aimed at finding the best drugs. Major projects were established in some countries, notably the United States, to test any substance (natural or synthetic) against a series of cells in the test tube that might give some clue as to anticancer activity. This is called "treatment-directed research." While that was going on, there was also a rapid and massive expansion in more basic research, for example, into the fundamental differences between cancer cells and normal cells.

Both types of research—treatment-directed research and basic research—made, and continue to make, progress. The problem was that the early spectacular results with the curable cancers could not be repeated in far advanced cases of the commoner types of cancers such as bowel, breast, or lung. Responses were seen, but cures were rare in other cancers if there had already been spread (metastasis). Over the last two decades, quiet, steady progress has certainly been made, even if it isn't newsworthy. For example, there have been advances in the treatment of breast cancer, some lung cancers, ovarian and colon cancers, and sarcomas, and overall cure rates have risen noticeably over the last two decades.

Appropriately, then, this type of research is still going on in a big way, and every few years a drug is discovered or invented that has several advantages over its predecessors. These drugs have steadily been introduced into clinical practice, but so far none of them has produced new cures in large numbers. From the patient's point of view, then, treatment has not yet altered dramatically. The chance of getting a remission is a bit higher (in some cancers a lot higher), but, apart from the rarer types of cancer that I mentioned above, the chance of cure if the cancer is advanced is not much different from what it was about ten years ago. So treatment-related research has produced many incremental advances but nothing to equal the dramatic effects of the early discoveries on what had been incurable cancers.

Advances in Understanding the Cancer Cell

Simultaneously with treatment-directed research, basic research was also proceeding on a large and ever-increasing scale. In particular, new tools were invented that allowed scientists to study the behavior of cancer cells in ways that had never been dreamed of before the 1950s. Here are just two examples out of literally thousands.

Monoclonal Antibodies In the best tradition, one scientist (working with a junior assistant) invented a technique by which cells derived from a mouse cancer could be altered to produce limitless quantities of a single, pure antibody. It was therefore possible to produce a large amount of an antibody that would attach itself to, for example, a component found in the lining of the ducts in the breast. This was a great improvement over the older method. In the old method, extracts of breast epithelium were injected into, say, a rabbit, and the resulting serum, which contained thousands of different antibodies, was purified by removing as many as possible of the unwanted ones. The invention of the monoclonal antibodies changed the whole approach to the study of tumor biology. For example, it allowed us to study cancer cells and to look for substances that were produced by or attached to the surface of the cancer cells but not by normal cells. In the early days, it was hoped that this would lead to the discovery of a true magic bullet that would guide drugs or other substances to cancer cells exclusively while leaving normal cells alone. As I illustrate below, sadly that has happened in only a few instances. Even so, the technique of producing monoclonal antibodies has opened whole new vistas of understanding tumor biology.

DNA Technology Another example is the way we are now able to study the genetic material of cells, the nucleic acid or DNA. As a result of some extraordinary technical advances in the study of DNA, we are now able to identify specific parts of the DNA that we call oncogenes (see Chapter 3) and that are somehow involved in the process of causing cancer. With many oncogenes it is now possible, in some research laboratories, to see if a particular cancer of the bladder or lung, say, has or does not have an excess of a particular oncogene or of some product of the oncogene. Again, as this research got under way, it was hoped that a treatment directed against oncogenes (or against the substances that they produce) might effect cures. That is still a possibility, but it may be some years away, because the process by which oncogenes are involved in carcinogenesis is very complex and still incompletely understood.

Current Limitations of Laboratory Research in Cancer

Thus there has been enormous progress in basic cancer research over the last forty years, and the pace has accelerated in the last decade. It would, in fact, be quite justifiable to call it an explosion of knowledge. These advances deserve the recognition and plaudits they receive. However, partly because doctors, researchers, patients, and media alike are buoyed up by that progress, it is difficult to get a balanced view of the current limitations of research. What I am about to say is not meant to sound negative; it is an attempt to look at not only the road we have traveled so far, but also the distance we have yet to cover. As oncologist Eugenie Kleinerman neatly put it, *"We're running a marathon, not a sprint."* The following examples give some idea of what that marathon is like.

We now have a very large number of ways of looking at cancer cells in the laboratory. We have thousands of different types of cancer cells growing in dishes, many of which can be grown and then cured in laboratory-bred mice. We also have thousands of different ways of looking at and testing those cells. We can look at the cells' growth, their ability to produce different substances, their sensitivity to some chemotherapy drugs and their resistance to others, the way they respond to growth factors, their genetic material including oncogenes and substances controlled by oncogenes, their ability to affect other cells (of the immune system, for example), their ability to damage membranes and invade, their structure under the electron microscope, and whether or not the cell surface has any of hundreds of different marker molecules on it. These are just a few examples of what can be done nowadays; the complete list of ways in which cancer cells can be tested would probably be longer than this entire book. But here is the snag: although this accumulation of experience is wonderful and commendable, the truth is that cancer in human beings is far more complicated than any laboratory system can ever be (at least in the light of current knowledge).

Cancer in human beings—*"cancer in real people,"* as one of my patients put it—is infinitely more complex than even the most sophisticated system we can devise in the laboratory because, for one thing, it involves so many different cells and systems. Cancer cells interact with the normal cells around them: they alter the immune system in ways that we can only guess at; they can avoid being killed by lymphocytes; they can persuade the body to produce blood vessels for the tumor; they can influence the growth of cells in the neighborhood and elsewhere in the body; they can produce substances that attack the "glue" between normal cells, and so on. Furthermore, they do all these things in three dimensions as a clump of cells that expands outward, whereas most of the time researchers in the laboratory test their ideas on cancer cells growing as a flat layer in a dish. Cancer is not like that in human beings. In fact, it has recently been shown that when cancer cells get together in a group or a clump they can do things (such as resist the actions of chemotherapy) that they could not do when they were arranged as a flat layer. So—and I am not saying anything that researchers are not already aware of—many of the ways that we study cancer cells in the laboratory do not give a very accurate picture of what cancer is like in people. It is as if the police wanted to study what happens in a riot when thousands of people, let's say, cause a disturbance at a public meeting. So the police take one person out of the rioting crowd, put that person into a prison cell, and carry out careful, long, and detailed interviews. Although that's a good way to start an investigation, it may not necessarily tell you very much about the behavior of the crowd, particularly about the things people do when they're in the middle of thousands of other people and are all in a belligerent mood. It's the same with cancer. Laboratory systems are a good start, but because cells growing in a dish are a far cry from tumors in real people, we should not be surprised when things that work in the lab do not work in real life. The two things are very different, and this is another reason for the large gap between laboratory and bedside.

Collaborative Optimism: How Research Is Reported

Let's turn now to the public relations aspects of cancer research. In order to explain why it is that so many "breakthrough" stories appear, I first need to explain how research happens and how it is funded.

In the United States, as in most countries in the world, cancer research depends partly on government support and partly on the generosity of individuals—in other words, true philanthropy. Every discovery leads to more questions that need to be answered, and doing that requires more researchers and more laboratories. Furthermore, as the techniques involved become more sophisticated, the costs rise. Thus all cancer research agencies are faced with requests for funds that increase in number and size each year. As an example, the National Cancer Institute has an annual budget of $2 billion, and this has barely kept pace with inflation over the last five years.

The way that all funding agencies decide who gets the money and who does not is a well-established, time-honored, and generally fair and equitable procedure. A scientist who wants to do research in a particular field writes an application for a grant (many laboratory chiefs spend more than 60 percent of their time writing grant applications) and sends it, for example, to the National Cancer Institute, the American Cancer Society, or a small number of private foundations. That grant application will be a long and detailed document setting out what the scientist has done so far in the field—his or her track record—the objectives of the research, the methods that she or he proposes to use, and all the details of it (including costs of laboratory materials, salaries, and so on). Usually grants arc awarded for a number of years (from three to five years is the typical range), so if the research does not work out, the granting agency is not committed to endless funding. By and large, this system is the best way of being fair. Even totally unknown and novice scientists can get funding if their ideas are good and if they have a clear idea of how to proceed. Yet the demand is so great that, on average, only one grant application out of every five is funded, and quite often researchers have to resubmit their proposals many times over a period of years to get funding. In some regions, state governments provide more steady support for university-based researchers, but even that practice has frequently been capped (that is, limited) in recent years. This means that donations to the American Cancer Society and to private foundations and cancer centers have provided support that in many cases has been absolutely critical for scientists.

This difficulty applies not only to laboratory research but also to the testing of new drugs and therapies in clinical trials (see page 233), for which funding is in an even more precarious state. Many clinical trials have been traditionally funded, at least in part, from the "profits" of academic centers. Now, with the advent of managed care, many managed care companies are refusing to pay for anything that could be regarded as "experimental," so it's uncertain how clinical trials will be funded in the future.

All of this means that over the last few years the number of researchers and scientists competing for funding has increased dramatically. Nowadays scientists cannot afford to be in the least bit vague about their proposed projects; they must be detailed and specific. Furthermore, *"Nothing succeeds like success."* So if a scientist has a good track record of productive research, by and large, his or her next project is likely to be weighed more favorably. Thus the pressure to achieve visible success increases year by year.

This competitive climate increases the pressure on the researcher and is one of the causes of overoptimistic reporting. If a scientist is telephoned by a journalist or a television reporter (who may need a sound bite or major breakthrough headline immediately), it is easy for the reporting to be overoptimistic and for the journalist to misinterpret (or even not ask about) how long it would take for this advance to reach the clinic. A good "major breakthrough" story is what the media want, and it is very difficult for a scientist to make sure that the limitations of the research are accurately reported. In fact, as the scientist has no control over the final article or film, it is impossible to ensure what the scientist might regard as a fair and balanced report. So "major breakthrough" stories can be generated very easily. Furthermore, even though one might think a splashy story might help a scientist in his or her next grant application, often it does the exact opposite—it jeopardizes the researcher's chances of funding. So inaccurate overoptimistic stories may well harm not only the public that reads them but also the scientist whose work is being described.

In any event, overoptimistic reporting leaves the patient with cancer with a strong impression that major changes in therapy and major advances in the treatment of cancer are just around the corner, when often, at best, they are many years or even decades away. When those promises show no sign of immediate fulfillment, there is often a sense of having been misled. Hence the common feelings of disillusionment or even skepticism that may greet the latest breakthrough headline.

It might be helpful to give two examples, in which I was involved personally, of research that might have worked out but didn't. I describe these projects to show how easy it is to greet research findings as if they hold the key to the future and how difficult it is to tell the story in a balanced and truthful fashion. Another advantage of using my own projects as examples is that I am certain that I will not be offending or upsetting someone when I explain the limitations of the project and the lack of success in terms of advances in treatment. After describing projects that yielded knowledge but not instant progress in treatment, I then give a few examples (out of thousands) of projects that are now going on all over the world and that might *or might not* lead to changes in treatment. In describing those projects, I must emphasize that it is quite possible that few (or even none) of them will yield revolutions in treatment. Yet I hope you will see that research along these lines is *still* valid and very important and thoroughly deserves the support and funding it gets.

Research That Might Have Worked Out but Didn't

Marrow "Clean-Up" In Chapter 5, I discussed the technique of autologous bone marrow transplantation (ABMT), which was invented as a way of giving higher doses of drugs to the patient in the hope that those higher doses would kill all the cancer cells and cure the cancer. In fact, the technique was first described in 1961 by a British surgeon who invented the method while treating African children who had Burkitt's lymphoma. The technique was largely ignored for some years, then rediscovered after the technique of donor bone marrow transplant had been shown by pioneers in the United States to be an important advance in the treatment of leukemia.

During the late 1970s and early 1980s, more and more researchers became interested in the use of high-dose chemotherapy with ABMT for the treatment of the commoner cancers such as cancers of the lung, breast, and ovary. However, there was a theoretical danger: because a portion of the bone marrow was removed from the patient *before* the treatment was given, it was possible that there might be cancer cells in the marrow. Thus when the bone marrow was given back to the patient, it might contain cancer cells capable of starting new tumors.

The cancer institute at which I did my research was devoted entirely to research into breast cancer (a very far-sighted choice in the 1970s), and one group at that institute had already shown that in patients with breast cancer there were small numbers of cancer cells hiding in the bone marrow. Sometimes they were there in very small numbers (5 or 6 cancer cells among 200 million marrow cells), but we all suspected that even that small number might be enough to start new tumors when the marrow was given back to the patient. The question was: while the patient was receiving the high-dose chemotherapy, could we do anything to the marrow to remove or kill the few cancer cells in it?

It took about two years to work out the best way of doing that. Eventually I found a monoclonal antibody that could be used to target the breast cancer cells, and collaborating researchers linked the antibody with a part of an extremely poisonous drug. This technique had been invented by another researcher, and it was in the true tradition of Paul Ehrlich's "magic bullet": the antibody-poison molecule was poisonous only to those cancer cells that were recognized by the antibody. This antibody-poison combination would, it was hoped, function like the magnetic mines used in the Second World War. The magnet attached the mine to the enemy's ship, and then the explosive in the mine did the damage. In fact, as only part of the poison was attached to the antibody, if any of it fell off during the treatment, it would not be poisonous to the normal marrow cells because it was like a mine without a detonator. Theoretically it was a true magic bullet, capable of killing the cancer cells while doing little damage to normal marrow cells.

I devised several systems of testing the combination to make sure it would kill all cancer cells and leave the normal marrow cells relatively undamaged. After all the testing was complete, our group tried the technique on a small group of patients (with their fully informed consent) who had recurrent breast cancer. Sadly, it did not turn out to be a major advance in treatment. The high-dose chemotherapy did not cure the patients of their breast cancer. If there was, say, a recurrence in the liver, that recurrence would get smaller after the high-dose therapy, but eventually it got bigger again. We had, as it were, cured the marrow, but the high-dose therapy did not cure the patient. The problem with high-dose therapy and ABMT was not the theoretical danger of reseeding the patient with cancer from the marrow but that the high-dose chemotherapy used in those days was no better at curing the breast cancer than ordinary doses. (I should point out that nowadays similar techniques are used in many centers for the treatment of different cancers, particularly leukemias, some of which *can* be cured by high-dose treatment. Furthermore, this type of treatment may also have some value in the treatment of certain carefully selected cases of breast and other cancers, and research is active in this area.)

Until our results were analyzed, this approach to breast cancer seemed like a very plausible and useful technique, which it might well have been. In fact, the head of our research group was interviewed by a newspaper during the research, and I heard him give careful and considered answers to all the questions. But that weekend the interview appeared as a "major breakthrough" story, complete with a graphic illustration of how the treatment would be given (this was about three months before we actually gave it). So, because the treatment seemed as though it *should* work, it was greeted as if it already had.

The various committees that considered our grant applications thought, quite rightly, that this was valid and potentially valuable research. The reviewing and funding process was quite correct and appropriate, yet in the end we failed to achieve any immediate advance in the *treatment* of breast cancer. So this is one answer to the question, *"What happened to that major breakthrough we heard about last year?"* The research was good—and one might even say the money was well spent—but, for reasons that could not be predicted at the time, the treatment did not work as we had hoped. Let me stress this point even more clearly: even though our work at that time didn't yield a cure for breast cancer, it was still valid and useful research, and it added to the accumulation of information about high-dose therapies. It was not a waste of money, time, or effort; it was a contribution to the way knowledge about cancer and its treatment is amassed.

Antibody-Guided Therapy Ever since the invention of monoclonal antibodies, cancer researchers have tried to use them to carry poisons (for example, drugs or radioactive substances) directly to cancer cells while keeping them away from normal cells. Hence the term "magic bullets" was quite appropriate. By the mid-1970s, researchers had already started using monoclonal antibodies (initially without a "warhead") and had achieved some dramatic successes in certain types of lymphoma. During the 1980s, monoclonal antibodies with various types of "warhead" were used in dozens of different types of cancer including cancer of the bowel, melanoma of the skin, cancer of the ovary, and so on. Like several researchers in various countries, I became interested in the use of monoclonal antibodies armed with radioactive iodine, which had achieved some impressive results in Britain when used to treat recurrent cancer of the ovary.

When ovarian cancer recurs, it may sometimes create a lot of fluid in the abdomen (ascites). In the early 1980s, some reports were published by pioneers in Britain detailing some very impressive remissions, with complete disappearance of the ascites, after the antibody-iodine combination was injected directly into the abdomen. Our group set about attempting to confirm those results, and I started collaboration with a pathologist named Pat Shaw (we got married during the project—another unpredicted outcome of research). Over the course of four years, our group tested various antibodies, assessed different methods of attaching the iodine, and then, having done all the routine tests on the material, gave various doses of the antibody-iodine material to patients (again, with their fully informed consent). Sadly, the results were disappointing. Out of the first twelve patients that we treated, only two had good remissions of the ascites. As part of the project, we had measured precisely what went on when we injected the antibody-iodine combination into the abdomen. Those results demonstrated that it stayed in the abdomen just as it was supposed to. Other studies that we did on the ascites, however, showed that most of the antibody-iodine combination was not sticking directly to the surface of the cancer cells but was binding to little fragments that the cancer cells had cast off into the ascites. It was as if we had dropped magnetic mines into the sea near the enemy ships, and the enemy had responded by throwing a large number of metal plates into the water as decoys, to which the mines attached themselves and exploded, doing little damage to the ships themselves. Of course we—and our patients—were disappointed, although there had been a small advance in knowledge. Again, the research was valid and useful. Even though it didn't produce a dramatic advance in treatment as we'd all been hoping, it did yield valuable information about some of the limitations to using monoclonal antibodies in treatment, and this form of treatment may have a role in certain cases (for example, of lymphoma, brain tumors, and earlier stages of ovarian cancer).

These two examples show how something that sounds promising may be thwarted by the unpredicted tricks by which cancer cells avoid damage from treatment. More than 90 percent of cancer research is like that. There are good grounds for thinking that an approach *should* work, but then, for reasons that cannot be predicted at the outset, it does not. In research, of course, the scientists learn from their failures, which is why cancer research yields advances in knowledge and understanding more often than advances in treatment. And *that* is one major reason why it sometimes seems as if there are so many breakthroughs and so little progress.

Research That Is Currently Interesting and Might or Might Not Work Out

To illustrate how difficult prediction of the future can be, here are some examples of approaches to cancer research that is going on at the moment. As you will see, for each one there are good and compelling reasons why it might produce some progress. At the present time, nobody can yet know which of these approaches will work and which will not. Hence the difficulty in predicting when progress will happen and what it will look like.

Chronobiology The hormonal environment inside the human body has various cycles of activity. In particular, there are monthly cycles in females (which cause monthly menstruation) and daily cycles in males and females. Many hormones—including growth hormones, "stress" hormones, and others—have their own particular cycle. For example, some may be at their highest levels in the early morning and their lowest levels at night. Some interesting data suggest that when cells become cancerous they no longer obey the same cycles as the normal cells, and this finding may possibly be used to advantage. This field is called chronobiology.

For instance, some data suggest that if a woman has breast cancer, the timing of the initial surgery—whether it is done in the first half of her menstrual cycle or the second—may influence the chance of recurrence. The data on this point are, at the moment, contradictory, with some studies showing one thing, other studies showing something else. As well as the monthly cycles, the time of day when different drugs are given may be important. For example, platinum drugs may be less toxic to normal cells when given in mid-afternoon. In theory, this means that it might be possible to give more of the drug with less toxicity to the patient.

This may be important or, again, it may come to nothing. At the moment, one can say that this is an area worth investigating, and that if it all works out, it might mean that we can give chemotherapy drugs more safely and with fewer side effects. There may even be a greater anticancer benefit if we give them at the right time of day; and we may also be able to improve the prognosis if we do breast surgery at the right point in the hormonal cycle. Only the accumulation of results from research that is going on now will tell us whether this works or not.

Antitelomerase As all cells reproduce themselves, the genetic material—the DNA—forms itself into chromosomes that are the shape of an *x*. The center of the *x* holding the two strands together is called the centromere, and the ends of the arms are capped with a structure called the **telomere**. The telomere is often described as being like the plastic cap at the end of a shoelace. Although we do not understand all the mechanisms involved, the telomere has an important role in limiting the number of times a cell can multiply before it dies. In other words, the telomere is part of the mechanism of the mortality—the limited life—of the cell. Cancer cells are able to escape from the control of the telomere, and one of the ways they do this is by producing an enzyme called telomerase. By using telomerase, some cancer cells seem to be able to increase the number of times they can multiply, and therefore they become immortal (or nearly immortal). The hope is that drugs that stop the action of telomerase might be useful in preventing cancer cells from becoming immortal and therefore bring them under control. This is a new field of research, so discoveries are being made rapidly.

Antiangiogenesis As a secondary tumor (a metastasis) develops and establishes itself, it somehow persuades the cells around it to provide it with new blood vessels that supply oxygen and nutrients for the growing cancer. This process, as mentioned in Chapter 2, is called **angiogenesis** (or sometimes angioneogenesis), and it seems to be an essential part of a cancer's ability to produce metastases. We are just beginning to learn more about this process, in

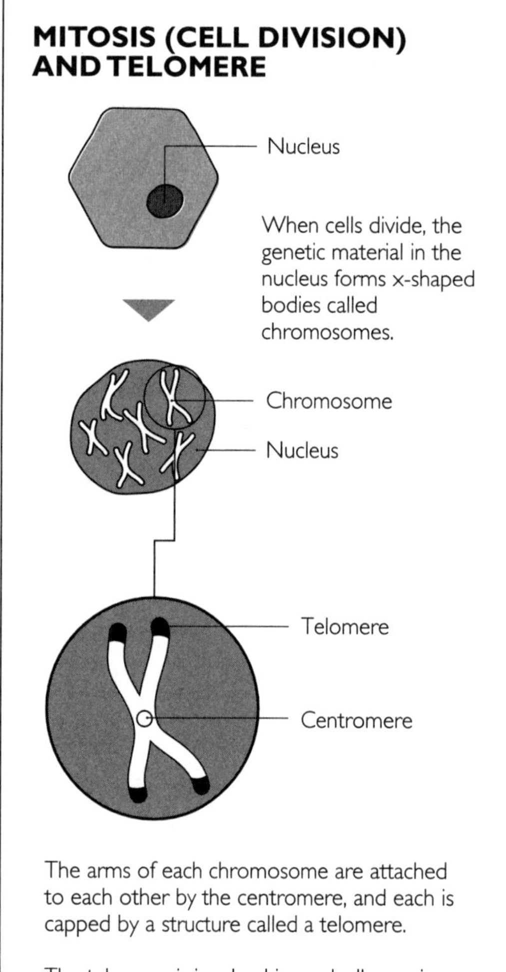

particular, we are beginning to have some clues as to what substances are used by cancer cells to send signals to normal cells and start the angiogenesis. If it were possible to block those signals, it might be possible to prevent cancer cells from establishing themselves in distant parts of the body and developing metastases. In other words, we could concern ourselves not with stopping the cancer cells from spreading but with preventing those cancer cells that have spread from becoming secondary tumors. If this approach works out, this might mean giving antiangiogenesis, say, injections or treatments for years and years after the cancer was first diagnosed and removed. Research studies on this basis are now under way. If it works, it will be a completely different type of treatment.

Antiadhesion Molecules As I mentioned above, cancer cells in clumps behave differently from cancer cells growing in a flat layer in a dish. For example, when there are clumps of cells, they organize themselves and may be capable of resisting or disposing of chemotherapy drugs. It may be possible to identify some of the cell-to-cell signals and "glues" that are used by the cancer cells in making clumps. If those substances could be reliably identified, it might be possible to produce other substances that block their action. If that could be done, we might be able to stop the cancer cells from clumping together, which in turn might make them weaker and easier to attack with drugs or other treatment.

Antioncogene Products and Gene Therapy Ever since oncogenes were discovered, it was realized that these specific portions of DNA were responsible for the production of some substance in the particular cancer cells in which they were found. We now also know that in some cancers the presence of a particular oncogene carries a worse prognosis than if it is absent. For example, in many cancers (in fact, in nearly a third of all cancers), there is an oncogene known as *ras* that has an important role. There is very active research going on into drugs that may interfere with the action of *ras* and stop the way it attaches itself to the cell membrane (which is part of the way in which it contributes to causing cancer). If substances are found that prevent the action of *ras* in human cancers, they may be useful in the treatment of cancer in the future. At present this, too, is an exciting area of research, but no one knows yet whether it will yield advances in treatment.

Another interesting approach is based on the fact that, in some cases of breast cancer, an oncogene called HER2/*neu* is found in abnormally high amounts and causes the cells to produce high amounts of molecules (receptors) that recognize and bind growth factors. The increased ability to bind growth factors then makes the cells grow and divide more rapidly. So when the HER2/*neu* oncogene is present in large quantities, it is associated with the cancer behaving more aggressively than average. Research is under way to test antibodies that bind the receptor molecule produced by the HER2/*neu* gene in the hope that they will block the action of the molecule and make the cancer more sensitive to chemotherapy.

Another related area is the possible use of tumor-suppressor genes. We know that some cancers are caused (or partly caused) by loss of tumor-suppressor genes (see page 26). In theory, it might one day be possible to insert a small strip of DNA to replace the missing gene. In certain circumstances, this might prevent the development of a cancer in someone who has a high risk of it. This technique may first be applied to conditions other than cancer, but even so, it is theoretically of value.

Growth Regulatory Factors We know that many types of cancer seem very responsive to substances that stimulate growth. Some cancers even have a special way of producing growth factors themselves, which then cause the cancer cells to increase their growth rate, just like a racehorse digging spurs into its own side! If we could accurately identify the relevant places on the cancer cell where the growth factors bind, then it might be possible to produce substances that block those areas and somehow cut the cancer cells off from the source of their own stimulation. This sounds much easier than it is in practice. There are also other approaches that may be useful. For example, there is a growth regulatory factor called p53 that is part of the growth-control mechanisms and has been shown to be abnormal in most cancer cells. It has recently been found that certain viruses can be produced that get inside only those cells that have an abnormal p53 system. Furthermore, those viruses may be able to damage and kill exclusively those abnormal cells, in other words, the cancer cells.

Another possible approach sounds at first paradoxical. The substance p27 is another growth-control substance and is also found to be decreased in certain types of cancer. It might be possible to restore the p27 within those tumor cells to normal (and "recontrol" the growing cells). However, another possibility is even more fascinating. Some cancer cells that are resistant to chemotherapy have been shown to have too much p27 when they grow in clumps. Thus the process of growing in a clump seems to be associated with going into a "resting" phase and becoming resistant to chemotherapy. It might be possible to decrease the function of p27 yet further in chemotherapy-resistant cancer clumps and thus speed up the growth of the cancer cells in order to make them more sensitive to chemotherapy.

Vaccines The word "vaccines" has been used very loosely for decades in cancer treatment. There are hundreds of complementary or alternative clinics all over the world where so-called vaccines are given. These usually consist of an extract of a cancer mixed with various substances. Without exception, those complementary types of vaccines have proved useless. However, there is now a growing interest in producing special vaccines directed against certain substances on the surfaces of cancer cells. The important thing is to select the right target on the cancer cell and make sure that the vaccine is effective in producing an immune response that deals with that particular target. The new generation of experiments and agents is still relatively young and clearly very interesting. Many years of research will be needed before we know whether this approach has value or whether cancer cells have the ability to adapt to the new immunization and avoid being damaged by the immune system. (As a matter of note, the older types of vaccinations do have a role. For example, worldwide immunization against hepatitis B, by preventing the long-term damage that occasionally follows the attack of hepatitis, would prevent cancer of the liver. Although this is not a common cancer in this country, vaccination against hepatitis B on a worldwide scale would save a million lives a year—the number of people who otherwise would have died of liver cancer.)

Genetic Identification of High-Risk Individuals

If we could reliably identify individuals who have an extremely high risk of getting a particular type of cancer, we might be able to recommend steps aimed at prevention or early detection. For example, if we knew which individuals had an extremely high chance of getting lung cancer if they smoked cigarettes, we could (perhaps!) work harder to educate them, help them realize that they were at high risk, and encourage them to stop smoking. If we could identify the women who were at particularly high risk of developing breast cancer (the BRCA1 and BRCA2 genes may help us with about 5 percent of all future breast cancer patients), we might be able to start regular mammograms at an early age or even discuss the possibility of preventive surgery. (This idea has been raised several times before, but we had no way of accurately identifying a very high-risk group.)

You can see how some early positive research findings might be greeted as major breakthroughs. Yet even if these approaches turn out to be of major importance, it will be several—probably many—years before the treatments are used in routine practice. This is partly because the process of testing a new treatment and assessing its impact on cancer is a long one. It takes several years to organize and carry out a clinical trial (see page 233) of a new treatment, and if it is the kind of treatment that may have a benefit in the long term, it may take even longer to see and quantify that effect. Hence whatever the promise of a discovery, the evaluation and assessment of its effect on cancer will almost certainly take many years.

Front-Page Stories

The increase in knowledge produced by new research techniques enabled many scientists working in basic research—and many physicians collaborating with them—to see the possible implications of their research. Many naturally became very excited about the possibilities. Unfortunately, although scientists gave carefully phrased interviews appropriately loaded with *"ifs"* and *"it might be's"* and *"perhaps in a few years,"* those statements were often stripped of such qualifying remarks before being passed on to the public. Television and newspaper items were often simple and easily intelligible stories about major breakthroughs that were just around the corner. As a result of that sort of coverage, the expectations of the general public have been raised higher and higher over the last twenty years (although, to be fair, they have been at a fairly high level since the end of the nineteenth century). A typical recent example was the discovery and first reports about the chemotherapy drug Taxol.

There is no doubt that Taxol is an interesting and somewhat unusual drug. It is derived from the bark of the Pacific yew tree, which in itself is newsworthy because widespread use of Taxol might threaten that species of tree with extinction. Early research reports, in the late 1980s and early 1990s, showed that Taxol could produce remissions in cases of cancer of the ovary where the cancer was already resistant to the standard therapy (platinum drugs). Somehow—no one is quite certain how this happened—this fact was taken up widely in the newspapers and even made its way onto television drama series. Taxol seemed to enjoy the status of a miracle drug—a major breakthrough. As later research results became available, it became clear that Taxol was indeed capable of causing a remission in platinum-resistant ovarian cancer, and that it produced remissions in about 30 percent or so of cases. The remissions lasted a few months to a year or so (which is, of course, not a trivial achievement in itself) but were not cures. Concurrently, other studies showed that Taxol could also produce remissions in some cases of drug-resistant breast cancer. In other words, Taxol was, and is, a useful and significant drug that deserves a place in the armory of cancer treatment, perhaps even in the first-line treatment of some cancers such as cancer of the ovary. However, as with all drugs, the exact place that it should occupy will be defined as the research goes on. How the story of Taxol became a "miracle breakthrough" story is unclear. Nevertheless, thousands of patients firmly believed that if they were given Taxol they would be cured (no matter what type of cancer they had) and that if they did not, they would die. The atmosphere of desperation is very difficult to describe or quantify, but the aura around Taxol made it very hard on patients (and also on their medical teams).

This unhappy episode in the history of the public relations of cancer treatment caused disappointment and mistrust all around (in the public, the medical profession, and the media). It is partly because the parties involved in media coverage are almost "preprogrammed" to make the stories as vivid and dramatic as possible that there has been such an erosion of confidence in the whole field of cancer research.

Too Many Breakthrough Headlines: A Personal View

In retrospect, it may have been a great mistake to treat cancer research as if it were a war that could be won in a few years if it was waged with enough willpower and enough money. In fact, the war on cancer does have an identifiable beginning. War against cancer was declared by President Nixon in 1971 as a deliberate public relations move. He officially declared the war and apportioned a large budget for the fledgling National Cancer Institute in Maryland to make sure that the war would be won. Many analysts believe that President Nixon was looking for an identifiable campaign, a crusade that would match the dramatic success of President Kennedy's objective of setting a man on the moon. Sadly, putting a man on the moon was, as one commentator put it, merely a matter of technology—brilliant and innovative technology, but technology nonetheless. In the case of cancer we could not even see our moon clearly, and at that time we had not even invented the cancer-treatment equivalent of jet engines, let alone rockets.

If you declare a war, you had better win it. In wars, most governments do not readily admit that they are not winning. They make overoptimistic speeches and ask for more resources and more cooperation and promise that victory is close at hand. That is what has happened, in a global sense, to the field of cancer research. In an attempt to keep public interest and enthusiasm high, researchers and the media together have been tempted into overoptimism and speculation. There is nothing wrong with this in itself. Speculation is a valid form of opinion, but it is not fact. Too often, however, a researcher's speculation is reported almost as fact—as if it had happened or was definitely about to happen, not as if it *might* happen. The person who pays the price for that overoptimism is the patient with cancer who wonders how the war is going and when it is going to be won.

It would have been better, in retrospect, if we had never compared cancer research to a war in the first place but had portrayed it as a complex system of researchers looking toward the same goal from hundreds of different directions. As I quoted Dr. Kleinerman earlier: it's not a sprint, it's a marathon, a marathon being run by thousands of diligent and careful collaborators all over the world. Too many comparisons to a war or to a sprint—and too many false dawns—are bad for credibility. We are all going to have to be more careful in avoiding excessive speculation and the overoptimism it can produce.

Instead of those surges of unrealistic reporting, often followed by a feeling of disillusionment, or even distrust, we need stories that accurately report some of the work being done by groups of steady and thoughtful people involved in steady and diligent research. Such research necessarily requires steady and secure funding. It may be true that breakthroughs in knowledge have not yet led to dramatic breakthroughs in treatment, but there has been no deception. Marathons last longer than sprints, and spectators who have been led to expect a sprint get impatient with marathons. Research is hard work, and it requires not only diligence but also talent, often found at only the larger research centers where a good number of scientists—a critical mass—can link up with each other and stimulate each other's work and thinking. What we need next is lots more of what we're building now: lots of talented and diligent researchers doing lots of work with lots of collaboration and a steady, secure supply of support and funding to keep it going.

LIVING WITH CANCER

10

What's in This Chapter

More than any other part of this book, Chapter 10 is intended almost exclusively for the person with cancer and her or his family and friends. I realize that it may seem presumptuous of me to attempt to summarize the major aspects of living with cancer in a single chapter (after all, numerous books have been written solely about this subject). Nevertheless, this book would be incomplete without at least an attempt to provide a few guidelines—again, background rather than foreground—to assist you in understanding what is going on, what is available to help you, and how you can ask for what you want and need.

Many people believe that the diagnosis is in itself a death sentence. Yet, as we saw in Chapter 4, that is untrue for a very large number of patients. As many experts have pointed out, "There are many more people living with cancer than there are dying of it." You may therefore find it very useful to have some practical hints and tips about how you can improve the quality of your life with cancer. To assist you and your family, therefore, the first section of Chapter 10 will deal with three of the most common and most distressing physical symptoms (pain, tiredness, and depression). Then follows a table outlining some of the most important medical emergencies, the symptoms you may notice, and what to do to get help. The next section is a brief summary of issues to do with sexuality. Following that is a section for people who will require a stoma (a colostomy, an ileostomy, or a urinary stoma) or who already have one. The fifth section deals with communication problems: your communication with your friends and family as well as your medical team. The sixth section includes some guidelines for your friends and family about how they can help you. The seventh section sets out a practical approach to spiritual issues, and the eighth section deals with issues in palliative care and at the end of life. As everyone knows, sometimes things go badly, and so I thought it important to include in this section of the book some guidelines and thoughts on how to make plans and how to cope should that happen.

Three Common Symptoms

Although cancer can, in theory, cause almost any symptom you can think of, some symptoms are much more common than others. In particular, pain, tiredness, and depression are very common with almost all types of cancer and sometimes may be almost overwhelming. Often, not knowing where the symptoms come from, what they mean, what can be done, and the resulting feeling of fear can aggravate all three symptoms and increase their negative impact on the person's quality of life.

As in so many difficult situations, the more knowledge there is, the less fear there is. Many people find that they can increase their ability to cope simply by knowing more about these symptoms, what assistance is available and what to ask for. Other problems that may occur in cancer are usually specific to the particular type of cancer, and they have been mentioned in the appropriate places in Chapter 4.

Pain and How to Cope with It

SUMMARY OF THE KEY FACTS IN THIS SECTION

- Pain occurs in about two-thirds of all patients with advanced cancer.
- Pain caused by cancer can be completely or mostly controlled in at least nine out of ten patients.
- Pain-killing medicines need to be taken regularly (usually every four hours). They are NOT addictive and do NOT shorten life.
- Side effects caused by pain-killing medicines are constipation and nausea (both of which can be controlled in the great majority of cases) and sleepiness (which usually wears off after two or three days).

The Most Important Features of Cancer Pain

Pain is the aspect of cancer that causes the most concern and fear. Many people think that if you have cancer, you are *bound* to have pain and that nothing can be done to relieve it. Both beliefs are completely unfounded: they are myths. First, pain does not happen to every person with cancer; in fact, it is a problem for just under two-thirds of people who have advanced cancer. Second, and even more important, if it does happen, cancer pain can be controlled (often *completely* controlled) in the great majority of cases.

Several other important points about cancer pain in general need to be emphasized.

First, there are different ways that a tumor can cause pain. Although it seems peculiar, in fact pain does not usually come from within the tumor itself. Rather, tumors may press on or interfere with adjacent parts of the body—a bone, a nerve, or the wrappings around the liver, for example—and so there may be pain originating from those organs or tissues.

Second, the diagnosis of the exact cause of the pain is very important in planning effective relief. In many cases your doctor will be able to find out what is causing your pain from what you tell him or her about it. This means that your description of the pain and your answers to your doctor's questions are very important.

Third, not only is there a great deal that can be done to relieve pain but also, in most cases, you the patient are a very important part of that process. Hence your understanding of what is going on (and your understanding of why the treatment is being given and how it is meant to be taken) are major factors in deciding whether the treatment will work and your pain will be controlled.

How Cancer Can Cause Pain

Tumors caused by cancer are, in themselves, usually painless. A tumor in the breast, bowel, skin, or almost anywhere does not usually hurt. That is what makes early diagnosis of cancer so difficult: because it is painless it may often go unnoticed in the early stages. Occasionally, if the tumor happens to grow in a certain way, or if the defense systems of the body react to it very strongly and make the area around the tumor inflamed, there may be pain coming directly from the tumor, but in most circumstances there is not.

In general, pain related to cancer is caused by a tumor pressing on or invading neighboring structures such as a nerve, the membrane covering a bone, the liver, or some other organ. For example, a tumor can irritate a nearby nerve in the same way as an inflamed disc ("slipped disc") in the back can irritate the sciatic nerve and cause the pain we call sciatica. Furthermore, the pain caused by irritation of a nerve may be perceived as coming from the area that the nerve is responsible for. Just as the pain from a slipped disc may be felt as if it had started in the back of the thigh, so may a tumor in the vertebral spine cause pain that apparently begins in the thigh, a tumor in the upper back cause pain that feels as if it is coming from the chest, a tumor in the diaphragm cause shoulder pain, and so on.

As well as irritating nerves, tumors may cause indirect pain in other ways. For example, a tumor might interfere with the normal function of part of the bowel. That might cause the bowel to go into spasm as it tries to move the contents of the bowel past the tumor. The person will feel spasms of pain that come and go in waves as the bowel tries to squeeze the contents past and then relaxes. Pain that comes and goes in that way is called **colic** or **colicky pain**.

In other places, a tumor might cause pain by stretching the covering of a bone, the periosteum. If a small tumor develops inside a bone, you may not feel any pain or discomfort at all. If the tumor grows larger, however, particularly if it started near the outer surface of a bone, it may stretch the periosteum and that stretching may cause pain. A tumor might also grow in a place in a bone that makes it easy for the bone to break, and that break might cause you pain.

The same is true in the liver. A tumor might develop in your liver and not cause any pain or problems at all. But if it is near the outside of the liver instead of in the middle, then, like a tumor in bone, it might stretch the covering of the liver and be felt as a discomfort or pain in the upper part of the abdomen on the right or in the center.

Another place where tumors can sometimes establish themselves is inside the head and skull. Again, small tumors may sometimes develop and not cause any symptoms. If they grow bigger, however, they may cause swelling of the brain around them and interfere with the wrappings around the brain, the meninges. This may cause a certain type of headache, which can be moderate or severe. It is often made worse by coughing or straining and is sometimes accompanied by blurring of vision or vomiting. (Once again, let me emphasize that **not every headache means a tumor in the brain**. In fact, recent research shows that among cancer patients the commonest cause of headache is migraine, not cancer.)

Diagnosing the Cause of Cancer Pain

Your Account of the Pain By far the most important step in most types of cancer pain begins with your doctor finding out from you all about the pain: where it is, what it feels like, how bad it is, what makes it worse, what makes it better, and some other aspects as well. To do that, your doctor will probably ask you a number of specific questions about the pain. Because your description is essential in planning the right treatment, it is important for you to try to answer the questions in as much detail and as accurately and honestly as you can.

In general, the following are the most important aspects of your pain that your doctor is likely to focus on:

Site Whereabouts in your body do you feel the pain, and does the pain seem to start in one place and then spread or move to another area?

Nature or Type of Pain What does the pain feel like? Is it a constant dull pain, a quick sharp pain, or does it come and go in waves (colic)?

Duration How long does it last—a few seconds or an hour or more? At what time of day or night does it come? Does it wake you from sleep or stop you from getting to sleep?

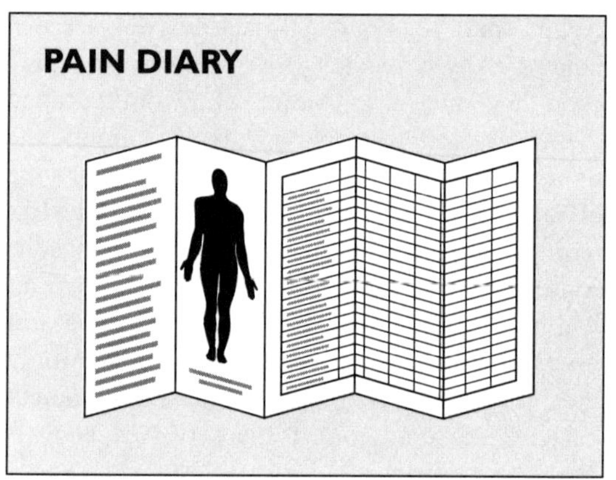

Things That Make the Pain Worse Have you noticed anything you do that makes the pain worse or that starts it off: activities such as bending over, lifting things, moving around, breathing in, coughing, eating meals, and so on?

Things That Make the Pain Better Have you noticed anything you do or take that reduces or relieves the pain: activities such as resting, avoiding certain movements, or eating small meals? Have any painkillers you have tried made the pain better?

Those are just some of the questions your doctor may ask you about your pain. You may also be given what is called a **pain diary** to help you record what is going on with your pain. There are many different types of these, but usually they have a diagram of the body so you can mark where you feel the pain or pains, if there are several locations. You can also record other aspects of the pain, such as what it feels like, when you felt it, and for how long.

Additional Tests As well as going over the details of the pain with you, your doctor may need to do some tests as well. These could include X rays (such as X rays of the chest or back), bone scans, ultrasound tests (which can show problems in the liver or the abdomen or lower down in your pelvis), CT scans, and in certain circumstances MRI scans. Any or several of these may be useful in your case. Your doctor will tell you exactly which tests he or she is recommending and what areas or problems the tests are best at showing up.

Because it can take some time to get all the tests organized and assess the results, it is customary to start treatment for the pain—with painkillers, for example—before the test results are in.

Members of Your Professional Support Team

A number of different people may be involved in your care, particularly in the relief of pain and other symptoms. The exact type and number of services available depends to some degree on where you live and how things are organized in your area. In general, however, looking after people with cancer these days usually means getting several different disciplines involved in providing a range of connected services. This is called the **multidisciplinary approach**, and it means that your medical team may include (in addition to your doctor) nursing services, social work services, psychology services, occupational therapy services, and so on. In areas where there are specialized nurses, often called **clinical nurse specialists**, your pain treatment (along with other aspects of your treatment) may be supervised by a nurse who visits your home or who assesses you regularly at the clinic or health center. There may also be a specialized **pain clinic** at your local hospital and pain control teams who supervise special pain treatments, such as the pain pumps that will be discussed below.

Thus the expertise available does vary from place to place, and you may wish to investigate what can be provided in your area. You may find that a lot of the questions you want to ask about the details of your treatment can best be directed, for example, to the nursing team.

How Cancer Pain Can Be Treated

The many different types of treatments used in the control of cancer pain fall into three broad groups.

First, there are treatments aimed at the tumor itself and that may decrease pain by causing the tumor to shrink, thus relieving pressure on a nerve or an area of periosteum. For example, radiotherapy is often used for tumors in bone or in other areas. In some circumstances a single lesion that is causing pain might be removed surgically if that is feasible. There are also some circumstances in which chemotherapy can be used to reduce pain. These types of pain-relief treatments are described under the individual headings in Chapter 4.

Second, there are treatments to control the pain itself: these include painkilling (analgesic) medications and some other methods as well. In this area there is a great deal of information that may be of help to you about the different painkilling medications, how to use them to get the most benefit, how to deal with any side effects, what other methods can help with pain, and so on. I give details of some of these treatments below.

Third, in some circumstances there are specialized techniques that can be used to control pain. I give a brief outline of the types of treatment available in this area. You will need to discuss the details of such treatment with your doctor.

Analgesics (Painkilling Medications): The Basic Principles The primary objective in prescribing and using analgesics is to get five aspects of the treatment right for you and for your pain:

- the **right medication**
- at the **right dose**
- on the **right schedule** (in other words, how often and when you take the medication)
- by the **right route** (by mouth, suppository, or injection)
- with **control of any side effects** the analgesics may cause.

There are many different analgesics, which fall into three main groups of increasing power, a sort of three-step ladder. The bottom step of the ladder

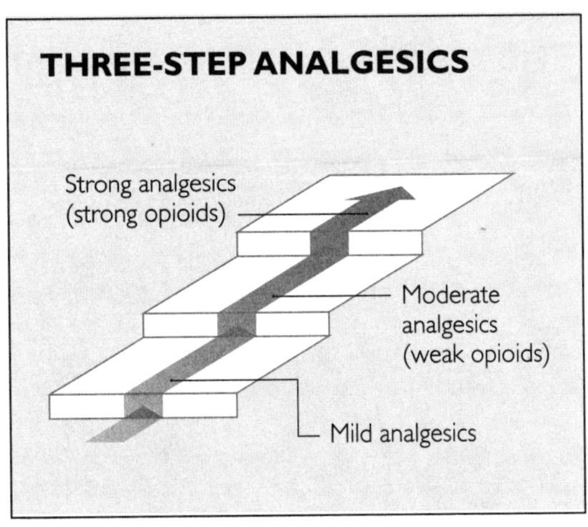

consists of the medications that are called **mild analgesics** such as **acetaminophen** (Tylenol is one brand name) and **ASA** (acetylsalicylic acid or aspirin). As the name suggests, these are medications that are used for the milder pains. The second step consists of **moderate analgesics** such as **codeine** and **anileridene**, which are stronger than the mild ones. The third step consists of the **strong analgesics** such as **morphine**, **oxycodone**, and **hydromorphone**. Because drugs such as morphine (and codeine) are similar to substances found in opium, all drugs with this type of chemical structure are called **opioids**. The moderate analgesics are often referred to as **weak opioids**, and morphine and hydromorphone are called **strong opioids**.

It is important to remember that not only is everyone's pain different, but everyone's perception of their own pain is different too. Some people may have what they regard as a small ache that is well controlled by mild analgesics, whereas another person with the same type and size of tumor in the same place might well need moderate analgesics or even strong ones. Your physician will try to match the painkillers not to the type of the tumor or the location of the problem, but rather to your pain. For that reason, you need to be as honest and specific as possible when you describe the pain.

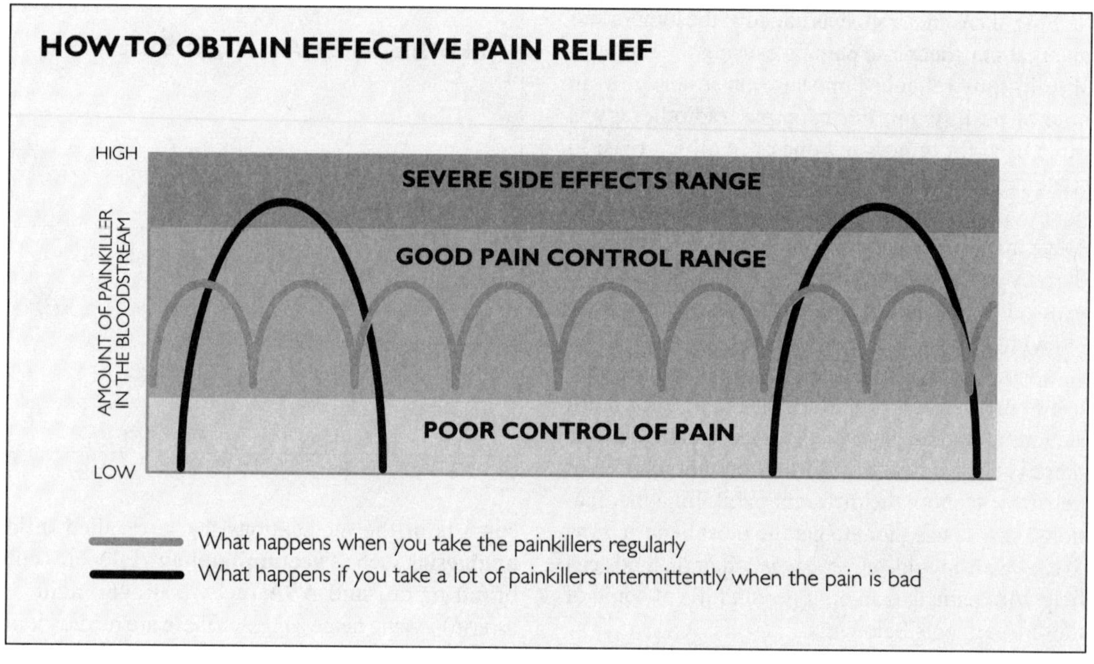

How to Use Analgesics If you have pain only occasionally, it may be fine, if that is what your doctor recommends, to take the painkillers only occasionally. But **if the pain is there most of the time or all of the time, you need to take your painkillers regularly** so that there is enough of the medication in your body to keep the pain under control. That means taking the dose of medication that your doctor recommends (no more and no less) and taking it regularly as prescribed. Taking your medication as instructed allows your pain to be controlled properly. Also, you will probably end up using fewer painkillers per day than if you wait until the pain really hurts and then take a lot of painkillers to try to switch the pain off.

The correct time interval depends on the actual medication that your doctor has given you. But **for most painkillers, except the slow-release ones, the regular doses should be taken every four hours**. This applies to the standard preparations of mild analgesics (such as acetaminophen), the weak opioids, and the strong ones. Unless you have been given slow-release preparations or have been given different instructions, you should take your regular analgesics every four hours.

The **slow-release preparations** just mentioned allow the drug to be released into you slowly from the tablet or capsule. Morphine and some other drugs are available in this form. These preparations should be taken **every twelve hours** (or, only if your doctor recommends it, every eight hours). The key is stability: if you take the medication regularly, your body gets a steady amount of the drug all the time, which means you'll get the best chance of good pain control.

In addition to the regular doses, your doctor may prescribe additional doses that can be taken occasionally if you have bad pain at one particular time. These are usually called "**breakthrough doses**," and the dose may be different from the regular dose. Some doctors, myself included, also advise some patients to take one and a half times their regular dose as their last nighttime dose taken at bedtime. With the higher dosage, they may be able to sleep through the night and not have to wake up to take further doses.

Myths about Analgesics First, many patients worry that if their painkillers are gradually increased in strength, they may become addicted or have their mental abilities impaired. Such stories are *not* true, and there is a lot of very good research data to prove that they are largely myths. The real situation is simple: if you have continuous or long-term cancer pain, then strong painkillers are *not* addictive, any more than insulin is addictive to someone with diabetes. You need the painkillers to keep the pain at bay. If the source of the pain is stopped by some other treatment (such as radiotherapy or surgery, if those are possible), then you will be able to reduce and even stop your painkillers.

Second, strong painkillers are not a sign that the end of your life is imminent. A lot of people think, *"If the doctor gives me morphine, that means I'm going to die soon."* This is also not true. Decades ago doctors gave morphine to their patients only at the very end of life; but for many years now, all doctors, myself included, prescribe morphine as treatment for cancer pain quite early after the pain starts if it is needed at that time.

Third, when prescribed in the correct doses and taken at the correct time intervals, analgesics will not turn you into a zombie or put you into coma! You may notice that you are tired or even very tired and sleepy for the first two days or so after you start, and again for another two days or so after the dose is increased, if an increase becomes necessary at any point. This may be due partly to your previous lack of sleep caused by the pain and partly to the medication. But after those two days, almost certainly you will not be sleepy or drowsy. From my own practice, I have dozens of photographs sent to me of patients out mowing the lawn, on vacation at the beach, playing golf—doing almost everything you can think of while regularly taking their analgesics (quite often morphine). Thus the myths about morphine or any other analgesics are exactly that—myths.

To put it simply, the myths and fears of cancer pain may actually make the pain seem to be worse; and, on the other hand, effective relief of pain will decrease the fear as well as controlling the pain. As the saying goes, *"Nothing succeeds like success."*

Route of Administration If it is difficult for you to take tablets or syrup—because of difficulty in

TWO COMMON TYPES OF PAIN PUMPS

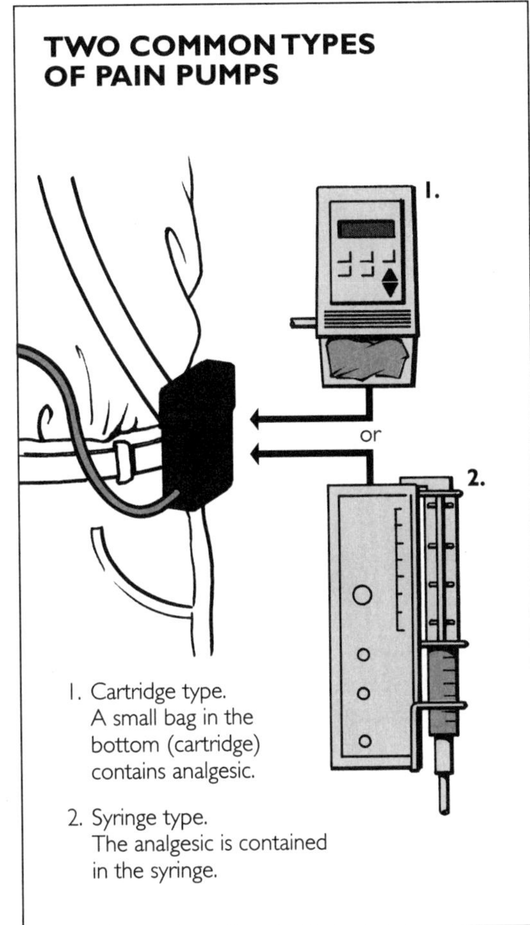

1. Cartridge type.
   A small bag in the bottom (cartridge) contains analgesic.
2. Syringe type.
   The analgesic is contained in the syringe.

swallowing, for example, or some other problem—suppositories can be used. There are several advantages to suppositories. First, you do not need to swallow them but instead simply insert them into your rectum after moistening them with warm water. Second, the drug in the suppository gets absorbed slowly and evenly over several hours. Third, you can put in one or two (or sometimes more) suppositories at a time, so you may be able to increase the dose if your doctor recommends it. For first-time users it is always a little unfamiliar and perhaps a bit embarrassing: but temporary awkwardness is far better than permanent pain. Other methods include patches that can be attached to the skin and that may also be very effective.

Pain Pumps Apart from these methods, if you need more analgesic than you can comfortably swallow or take by suppository, your doctor may recommend that the painkiller be given by slow steady injection under the skin (or sometimes into a vein) using a device called a pain pump. Some types of pain pumps are very sophisticated, and there are several models available, but they all work in similar ways. The analgesic medication is put in a small plastic bag inside what is usually called a cartridge, or, depending on the particular pump, it is loaded in a syringe. The pump then slowly pumps the medication out through a thin plastic tube. Your nurse or doctor will put a fine needle under your skin, usually on the abdomen or thigh. The needle is so fine that you will hardly feel it as it goes in, and once it is in place you won't feel it at all. The pump then gives you a steady dose of medication, usually for several days or a week. Most pumps have a button that can be pressed if you need extra doses of medication (breakthrough doses) if the pain is particularly bad at a certain time.

Side Effects of Analgesics There are three major types of side effects that you may get from analgesics. All of them are more common with the strong analgesics, but you may get them even with the mild ones, so it is worth my explaining the details here. They are nausea, constipation, and drowsiness.

Nausea is actually quite common and occurs in about half of all patients on analgesics. Antinauseant medications are usually very effective, and your doctor might well recommend that you take antinauseants either with your analgesics or perhaps twenty minutes or so beforehand. Many antinauseants are available as suppositories. If you do experience bad nausea, it may be helpful to put in an antinauseant suppository, wait until your nausea improves and then take your regular dose of analgesic.

Constipation is also very common. In fact, with painkillers from codeine upward, including morphine and hydromorphone, constipation is almost inevitable. Many doctors—again, myself included—routinely give laxatives with analgesics because constipation is so likely. There are many different types of laxatives, but generally doctors give a stool softener for you to take several times a day, plus something for you to take to stimulate the bowel into moving if you have not had your bowels open for two or three days.

Drowsiness may occur when you first take the stronger analgesic and again for a few days after the dose is increased, if that's needed, but usually the drowsiness wears off after a few days. Please note that you must not drive (or do anything potentially hazardous to you or other people) if you are feeling drowsy. If in doubt, ask your doctor.

Use of Other Medications Analgesics can be given together with other medications to help control pain. For instance, drugs that reduce inflammation (anti-inflammatories) or steroids can be used together with your painkillers. It is very important to make sure you understand what is being prescribed for you—what each medication is for and how it is meant to be used. If you are not sure, please do ask: it is better for you and for your doctor if all the details are clear.

Nonanalgesic Measures A few other things may be helpful in reducing your pain or allowing you to live with it more easily if it can't be controlled completely. These techniques vary in their effectiveness, but some people find some or all of them very helpful.

One of the most valuable in helping you cope with pain or any other symptom is counseling and support. Depending on what is available in your area, there may be psychotherapy services, or there may be support groups consisting of other patients dealing with the same problem. I deal with this topic more fully later in this chapter.

Then there is acupuncture, the traditional Chinese technique of putting needles in and either twiddling them or applying very small electric currents to them. This helps with pain in quite a few people. Relaxation techniques may be helpful, too. Usually that means getting a tape of a relaxation session and listening to it regularly. Biofeedback techniques, in which you teach yourself to relax, may be useful. There are also little devices that generate weak electrical currents to stimulate nerves in the skin to "distract" your nervous system from the cancer pain. These are usually called transcutaneous electrical nerve stimulators or TENS devices. Any or all of these may help you: they do not help everyone, but they may be useful in certain cases.

A Caution about Massage and Manipulation

One brief note of caution: do not take any chiropractic manipulation, shiatsu massage, Rolfing, or any procedure that involves being physically manipulated by someone until you have cleared it with your doctor. In cancer, there are situations (such as weak bones) that might be made worse if the person who manipulates you does the wrong thing. So check first.

Treatment of Particular Pain Problems

If your pain is not well controlled by any of these measures, one or two other procedures may occasionally be used to control pain, if they happen to be appropriate or feasible in your case.

Nerve Block If the pain is coming from a specific nerve, that nerve may be blocked with an injection given into or near the nerve. (Usually this will be done in a pain clinic or by an anesthetist.) The procedure may cause numbness in the area or weakness, so the potential benefits and risks will need to be discussed with your doctor.

Cutting a Nerve In the same way, it is occasionally possible to cut a nerve that is causing severe pain. Sometimes it is possible to interrupt the nerve by surgery where it joins the spinal cord.

Epidural Injections It is also possible in certain circumstances to put analgesics directly into the area around the spinal cord—the epidural approach—with a thin tube (a catheter).

If one of these special procedures is needed or is appropriate in your case, your doctor will discuss the details with you.

Tiredness

Tiredness, even exhaustion, is very common with any serious illness. It is common with cancer as well, particularly during and after therapy (chemotherapy or radiotherapy especially). Many patients find that when they are exhausted they may have to spend most of the day in bed or in a chair. While that in itself may not be distressing, many people also find that when they start to move around more and do light chores, their abilities and stamina are drastically reduced. Typically they may start a task—say, doing the dishes—and discover after a few minutes that they are exhausted and cannot continue. This is often very depressing and sometimes alarming. Let me emphasize that tiredness of that type is very common indeed. If it happens to you, think of it as "normal in the circumstances" and do not feel distressed or depressed. Try to accept it as a limitation, and work within those limitations. You may well find, as time goes on, that you can do a bit more. If so, that is good. But do not feel too discouraged at being limited in your exercise capacity. It is very common.

Work The same is true of work. You may find that you can return to work part-time and doing so may give you a feeling of support and of "being back in the swim of things again." On the other hand, you may find that you are rapidly exhausted, and you may then worry that your colleagues at work will think less of you. Again, take things one step at a time. If you can work for only a couple of hours or so, accept that and be honest with yourself (and your colleagues) about it. Do not push yourself to the point of collapse, as this will make you and your colleagues alarmed and despondent about the future.

Depression

SUMMARY OF THE KEY FACTS IN THIS SECTION

- Depression is very common in patients who have or have had cancer, including people whose cancer is in remission or even cured.
- Depression is relatively easy to diagnose using internationally agreed upon criteria.
- Once diagnosed and treated (with antidepressants, counseling, or both), it can be completely or mostly relieved in more than three-quarters of cases.
- No one should say (or think), *"Well, who wouldn't be depressed: the diagnosis is cancer."* For all cancer patients, depression is not only one of the most common problems but also one of those most easily fixed.

Most Important Features

Everybody gets a bit depressed at some time. We all have "bad days," "horrible Mondays," or some time when we feel blue or low in spirits. Usually such moods improve after a few hours or a day or so. Those feelings are not true depression. Depression is different: it is an illness in which a person's mood not only goes wrong, making him or her feel very low in spirits, but also stays that way and adversely affects the person's life. Thus depression is not the same as an occasional, short-lived mood of sadness. In depression, those low feelings are severe. They are not affected by what happens to you, they interfere with your ability to lead your normal life, and, most important, they do not go away even after several weeks. That is depression, and it is very common in any person who has or has had cancer, even though the cancer may be in remission (or even cured).

Depression is an illness that can be treated very successfully. Hence nobody with cancer should be told that, *"Anyone in your position would feel depressed."* **If you have depression (as defined below), then it can and should be treated.**

Diagnosis

The diagnosis of depression is really based on what you tell your doctor about your feelings and how your life is affected. There is no blood test or X ray that can be done to diagnose the condition, so that your doctor depends on your story to make the diagnosis. The symptoms of depression have been agreed upon internationally, and I give a brief summary of them in Table 10.1.

As Table 10.1 indicates, the key feature of depression is that you experience several symptoms nearly all the time for at least two weeks, and one of those symptoms has to be either a depressed mood or taking no pleasure in life. If one of those two symptoms is present, plus four of the other seven symptoms in the table, then the diagnosis is depression. It is a second illness that you have (in addi-

TABLE 10.1: SYMPTOMS OF DEPRESSION

IF there is no physical illness of the brain or psychiatric illness,

THEN depression consists of **five** of these symptoms present for **two weeks** (one of them must be item 1 or 2).

1. **Depressed mood** every day for most of the day.
2. **Very little interest or pleasure** in most activities nearly every day for most of the day.
3. **Noticeable weight loss or gain** or a major change in appetite.
4. **Sleep disturbance:** not being able to get to sleep or waking early or being very sleepy nearly every day.
5. **Feeling agitated or feeling slowed down** nearly every day.
6. **Feeling excessively tired** or lacking in energy nearly every day.
7. **Feeling worthless or guilty** nearly every day.
8. **Feeling unable to concentrate or make decisions.**
9. **Having frequent thoughts of death or suicide.**

tion to the cancer), and, most important, it can be treated.

Treatment

There are two basic approaches to the treatment of depression, and they can and often should be used together. There is tablet treatment with antidepressants and therapeutic dialogue with a therapist (a counselor, psychotherapist, psychiatrist, or other trained person).

These are not alternatives to each other. It is not a case of "either-or"; both can be used together and often are. It is true that some people with milder depression will improve with psychotherapy alone, for example. If you do need medication, however, it will work better if you also have some "talk"—about the drugs, about why they're being recommended, and about why you personally will benefit from them—with whoever prescribes them. You will get better more quickly if you are clear about why you are being given the tablets and what they are likely to achieve for you and if your progress is being monitored.

Therapeutic Dialogue For the nonmedication therapy of depression, there are many different options. Depending on the services available in your area, it may be that all that is required are several thorough discussions with your own doctor (particularly if she or he has been trained in counseling techniques) about your situation and how you are coping with it. There are also psychotherapists who have been trained to do this, but they are not usually medical doctors and so in most cases cannot prescribe medication for you in addition to the therapy. There are also psychiatrists—who are medical doctors and therefore can prescribe—who have been trained in this kind of therapy. Yet another alternative might be to participate in group therapy with other people with similar problems.

If you are wondering what sort of therapy to choose, a lot will depend on the kind of person you are. Some people feel much better in groups because they feel less alone and can see things more clearly when other people are describing them. Others feel very shy and cannot deal with the presence of other people. To help you decide, you may wish to start by talking it over with your family doctor or whoever has diagnosed your depression. Even though you may feel discouraged and may be thinking *"Why bother?"* that feeling or mood may itself be due to the depression, so do try to find out what is available in your area. If need be, get someone to help you do the phoning; it can really pay off.

Antidepressant Medications Antidepressant medicines have changed dramatically over the last few years, with great benefit to the patient.

There are now many different types of drugs that are highly effective against depression and that can dramatically change the way you feel. These medications help to reduce psychological distress—what one patient described as *"what I feel when my mind hurts."* Antidepressants do not change the world, nor do they change your thoughts or your personality; but they do change what you *feel,* and they reduce the amount of worry and distress that the world causes you.

Types of Antidepressants There are basically four different groups of drugs, which work in different ways to change the chemicals within the brain and nervous system. The four main groups are the **tricyclics**, the **tetracyclics**,* and two others that are real mouthfuls, the **SSRIs** (serotonin specific re-uptake inhibitors) and the **MAOIs** (monoamine oxidase inhibitors).

* Tetracycli*cs* are antidepressants that have no connection with the antibiotics called tetracycl*ines*.

Principles of Taking Antidepressants

Two general rules are very important.

Take Them as Prescribed and Regularly Take the tablets just as they have been prescribed, every day (or night), whether you are sleeping well or not. That's really important. You will probably find—usually in the first week or even less—that if you have been sleeping badly, your sleep pattern will improve. When that happens, you should not stop taking your antidepressants (that is, you should not take them only if you have sleep problems). Antidepressants really work only when they achieve steady levels in your bloodstream, and that cannot happen unless you take the tablets regularly.

Complete the Course Most people need antidepressants for a moderate amount of time, usually several months (at least three or four). Sometimes when the treatment is stopped after four months, you get depressed again, and some people need antidepressants on a long-term basis. If so, fine. It is not a reflection of personal weakness; it is just the way your brain chemistry is.

Antidepressants Are Not Tranquilizers and Are Not Addictive Antidepressants are quite different from tranquilizer medications and work in a totally different way. Many tranquilizers, as you may be aware from stories in the media, may be addictive after even a few weeks, and patients often have real difficulty in getting off them. Antidepressants are completely different and are not addictive.

Side Effects The main side effects are a dry mouth and feeling a little sleepy in the morning. If you are using the SSRI group of drugs, however, you may not experience either of those symptoms, although those medications may not be suitable in every single case. The MAOI antidepressants are somewhat different (though they are recommended relatively rarely these days). There are several foods that it is very important not to eat, and other medications you must not take while you are on MAOIs. So if you have been prescribed MAOIs, ask your doctor or your pharmacist for a complete list of the precautions and the things you must be careful of.

Emergencies and When to Get Urgent Help

Table 10.2 provides a list of some medical emergencies that may happen to cancer patients, particularly if they are receiving treatment.

This is only a brief list, so **if something very serious happens suddenly, even if it isn't listed on this table, please seek medical advice immediately. Common sense is also very important.** If things are suddenly deteriorating for you (or for the person you are looking after) and you cannot make contact with your local doctor for some hours, go to the nearest emergency department.

With those two notes of caution, I have listed some of the more common problems that can occur suddenly. For each one I have put in the most common type of cause or causes, though of course there may be other causes in your particular case.

Sexuality*

I have deliberately set the topic of sexuality apart from the section on the physical aspects of cancer because sexuality is much more than a physical issue. For many people, sex is an extremely important component of their relationships, but it is a subject that is rarely talked about openly and candidly. Most of the time, this does not matter. When a serious illness affects one partner, however, it does matter. In fact, specialists in this subject have found that sexual problems are almost universal among cancer patients who were sexually active at the time of diagnosis. Most of us in the health care professions did not realize how common these problems are because we didn't ask!

Why Sex Is So Important As we all know, the sexual urge is a powerful one for the majority of people. In fact, it is one of the few urges that is powerful enough to be an antidote to pain and misery, at least some of the time. For the patient, sex may sometimes be the only readily accessible means of escape, albeit temporary, from the world of worry and misery that seems to enclose her or him. Furthermore, sex is not only a means of escape, it is also a route to human contact and intimacy. Because it is a normal activity, it may also be an important means for the patient to feel like a normal human being.

Causes of Sexual Problems Although there are many different factors that can cause sexual problems, it may be useful to divide them into three groups.

Physical Problems First, there may be physical sexual problems created by the disease or its treatment. For example, pelvic surgery as part of the treatment of bladder cancer may cause failure of erection. Similarly, pelvic radiotherapy or surgery in gynecological cancer can sometimes cause physical problems such as discomfort during penetration. Urinary catheters or conditions affecting the back or hips are other examples. Any of these may impede or prevent the couple from having sex when they wish to.

General Reactions to Stress Second, as everyone knows, stress often causes sexual problems and vice versa. Obviously the diagnosis of cancer in one partner is going to affect the relationship in a major way. Often it may be the biggest strain ever

* Some of this section is adapted from a previous book of mine, *I Don't Know What to Say: How to Help and Support Someone Who Is Dying* (New York: Vintage Books, 1989).

TABLE 10.2: MEDICAL EMERGENCIES		
SYMPTOM OR PROBLEM	**POSSIBLE CAUSES**	**WHAT TO DO**
Fever of 38°C (100.4°F) or more or fever with shivering	Infection, particularly if patient has had chemotherapy recently	Contact hospital. Medical advice should be obtained within a few hours.
Sudden shortness of breath	Infection (pneumonia), blood clot (pulmonary embolus), fluid around the lung (effusion), or other problems	Get medical advice within a few hours. If breathlessness is so bad that the person cannot speak or if there is blueness around the lips, go to emergency department at once.
Coughing up blood	Blood clot, tumor, infection, or other causes	If not profuse blood loss, then medical advice needed in a few hours.
Vomiting material that looks like coffee grounds	Bleeding from the stomach, esophagus, or duodenum	Get medical advice within a couple of hours. If patient starts feeling dizzy or faint, go to emergency department at once.
Passing jet-black, tarry stools	Bleeding from the lower bowel	Get medical advice within a couple of hours. If patient starts feeling dizzy or faint, go to emergency department at once.
Large bruises or purple spots in the skin	Bleeding in the skin—may be due to low platelets (particularly after chemotherapy or if there is a marrow problem)	Get medical advice within a few hours. If patient starts feeling dizzy or faint, go to emergency department at once.
Bleeding from nose or mouth	Low platelets (particularly after chemotherapy or if there is a marrow problem)	Get medical advice within a few hours. If patient starts feeling dizzy or faint, go to emergency department at once.
Inability to pass urine	Sudden problem in the spinal cord or a problem in the pelvis	If no previous problems with the bladder, seek medical advice immediately. If accompanied by numbness or weakness in the legs or buttocks, this may be urgent: get immediate advice or go to emergency department.

TABLE 10.2: continued		
SYMPTOM OR PROBLEM	**POSSIBLE CAUSES**	**WHAT TO DO**
Inability to walk	Sudden problem in the spinal cord or a problem in the pelvis	If no previous problems with walking, seek medical advice immediately. If accompanied by any problem in passing urine, this may be urgent: get immediate advice or go to emergency department.
Sudden swelling of face, arms, or upper chest	Problem in the mediastinum causing obstruction to large veins there	Get medical advice in a few hours. If there is shortness of breath, go to emergency department if you cannot contact a doctor soon.
Severe abdominal pain (for several hours)	Obstruction of bowel	If severe, report to medical team. Go to emergency department if cannot contact team.
Protracted vomiting	Effect of chemotherapy (if after a treatment), bowel obstruction, or high calcium levels in blood	Contact medical team. If unable to hold down even small amounts of fluid, go to emergency department if cannot contact team.
Sudden paralysis of one side	Stroke or tumor (other causes are possible)	Report to medical team.
Seizures	Problem in brain or problem with certain blood salts	If person has never had a seizure before, get medical advice immediately, at emergency department if necessary. If seizure is a single convulsion and patient is already on anticonvulsant medicine, wait for patient to recover. If there are continuous seizures, get patient to emergency department at once.
Sudden loss of consciousness and person cannot be roused	Several, including problems in brain, too much analgesic, excess calcium in the blood, and many others	This is a coma and needs emergency attention. Take patient to emergency department immediately.

put upon the relationship up to that time. There is the fear of the disease, the fear of the treatment, the uncertainty about the future, and many other important factors. Just like any major stresses, such as unemployment or bereavement, these may seriously and adversely affect sexual libido (in either the patient, the partner, or both). Furthermore, depression, which, as discussed above, is common among cancer patients, very often decreases sexual libido. In fact, loss of interest in sex is one of the hallmarks and diagnostic features of depression.

Specific Interpersonal Problems In addition to the physical and general stress problems, there are often many other problems associated with the disease or its treatment. In each relationship, one or more of these factors may turn out to be significant.

Physical Symptoms Symptoms such as nausea or pain may make it impossible for the person to be interested in sex. Headaches are particularly likely to do this because the pain becomes worse during sexual excitation.

Perceived Attractiveness Problems with perceived attractiveness are common and may affect sex seriously. For example, a mastectomy may cause a woman to perceive herself as mutilated and sexually unappealing (even if her partner genuinely does not agree). A stoma may do the same, as can hair loss following chemotherapy. These problems are often quite severe and may be difficult to talk about at first.

Social and Status Changes Chronic illness of any sort, particularly if the future is somewhat uncertain, may cause the patient to be put on disability insurance, for example. If the patient was formerly the breadwinner of the family, this change may have marked psychological fallout and may cause considerable tension between the partners.

Other Interpersonal Issues There are many other issues that may have been only partly resolved and may have lain dormant before the illness but that now surface and create tension, for example, the attitudes of either partner to illness itself, to the possibility of dying, to religious factors, to ways of dealing with physical symptoms within the relationship, and so on. Then there are concerns that the partner might have about the patient, such as fears of hurting the patient during sex or even fears of catching the cancer.

There are therefore a large number of factors to do with the illness and its treatment that may affect sex within the relationship and may often stop most sexual activity altogether. This requires some attention if it is not to undermine most of the other aspects of the relationship.

Getting Sex Started Again Starting sex again is never easy. But if this is what the patient wants, then it is very important for you both to try to discuss it. If you do not, the patient will feel rejected and isolated. As one of my patients said, *"For a time I was a sexual pariah."* You may find that the following guidelines will give you a practical approach to restarting.

You Must Talk about It In my experience, somebody facing an illness such as cancer usually wants intimacy and human contact from the partner even more than sexual gratification itself. So if one of you cannot actually manage to join in sex, then do not make up an excuse. Making up a spurious excuse will simply add an air of dishonesty to an already tense situation. You should be prepared to talk about it and listen. If you feel tender toward the other person and want to be intimate but cannot show those feelings sexually, then it is really important and helpful to say so. Very often that expression of tenderness and concern will itself be helpful.

Make Plans Making and discussing plans about sex is something that most of us do not normally do, and most of the time we do not have to. When there is illness, discussion may be necessary, however awkward and embarrassing it is at first. You should try to be quite specific about what you can do and are prepared to do. Often a cuddle or a hug will achieve a great deal, and if you have discussed it in advance will not cause distrust or guilt if things go no further at that time. One of the most common problems is what to do if the patient is in the hospital. A decade ago, most hospital authorities had a pretty clear idea about what couples were supposed to do about intimacy in a hospital: nothing. Nowadays most hospitals will allow a couple some privacy, so do not be afraid to ask. Other problems that you can sort out include where you should sleep. If the patient has physical symptoms that cause disturbance in sleep, it may be easier for you to sleep in separate beds for part of the night. Again, if you talk about this, you will find that it need not lead to feelings of rejection or guilt.

Take One Step at a Time Particularly if you had a healthy sex life before the illness, you might have the feeling that you ought to be able to get straight back to normal. Usually that will not happen, and if you were expecting it you might feel discouraged. So do not be afraid to take it slowly and start with simple cuddles or hugs, increasing gradually to a greater range of sexual activities. Also be aware that physical problems might make it important for you to change the positions of sexual intercourse. This also requires discussion, planning, and a gradual approach.

Get Help If You Need It You may find that you cannot make progress in addressing sexual problems. If that happens, do not be afraid to ask for help. There are many sexual counselors available, and a small amount of counseling and help can make a very great difference.

COLOSTOMIES AND OTHER STOMAS

Being told that you are to have a colostomy (or ileostomy or a urinary stoma) is almost always distressing. Most people have an immediate fear that they will no longer be able to do anything they enjoy or value and that their entire life will be spent in a prisonlike existence. Fortunately this is totally untrue. For the majority of people with stomas, life is normal or near normal for most of the time. The following facts and guidelines may help you speed up adjustment and shorten the time of shock and distress that almost everyone goes through.

What Is a Stoma?

A **stoma** is an opening created by an operation in order to allow the body's waste products (either bowel contents or urine) to be excreted when the usual passage (in other words, part of the bowel or part of the urinary system) has been removed or cannot serve that purpose normally.

There are three types of stoma, and each is named for the part of the body in which it is situated. Thus, if there is, say, a cancer in the large bowel (colon) and part of the bowel has to be removed or bowel contents have to be diverted around it, the stoma is created in the colon, and that is a **colostomy** ("colon" + "stoma"). If the whole of the colon has to be removed, or if no part of it can safely carry bowel contents, the stoma is created in the small bowel (the ileum), and that is an **ileostomy**. If the problem is not in the bowel but in the urinary system—if, for example, there is cancer of the bladder—a stoma may be created to carry urine, and that is a **urinary stoma** or **urostomy**.

In all three situations the basic principle is the same. The objective is to allow you to get rid of either bowel contents or urine without pain or hazard when the usual means of doing that (excretion via the anus or the bladder) is no longer possible (because part of the system has been removed) or

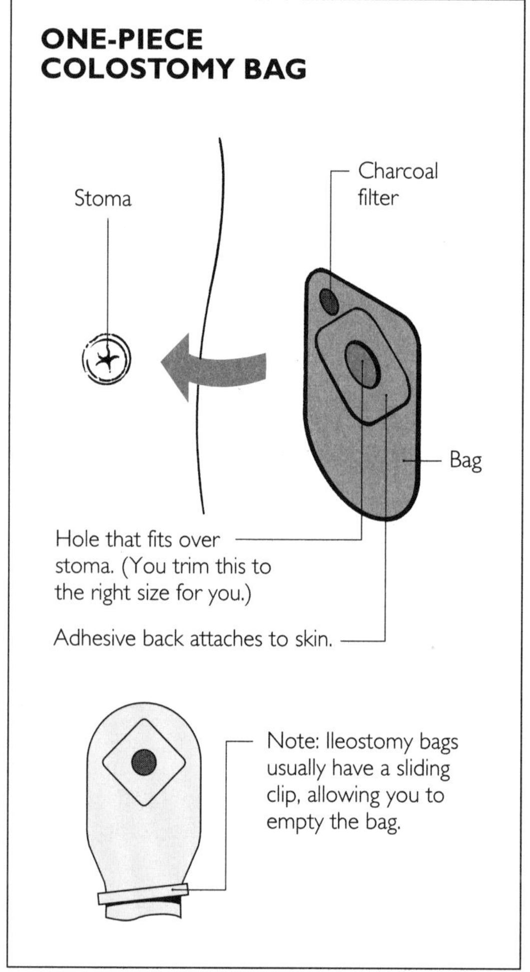

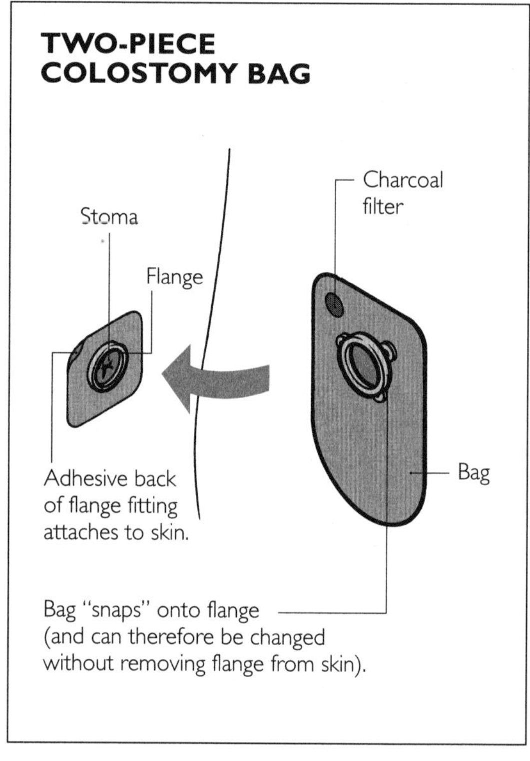

is hazardous or painful (for example, if the bowel is partly obstructed so that there is pain when bowel contents go through it).

How Stomas Work

In all cases the stoma consists of a small opening on the skin of your abdomen. At the time of the operation, your surgeon will attach a healthy part of your bowel (or urinary system) to the opening so that bowel contents or urine pass directly from the body through the opening in the skin and into a bag that attaches to the skin by removable adhesive. The bag fills up gradually with bowel contents or urine, and you are able to empty the bag yourself (as described in the next section).

Care of a Colostomy

With a colostomy the bowel contents that reach the colostomy bag are usually similar in consistency and color to normal stool, although they may in some cases be more liquid. Depending on how much of your colon is left in place, you will find that the colostomy acts (that is, produces stool) once or several times a day. Like any person's bowel habit, the number of times and the consistency of the bowel contents depend on what you eat. After a few days or weeks, you will learn which foods produce normal stool and which ones are likely to produce fluid stool, excessive gas, or too frequent actions. It is worth discussing this with the medical and nursing teams. Usually there is a clinical nurse specialist, or stoma nurse, associated with the hospital or clinic who will provide you with lists of foods that are usually well tolerated and ones that are often associated with excessive gas or fluid stool. In any event, you will find after a few weeks that you can predict your colostomy's behavior (just as we learn to predict our normal bowel habit).

With respect to changing the colostomy bag when it is full: in general, there are two main types of bags and fittings in use nowadays.

In one type the bag attaches directly to the skin around the stoma, so that you change the bag by peeling it off the skin and putting a new one in its place. This type is usually called a **one-piece** colostomy bag.

In the other type there is a special ring of pliable rubbery material that you attach to the skin around the stoma. This ring, called a **flange**, has a snap fitting attached to the outer part of it onto which you snap the colostomy bag (which, of course, has its own special snap fitting that fits the flange). This type is called a **two-piece** colostomy bag. Its main advantage is that you do not need to worry about the skin around the stoma except when you change the flange (usually once a week or so), so you can change the bag when it is full very quickly because the snap fittings are so convenient.

The question that almost everybody asks is: Is there any smell? The answer is that there is some smell when you change the bag, in exactly the same way that there is smell when you go to the toilet in the usual way! During daily use, once your colostomy has settled into its routine, there will be no (or very little) smell.

Care of an Ileostomy

With an ileostomy the bowel contents are more liquid than with a colostomy. In some cases the ileostomy may act continuously during the day; in other cases there may be distinct actions. As with a colostomy, after a few weeks you will learn to predict how your ileostomy is going to act, how it is influenced by your diet, and so on.

Again, as with a colostomy, there are two types of fittings: a one-piece fitting in which the bag attaches to the skin and you change the whole thing; and a two-piece fitting in which there is a flange attached to the skin and for most of the time you change the bag only, by means of a snap fitting to the flange.

In some cases it may be possible to empty the ileostomy bag rather than change it; if that is possible, your stoma nurse will discuss the advantages and disadvantages of doing that.

Care of a Urostomy

A urostomy carries urine, and the bag fills steadily throughout the day. Usually the urostomy bag can be emptied (and does not need to be changed) by means of a tap or valve at the bottom of it. Because they are drainage systems for urine, normally urostomies do not produce any smell.

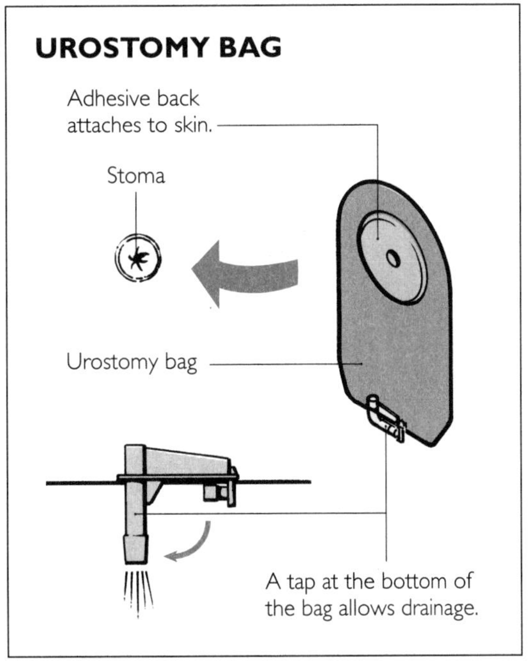

Living with a Stoma

There is a videotape on stomas that is part of the *What You Really Need to Know about . . .* series listed in Appendix C (see page 340). It consists of interviews with three people who have stomas and with a stoma nurse, and it covers a large number of topics, including diet, sexual activity, the types of fitting available, and so on. The video also includes an excellent demonstration by one of the people, Susan, of how to change a stoma bag quickly and easily.

As you can see on the videotape, stomas of all three types can be undetectable by other people in daily life. There are two key points to living a normal life with a stoma.

Learn the Best Technique of Changing the Bag/Fittings Although many people are naturally a bit worried about that to start with, as you will see on the video, the routines are very simple and, once you have got them right, become part of your daily routine. After all, as one of my patients said, we all had to learn how to go to the toilet; now stoma patients just have to learn a different way of doing the same thing.

Find the Best Diet and Stick to It Most of the Time (for Colostomies and Ileostomies) Of course, you will want to eat a variety of different foods, and you should. But generally you will find that some foods are best avoided or eaten in small quantities. Provided that your diet is fairly consistent, you will find that your stoma is predictable, and that predictability is what gives you confidence and a sense of security about living with a stoma.

Effects on Your Sex Life

Everyone wants to know how or if a stoma will affect his or her sex life. It has to be said that sometimes the surgery or treatment needed for the original cancer may affect your sex life. So, for example, many males with bladder cancer may find that they are unable to sustain an erection after the surgery. If the disease or treatment has not affected your sexual functioning, however, the stoma need not do so either. In the video, you will find that Susan's description of how she discusses the stoma with a sexual partner is very useful and very practical. Furthermore, as you will see from the interviews and photographs, a stoma need not adversely affect your attractiveness.

COMMUNICATION SUGGESTIONS FOR THE PATIENT: HOW TO TALK WITH OTHER PEOPLE*

What's in This Section

Almost everyone who has been told that they have cancer finds it very difficult to discuss what is happening to them and how they feel. They may find talking about it awkward and embarrassing (or uncomfortable and even painful) not only with friends and family but also with the nurses, doctors, and other professionals looking after them. In this section I try to help you overcome some of those difficulties by offering some simple guidelines and hints that will make it easier and less uncomfortable for you to ask for what you want and need and to talk about what you are feeling, if and when you want to. The discussion

* The text of this section is adapted from the booklet *Who Can Ever Understand? Talking about Your Cancer,* written by John Elsegood and me and published in Britain by the British Association of Cancer United Patients (BACUP). The phone number for BACUP in Britain is 0800-181-199 and the address is 3 Bath Place, Rivington Street, London EC2A 3JR, United Kingdom.

may also help you understand why your friends and family (and perhaps even your medical team) may find talking awkward, and how *you* can help *them,* even though they may feel that they should be helping you.

I should stress that there is no single "correct" way to do this. There is no One True Method or magic formula that you have to stick to, forsaking all others. A book like this can offer guidelines and objectives or aims, but how you achieve those objectives and how you fulfill those aims will depend very much on you. It will depend partly on your own style—on how you communicate with those around you—and also partly on the people around you. Don't be worried if the examples or illustrations I give do not fit in with your own style. There is no universal script that everyone has to follow.

Why It's So Difficult to Talk about Cancer

Even if it is not a medical and life-threatening crisis (and often, as you have seen in earlier sections, a new diagnosis usually is not a medical emergency), the moment when you are told you have cancer is almost always a moment of deep psychological crisis and distress. In fact, most people say that they have never faced a bigger and more daunting challenge. When most of us look back at the various crises we have been through (marital problems, financial problems, job problems, or problems with family members or children), most of those seem relatively insignificant compared to facing the diagnosis of cancer. Many people become almost paralyzed mentally and emotionally by the news, and it is worth spending a moment or two thinking about why that is. Understanding a problem is the first step in dealing with it. Perhaps we can best think of these effects under two headings: your feelings and the feelings of other people.

Your Feelings

Shock and Disbelief As a patient put it: *"When I heard that word 'cancer,' my mind went completely blank. I don't think I heard a single word the doctor said after that."* Her response is probably very similar to most people's initial reactions. When you first hear that you have cancer (however positive the future might be), it is very common to experience very strong feelings of shock and disbelief. The *fact* of cancer (as a reality, something that is actually happening to you) is something that most of us are really unprepared for. Even if we have been fearing that our problem is cancer (a thought that goes through most people's minds), the moment when that fear is confirmed is still very traumatic. There are many aspects to this feeling of shock: the common perception of cancer as a serious and perhaps fatal disease, the feeling of being invaded by a mysterious and alien enemy, the possibility of aggressive and unpleasant treatment, the fear of being in pain or being rendered useless (physically or emotionally), the fear of being a burden to one's family, anxiety about loss of earning capacity, social standing, and so on. In fact, the list of things that we each fear about cancer is probably unique: each person's list is probably different from anyone else's and is therefore a highly personal "recipe" of anxieties and concerns. But whatever is on that list, it almost always adds up to a sum of concern and fear that is, in total, shocking and deeply distressing. So shock and disbelief are the most common first reactions.

Denial In quite a lot of people, that feeling of disbelief is accompanied by a desire to shut out the news—to deny it. This reaction is called (logically enough) denial. There is a lot of material written and broadcast about denial that suggests it is somehow harmful and must be confronted and broken down at once. In my view (and in the view of many other professionals experienced in this area), that is simply not true. Many people use denial as a perfectly normal and valuable method of dealing with very threatening or overwhelming news *when they first hear it.* Denial is a normal human coping strategy that allows you to take serious news on board without having it swamp you totally. It is only when denial is prolonged, continuing for many weeks or months, and causes a breakdown in communication between patient and family (or patient and health care team) that it becomes a problem. So if you come to realize that you are using denial (or if someone close to you points that out to you), you do not need to chastise yourself or feel that you must hurry to overcome it. It may well be a normal reaction that in time (a few days, perhaps, or a couple of weeks) will allow you to accept the news and deal constructively with it.

Awkwardness Apart from shock, disbelief, and denial—all of which make it difficult for you to talk about your situation—another factor is that you may not be *accustomed* to talking about deeply personal and intimate matters. In fact, many people aren't. In a lot of families and friendships, deeply intimate concerns simply are not talked about or, if they are talked about, are not talked about easily and supportively. If that has been your pattern in the past, then of course you are going to find it difficult if you want (or need) to talk about your feelings at this moment of crisis. Again, being aware of this will help you a bit.

Guilt and Other Feelings There are other feelings inside you that may make you want to withdraw and withhold communication from the people around you. You may feel guilty and think that in some way you have brought this on yourself (that is also a very common feeling). You may be unsure and embarrassed about how you will react when you talk to other people. You may be afraid that you will cry (which, actually, is almost never a catastrophe—it usually allows easier communication rather than making communication more difficult). You may be worried about how your friends or family will react. Will they withdraw from you? Will they judge or condemn you? Will they blame you? Or you may be worried about the effect that talking about the disease will have on its progress. Some people have an almost superstitious belief that talking about future possibilities can cause those things to happen. For example, some people are afraid that if you openly discuss your concern that the treatment might not work, that in itself might cause the treatment not to work. Of course, such a belief is pure superstition but one that is held by many people (who are naturally very vulnerable at this point). Then there are other worries: that talking about things may change patterns within the family; that you will alter the ways that you have talked with each other for many years. (This, by the way, can happen, and when it does it almost always brings tremendous improvement and is a great relief to all concerned.) Finally, there is the natural reluctance that many of us feel about talking about our own needs and wants. We are brought up not to be pushy or demanding about what we want. You need to remember that once a diagnosis like cancer has been given, the people around you want to help and want to give you what you need. Thus you may have to overcome some of that inbred reticence and say what it is that you need or want. You will be surprised to learn how many people are really quite glad to be told clearly what your needs are.

Other People's (and Society's) Attitudes

When it comes to the people you want to talk to, you may be worried that they are a bit uncomfortable talking about these things, and you are probably right. The fact is that we are living in a society or an era in which serious subjects such as cancer (or serious illness in general) are not really regarded as legitimate subjects for ordinary, everyday conversation. It is not the fault of your friends or family—and it is certainly not your fault—it is just the way things are at the moment. There are signs that things are changing, and our society is slowly getting more accustomed to talking about serious personal subjects, particularly if they involve the health of one of the participants. But at the moment, there is a partial social taboo in operation, and nobody feels very comfortable talking about cancer.

It is also possible that the people around you may have no idea what to say (in fact, they probably are genuinely lost for words), although they may feel that they *ought* to know what to say. They may want to help you and believe that there is a magic formula phrase that would make you feel better if they only knew what it was. Rather than face you without that imagined magic formula, they may avoid you altogether. They may have no experience to guide them: never having had a serious or threatening illness or never having known anyone who did may make them unsure of themselves and also unsure about how to ask you what you want. They may also be worried about how you would react, afraid that they will not know what to do if you cry and so on. In what follows I discuss how you can help your friends and family to overcome these anxieties, thus helping them to help you.

The Benefits of Talking

If talking is so difficult, why bother? Why is it worth talking about what's going on if it makes you feel uncomfortable and may make your friends uncomfortable? Well, there are many things to be gained, and a lot of them will do a great deal to help you through any uncertainties or difficulties that may lie ahead. Perhaps these are best thought of under two headings: things that give you support and things that enable you to get control over your situation.

Benefits of Talking That Give You Support

First of all, we obtain comfort from communicating deep feelings. As a species, humans seem to be programmed to get comfort from talking to each other, most important, perhaps, because we often find that when our fears or concerns are voiced, somehow they are put into perspective by the process of articulating them. That is probably the basis of the old proverb *"A sorrow shared is a sorrow halved."* Second, if there are unresolved questions—things that you have been thinking about and about which you cannot make up your mind—you may find that you have already decided on the answer without being aware of it but only realize you have done so when you put the question into words. In short, talking about something often teaches you how *you* feel about it. Third, if your listener hears your fears or concerns and then simply stays with you (thereby showing that you are not being rejected), that also changes your attitudes to what you had been thinking or worrying about. It makes you feel that your fears or worries are "normal": if your friend can hear about them and not run away, then perhaps these fears are not as bizarre or strange or ugly as you feared. There is also the fact that talking about a fear or a worry often prevents it from growing larger in our minds. Often, as we mull things over, a fear or concern becomes magnified, assuming threatening, even overwhelming, proportions. Once the fear or concern is out in the open and is being discussed, that process of amplification often stops.

Finally, and this is difficult to express clearly, discussing something we feel deeply about produces a particular form of psychological intimacy. Perhaps the right word is "contact." In any case, a conversation about something important or personal produces a bond between the participants that is valuable in itself.

Things That Help You Feel in Control of Your Situation

We would all like to have control over our health and over any diseases that threaten it. If we can't have that, then most of us would like to have control over the treatment. And if *that* isn't possible, we would at least like to have control over the information about our situation. Unfortunately when the diagnosis is cancer, it feels as if we have little or no control over the disease or its treatment. And it is true that in many situations the number of treatment options are very limited. There is often one treatment plan that offers a chance of improvement and no real or viable alternative. Of course, you can always decide not to have any treatment: sometimes that is the right decision. Often, however, it is not. Thus the feeling *"I haven't got a choice really"* is very common. It is also very unpleasant and leads to a sense of powerlessness and then resentment. Information can help you deal with those feelings. The more information you have about your situation, the more you will feel involved in your own care and (at least partly) in control. Thus you will benefit from discussions with your medical team and then from talking with your friends and family about what you have learned (and perhaps what they have learned) from those discussions. To use an adage from the business world, *"Knowledge is power."* The adage is true: knowledge of your illness and its treatment gives you some form of power.

Those are just some of the benefits of talking about the subjects that worry you. Now let's discuss how you can make the conversation easier.

Who Is the Best Person to Talk To?

In an ideal world, each of us would have a close and confiding relationship with our spouse or partner. We would also have a reasonably wide circle of close and supportive friends with whom we could discuss our innermost feelings and apprehensions without fearing that we would be judged or rejected. That is the ideal. For a few lucky people, the ideal is a reality. Most of us, however, have something a bit less perfect than that, and some of us seem (at first) to have no one we can talk to. The first question is: If you want to talk, who is the best person to talk to? The first part of the answer is: To whom did you speak about your biggest worries before this? If there is someone to whom you've always confided your most serious worries or problems, then of course that person should be at the top of your list now. If you have not previously had a close confidant, try to ask yourself this question: *Who is the person that I could imagine would make me feel most comfortable talking about difficult problems?* It might be anyone. There's no universal "best person." It may be your spouse, your closest friend, your mother, sister, brother, priest, or even somebody you quite like but haven't (until now) been on close terms with. In fact, sometimes people with cancer find it rather daunting or intimidating to talk to close family about it and actually find it easier to speak first to someone else (even someone not particularly close, such as a business partner or an acquaintance; see Table 10.3).

If you simply have no idea whom to talk to, discuss the problem with your doctor or nurse or someone else on your medical team. There may be counselors or therapists within easy reach who can help you identify the most appropriate person in your circle. There are also support groups in most districts nowadays. Support groups consist of people with cancer, usually under the direction and leadership of a health care professional. The other members of the group may be in a similar position to you or they may not. It is quite usual to have people with different types of medical problems attending the same group. You may find this useful in broadening your experience and helping you to see your own problems from a different perspective, or you may not. Some people find groups extraordinarily helpful and form bonds with other members that are deeper and more significant than almost anything in their past. Other people are embarrassed or uncomfortable talking about personal issues with strangers; so if groups are not your style, don't worry.

How to Ask for What You Need or Want

When you've identified the person with whom you stand the best chance of having supportive conversation, what happens next?

First of all, having cancer does not prohibit you from talking about anything else. Most people find it quite normal to talk about the minor aspects of

TABLE 10.3: SAMPLE MODEL FOR CHOOSING A CONFIDANT

TYPE OF SUPPORT	NAMES (FILL IN)	TYPE OF SUPPORT	NAMES (FILL IN)
People who make me feel good about myself		People who help me to see all sides of a situation when I'm making a decision	
People who help me to cheer up		People who have the same interests and hobbies as me	
People who help me to feel positive about my future		People I can reminisce with	
People I can talk to about my physical symptoms		People I can talk to about spiritual matters	
People I can talk to about my emotions		People who give me sound advice about legal matters	
People I can talk to when I'm frightened		People who give me sound advice about financial matters	
People I can cry with		People who give me sound advice about insurance matters	
People I can rely on in a crisis		People who give me sound advice about employment matters	
People I can be quiet with		People who are frank with me about my illness	
People who are good listeners		People who give me clear explanations about my illness and treatment	
People I can be totally myself with		People who are coping well with cancer	
People who give me honest criticism when I need it		People who benefit from talking to me	

everyday life as well as the major issues confronting them, so don't feel constrained. Talk about the day-to-day things if you want to, when you want to.

When it comes to talking about your health problems, however, some of the following ideas may make the conversation easier.

1. If possible, **try to decide which things are most important** to you and are the things that you really want to talk about. Quite often you will find that there are only two or three things that you really want to discuss. If so, that is fine.

2. In order to introduce the topics that matter to you, it may be helpful if you can **give a headline first**. It may be something like: *"Look, I want to say a couple of things that are on my mind. Is that okay with you?"* The advantage of doing that is that it alerts your listener to the fact that what follows is something that really matters to you.

3. As you talk about the things that concern or worry you, **try to be specific**. You may find it is easier to take that in stages. You can start off talking about awkward subjects with generalities (such as *"Can we talk about the way things are at the moment?"*). That may make it easier to move to more specific areas (*"Look, I'm just not sure how long I'm going to be in the hospital this time."*). If there is something you've been thinking about or worrying about a lot, it's perfectly okay to say so (*"For the last few days, I've really been wondering about . . ."*). That way you'll ease your way into important topics, and your listener will be helped to focus on what it is you want or need.

4. As the conversation continues, when you're doing the talking it's a good idea to break up your own speech to **see if the other person is following you**. You can use any little phrase you like to do that (*"Do you see what I mean?"* or *"Does that make sense to you?"* or the more universal *"Are you with me?"*).

5. Toward the end of the conversation, **try to make sure that what you've said has been heard**. If you have asked for some things to be done, for example, it's worth summarizing (*"So you'll call your mother about next weekend and also ask Dorothy to pick up the children on Friday."*). After you've covered the main topics, don't feel embarrassed about going back to small talk (*"Let's talk about some little things. I like talking about small things, ordinary things."*). As someone once said, *"Small talk is the mortar of human communication."* It's true: the heavy bricks of important issues would just collapse without normal human chatter in between.

6. *Humor:* A lot of people ask whether humor is a good thing to use when talking about tense issues and subjects. The simple answer is: If humor was useful to you before you were ill, it will be useful to you now. Humor is primarily a coping strategy: it helps the user to draw a frame around something that is threatening and, by laughing at it, reduce its importance and the size of the threat. If humor has been part of the way you have coped with threatening crises in the past, it will help you now, and you needn't be afraid of its effects. If on the other hand you have not used humor for this purpose in the past, this may not be a good time to start doing so (despite what Norman Cousins implied in his book *Anatomy of an Illness*).

Those are some guidelines for keeping a conversation relatively comfortable. Now let's discuss how you can bring your own feelings into it.

How to Talk about Your Feelings

Most of us are not accustomed to talking about our own feelings. If we try it, we often feel a bit awkward. There are some people who don't have difficulty, but most of us do, and for most of the time that doesn't matter. But when something serious happens—such as an illness, and particularly a diagnosis of cancer—most people find that, although they do want to talk about how they feel, they are not used to it and so feel a bit clumsy. That is normal!

The first point about expressing feelings is that if you (or your listener) have strong emotions that are *not* talked about, you won't be able to talk about any subject easily. An emotion that nobody acknowledges has a paralyzing effect on all conversation. If you are feeling angry, embarrassed, or very sad (or if your listener is feeling one of these emotions), until one of you acknowledges that fact, your conversation will feel very sticky. Both of you will be preoccupied and will not be listening. The moment one of you acknowledges the emotion (*"I'm sorry I seem in such a bad mood today, but I've just been told that . . ."*), you will suddenly find communication much easier. Acknowledging the existence of an emotion partly neutralizes the paralyzing effect that it can have.

Here are some practical guidelines.

1. Always **try to acknowledge any strong emotion**, whether it's your own or your listener's.

2. Always **try to describe your feelings rather than simply display them**. There's a great deal of difference between saying, *"I'm feeling really angry today because . . ."* (which starts a conversation) and simply showing your anger by being curt or rude (which stops conversation).

3. **You are perfectly entitled to feel any way you like!** The way you feel is the way you feel: emotions are not right or wrong. It is only if you try to cover up any strong feeling that you have that problems really become unsolvable.

4. **Don't be afraid to tell the other person how much she or he means to you.** Again, in our daily lives we don't often do that. But when there is a crisis, it's really worthwhile explaining to the other person how you feel about them.

5. **Don't be afraid to acknowledge uncertainties.** If you don't know how you feel, or if you don't know what is going to happen or how you are going to cope, you should say so. More harm is done by pretending that you do know than by admitting that you don't.

6. **There are many occasions when words aren't needed.** Holding someone's hand or hugging or simply sitting together in silence can often achieve as much or more than words, once you are both clear about the situation.

7. **Everybody has some regrets** (despite what it says in pop songs!). Don't feel that you are not allowed to express any regrets you feel. More than any other emotion, regret is reduced when it is shared and may even prove a durable bond between you and your listener.

8. Finally, and this is a really important point, **never be afraid to cry**. Crying is not a sign of weakness; it's a sign of sensitivity and of the emotions you feel. Almost everyone will feel flattered that you feel close enough to them to cry in front of them if that's what you feel like doing. So if you do feel that way, don't think you are supposed to bottle it all up.

How to Respond to Other People's Reactions

Strangely enough, even though you are the person facing the diagnosis of cancer, you may have more difficulty in dealing with your friend's emotions than with your own. This is because, as I said earlier, when people are unable to cope with their own emotions, they tend to avoid the situation altogether. So your friend might be very tempted to stay away from you rather than face the fact that he or she has strong emotions but doesn't know how to deal with them. Here are the most important guidelines for helping both of you.

1. **Always try to acknowledge your friend's feelings.** If you are a good guesser, you may be able to

identify your friend's emotion and what caused it. You might say something like, *"You look as if you're feeling really uneasy when I talk about the cancer,"* or *"I guess coming here makes you very upset."* In an ideal world, of course, this wouldn't be necessary. Your friend would be able to explain what he or she was feeling and then bring the focus to you and what you want to talk about. But this isn't an ideal world, so you may have to do some of the groundwork to get the support you need.

2. **Don't be afraid to acknowledge how you feel** at the same time: *"This is making both of us feel awful,"* or *"I know you're worried about what's going to happen next, and so am I."* The more you are each aware of your own feelings and the other person's, the better the dialogue will be.

3. **If you get into some form of conflict** (and that happens quite often), see "Hints for Resolving Conflict" below.

4. **If the other person is your spouse or sexual partner**, don't ignore the subject of sex. The part of this section headed "Sexuality" gives specific suggestions for how to approach the topic (see page 287). If you have had an active sex life until the illness, it will almost certainly be affected by the diagnosis; it almost always is. There are many elements that come into play: fear of the illness and of the treatment, resentment about the illness, change in physical appearance, embarrassment, feelings of disgust, and so on. All these tend to make both partners withdraw from each other physically and feel shy and awkward. Quite often, sex may stop completely, often at a time when you most need to be reassured and cuddled. If that happens, you must say so, as coolly and calmly as possible. Try to explain your needs and wants and to discuss what can be done by either or both of you. Of course it's embarrassing to talk about these things, but a very small amount of dialogue makes a great deal of difference, whereas ignoring the subject and (literally) turning your back on it will cause serious resentment and mistrust on both sides.

How to Tell Other People

One of the most awkward and difficult aspects of being ill is the necessity to tell friends and family about the illness. Most patients feel (as all of us would in those circumstances) that they won't know where to begin. If the person is your spouse or partner or a close friend, it is usually possible to have her or him present when your doctor talks to you: that way you both hear the same thing. If your friend cannot be present, and you must tell her or him on your own, you may find the following guidelines useful.

1. Try to get the physical setting right. That means making sure the television is turned off, the door is closed, that you can each see the other person's face easily, and so on.

2. Signal that you're introducing an important subject; don't just start off baldly. Try saying something like: *"I think it would be best if I tell you what's going on. Is that okay?"*

3. If you think your friend knows some of what has been happening, then it can be quite useful to start by asking what he or she knows before you go over ground that has already been covered: *"You probably know some of this already, so why don't you tell me what you make of the situation so far, then I'll take it from there."*

4. It often helps to start with a preliminary statement, a warning shot. For example, if the situation is serious, you can say: *"Well, it sounds as if it might be serious"*; or if it's worrying but sounds as if it will be all right in the long term, you can say that.

5. Give the information in small chunks, a few sentences at a time, and ask your friend if he or she understands what you're saying before you con-

tinue. You can use any of several little phrases for that purpose: *"Do you see what I mean?" "Do you follow me?" "Is this making sense?"* and so on.

6. There will often be silences, but don't be put off by them. You or your friend may well find that just holding hands or just sitting together in the same room seems to say more than any words. If you find that a silence makes you feel uncomfortable, the easiest way to break it is with a simple question such as *"What are you thinking about?"*

7. When you tell someone close to you that something serious is wrong with you, he or she may feel very low and depressed in sympathy with your situation. You may therefore feel that you ought to try to be positive and upbeat in order to relieve your friend's feelings. If the facts of your situation support that, by all means do so. But if there is a great deal of uncertainty or worry about the future, you shouldn't feel that you need to hide the fact from your friend in order not to hurt her or his feelings. **Try to stay as close to the real situation as you can.** It may be painful for your friend at this particular moment, but if you paint an overly rosy picture that proves to be false, your friend will be much more disappointed (and even feel hurt) later on.

You'll find that these principles will make what is always a difficult conversation a bit less awkward. It's not really fair that you should have to do so much, particularly at a time when your needs are so great and many, but it often happens like that. By following these suggestions you can leave your friend much better equipped to give you support in the future.

An Important Topic to Talk About: Who Should Be Your Health Care Agent?

As you talk with your family and friends, you should seriously consider appointing one person to be your health care agent. Then, if you are ever not able to make health care decisions for yourself, even for a brief time, someone you know and trust will have full authority to make decisions for you. Appointing an agent is one of those tasks that everyone, not just people with cancer, should consider doing.

Once you have chosen an agent, you should talk with that person and let him or her know how you feel. Talk about your *values*: Is it important to you to consider all options for treatment? To act according to your religious beliefs? To have quality time? Talk about *how you would like to live*: Is it important to you to be free of pain? To be able to take care of yourself? To avoid life-prolonging measures depending on your quality of life?

Next, complete a Durable Power of Attorney for Health Care form. This is the form that makes someone your legal health care agent. Many such forms are available (contact your local services for more information) and you should check your state law to see if your state has special requirements or requires a special form. (In some states, you can write to the state attorney general's office and they will send you a form to complete.) Once you have completed the form, give it to your doctor and to the person you have appointed to be your agent.

Talking with Doctors and Other Health Care Professionals

It would be unrealistic to expect conversations between patients and their doctors, nurses, or other health care professionals always to go smoothly. Feelings often run high on both sides (they shouldn't, but they do). Here are some ways you can increase your chances of getting what you want and need.

Talking about Your Symptoms

There will often be occasions when you are asked to describe your symptoms: pain, nausea, shortness of breath, or some other medical problem. To do this efficiently is actually quite difficult! Here are a few pointers that may help.

1. As you describe the medical problem, **try to be as factual as you can**. It's very easy to exaggerate the pain or nausea in order to convince the doctor. As a patient, one often feels that somehow this will

produce better or more immediate results. Or you may be tempted to underplay the symptoms so as to appear stoical. If possible, ignore both temptations and try to describe the medical problems in as factual and neutral terms as you can. It's not easy, but if you do that, you will end up with your doctor or nurse supporting you and on your side. If you try to overplay or underplay your problems to a great extent, your medical team may become alienated and be less willing to help you. In an ideal world, that wouldn't happen, but because you and they are human beings, it can! As far as possible, then (as the saying goes), "play it straight." You don't need to try to impress your doctor with either the severity of your symptoms or your own personal courage.

2. **Use your own language.** Your doctors or nurses may use medical jargon, but you don't need to. There's nothing wrong with using your own words to describe the problem. In fact, using jargon that you only partly understand might cause difficulties by giving the wrong slant to your problem.

3. **When you're embarrassed, don't hesitate to say so!** We all find certain kinds of medical symptoms and problems embarrassing: they're very often the kind of personal matter we don't talk about to someone else. So when you start talking about something that is embarrassing, just say so (*"I'm sorry . . . this is embarrassing to talk about"*). Remember, emotions that are acknowledged are partly neutralized.

Asking for Information

When it comes to getting information from your medical team, you may find that your own feelings and fears make it difficult for you to ask the right questions and to remember the answers. The following suggestions may be helpful.

1. **Try to think of the most important questions** before the discussion with your doctor.

2. To help you remember the important points, **jot them down on a slip of paper** to take with you.

3. It's also a good idea to **take a friend or relative with you**. Often the other person can remember things the doctor said that you later forget and the questions you wanted to ask but haven't got around to yet. Every health care professional knows how difficult it is to understand and retain information when it is serious and when it is about you. Nowadays nobody will mind your using such aids to help you understand your circumstances.

4. **Remember that this is not your only chance to ask questions.** Sometimes there won't be advance notice of an important subject (you may hear bad news quite unexpectedly, for example), but even then, there will always be another interview at which you can ask for clarification. No matter what the circumstances, if you're not clear about what you've heard, don't hesitate to ask for clarification. So, once your doctor or nurse has answered your questions, it's not a bad idea to restate what you've heard: *"So you're saying that . . . ,"* or *"If I've got that right, you mean that. . . ."* In this way, you make it clear what you have understood and often encourage your doctor or nurse to explain things clearly and intelligibly.

5. Often, definitive answers are not possible. **Try to accept that uncertainties are common**, particularly with questions about the future. When the conversation is about very serious matters that threaten your health or your view of the future, it's easy to imagine that your doctor or nurse knows what is going to happen but for some reason will not tell you. Usually that's not the case. If a type of treatment has, let's say, a 40 percent chance of success (and therefore a 60 percent chance of not working), very often there is no way of predicting whether you in particular will be in the more fortunate 40 percent group or not. It may well help you come to

grips with the situation if you can understand how progress will be measured (*"So you'll decide from the X rays if the treatment is working. . . ."*). But with cancer therapy, there is very often a lot of uncertainty. Uncertainty is extremely unpleasant and difficult to cope with, but it exists, and it doesn't mean your doctor is holding out on you!

6. If you feel doubt or dissatisfaction with your health care team or one member of it, try to **express those doubts as diplomatically as you can**. I say that not to save my own skin (or at least not *merely* to save my own skin) but to encourage you to get better service. Most doctors and nurses—like all human beings—respond to constructive criticism well and react to destructive criticism either defensively or angrily. If you are able to voice your criticisms in a balanced manner, you'll find that you are much more likely to get your needs met.

Getting a Second Opinion

If you have any doubts about your medical situation, if you do not fully understand what your doctor is saying, or if you are not sure that his or her view of the situation is the only option, then a second opinion may be a great help to you. But do keep the following points in mind. First, it will be helpful to your doctor if you inform him or her that you would like a second opinion. This is not merely a matter of etiquette and politeness. It is essential because your doctor will need to send a summary or copies of your case record to the other doctor. Without actual details of your cancer, the tests that you have had, and details of any previous treatment, the doctor who is giving a second opinion will be unable to comment usefully. So do make sure you tell your first doctor that you would like a second opinion.

The second point is this: if the second opinion is the same as the first, stop and think. There is a considerable temptation to shop around and see many doctors until you find one who says what you want to hear. Usually that does not happen. In fact, very often the act of seeing many doctors is really an expression of denial, an effort to resist the diagnosis or the view of the future. If you hear the same thing from more than one doctor, it may be helpful to you to reflect on what that means. Some people become deeply distressed. In such a case, you might do better to seek help to reduce the distress (further discussion with your doctor or counseling perhaps) rather than go on what may turn out to be a deeply disappointing and frustrating quest.

Talking with Children

Talking with children about your illness—or about the child's illness if a child happens to be the patient—is extremely difficult. We all think of childhood as a time of innocence and freedom from pain and guilt, and we all hope that unpleasant or painful facts will never confront our children (or anyone else's) until they are older and have what we think are adequate coping skills. Unfortunately, serious illness can come to people at any age. Often, having to tell children what is happening is the most awkward and painful part of the illness. The following guidelines may help you a little.

1. **Ask yourself if you would like some help** with it. Very often, having a health care professional—a doctor, nurse, therapist, or social worker—present at such a difficult interview can be very helpful. I have conducted many interviews like this, and it is helpful because the child can often focus any anger or resentment on the professional instead of on the parent. The professional becomes a sort of lightning rod, and that may reduce the burden on the patient. Also there may be questions that are technically very difficult to answer, and again, the professional can relieve you of some of that. It is worth thinking about this option and discussing it with your health care team.

2. **Pitch the information at the child's level of understanding**, not the child's age. Children differ enormously in what they can understand and what they can't. Some five-year-olds can understand concepts that escape other children of ten. Check as you go along to see what the child is understanding and tailor what you say to that.

3. **Be prepared to repeat the information.** Children usually ask for important information to be repeated, perhaps several or many times. If the subject is painful to you, you may be tempted to stop the conversation (*"I've answered that three times already—that's enough now!"*). But when children ask for repetition, it's not because they are stupid or malicious; they simply need to check that you really meant what you said. Try to be more patient than usual and go over the ground again, keeping your answer consistent with what you said last time.

4. Be aware of what is known as "**magical thinking**." Children almost always feel very guilty when things go wrong around them and often feel that in some undefined way they are to blame for the situation. This is called magical thinking (*"If I'd cleaned up my room like Mom told me to, she wouldn't be sick now."*). It's important to make sure the child understands that the situation is not his or her fault. It's often worth building that into an overall statement such as, *"This is just one of those bad things that happen occasionally, and it's nobody's fault. It's not my fault, it's not the doctor's fault, and it's certainly not your fault—it's just a piece of really bad luck."*

Explaining difficult or threatening facts to a child is always painful. These guidelines may help a bit, but don't hesitate to ask for whatever help is available to you.

Hints for Resolving Conflict

When the diagnosis is cancer, for the reasons I discussed at the beginning of this section, the emotional atmosphere is tense and conflict is common. It may be conflict with your friends or family or (probably more likely) with some member of your health care team. A lot of complaints may later turn out to be justified, and many problems may be fixable (particularly if you are able to raise the issues relatively calmly). Nevertheless, many patients find themselves getting almost uncontrollably cross or angry with friends or the health care team. Some of this anger can be attributed to the basic human tendency to blame the messenger for the message. Somebody tells you that you have cancer; you find it difficult to focus your anger on the cancer itself, so you focus it on the person who tells you. This reaction may go along with the feeling of unfairness that you should have this disease when the other person seems to be getting away unharmed. Whatever the reason for the conflict, you may find the following guidelines helpful in dealing with it.

1. Whenever possible, **try to describe your feelings rather than display them**.

2. As emotions rise, **try to acknowledge all emotions**, whether they are yours or the other person's.

3. **Try to "disinvest" in the outcome** of the argument. In other words, try (although it's not easy) not to feel that your worth as a human being is tied to the outcome of the dispute. It's easy to imagine that if you win, you are a wonderful person and if you lose, you are not. That is untrue of almost every conflict known to humankind. Try to remember that you are still a perfectly satisfactory person even if you lose this argument.

4. With an issue or area over which you simply cannot agree, try to define the area even though you can't resolve it. In other words, aim to "agree to disagree" on a particular issue.

5. **Talk the dispute over with someone else.** As you describe it, try not to turn the other party in the dispute into a monster. In other words, try to "demonstrify" the other person as you describe the dispute. That way, you may see a way out of the argument simply by describing it, as it were, from one step back.

Conclusion

Serious illness is always perceived as a threat to health and life, and we all feel at first that what we want to do is to shut out the whole thing from our minds and, as it were, pull the bedclothes over our head in the hope that the problem will go away. Sadly, that is not usually a helpful thing to do, either for you or your friends. The suggestions given above may help you make and maintain real contact with your friends at a time when the illness itself threatens to pull you away from each other. You will be quite surprised at and pleased with the changes that can be brought about by the relatively simple techniques of talking and communicating described above.

Even more important is the psychological bond that can be created between you and your friend or friends. The closer you are to someone, the more meaning you will both see in your life and in the way you lead it. Although it may sound odd at first, several patients have said to me that being diagnosed with cancer had some unexpected benefits. For some people, a crisis or a challenge can often help them sort out what really matters in their lives—decide who is a real friend and who isn't, who really matters to them and who is just an acquaintance.

Of course, everyone who has cancer would much prefer not to have it or to be cured of it. Often that can be achieved, but even if it cannot, the contact between you and your friends can be, and often is, an extraordinary and moving proof of the value of human companionship.

COMMUNICATION SUGGESTIONS FOR FRIENDS AND FAMILY MEMBERS: HOW TO LISTEN TO AND TALK WITH A PERSON WITH CANCER*

Not Knowing What to Say

Everyone feels somewhat stuck, sometimes almost paralyzed when a friend receives some bad news (even if things later work out much better than we feared at first), and we all tend to feel that we don't know what to say.

To make things worse, we probably think that there are things we *should* be saying or doing that would automatically make things easier for the person with cancer if only we knew what they were. That is the problem that this part of the chapter addresses.

Perhaps the most important thing to realize is that there are no magic formulas or phrases or approaches, no "Correct Thing" to say or do that covers all circumstances. There is no magic set of words or attitudes, no Universal Phrase that everybody but you knows. If you really want to help your friend, your own desire to help is the really vital ingredient, not some perfect script that you're supposed to follow word for word.

Another important point is that it's not what we *say,* it's how we *listen.* Sometimes the single most important thing you can do for your friend or relative with cancer is to listen. Once you've learned a few simple rules of good listening, you can be of great help and support, and communication will improve from there on. The secret is to start. Learning how to be a good listener begins with understanding

* Some issues and topics in this section repeat what was said in the previous section. I am assuming that most readers will read one or the other. If you happen to read both, I apologize for the repetition.

why listening (and talking) are so valuable, as I discuss in the next section. (The suggestions are summarized in Table 10.5.)

Before we can listen effectively, however, we need to recognize the unique atmosphere of dread and foreboding associated with the word "cancer" in our society. It is true that large numbers of patients with cancer will be completely cured, and that number is increasing slowly and steadily all the time. Nevertheless, for many reasons and despite those good statistics, the word "cancer" has a more paralyzing and numbing effect than most other diagnoses; that's why a book like this is needed more often when the diagnosis is cancer than with many other diseases.

Why Talk, Why Listen?

You want to help, but you're not sure what is the best thing to do. Well, perhaps the most logical place to start is with what you're trying to achieve for your friend—the objectives of conversation and dialogue. There are three excellent reasons for talking (and, of course, listening).

1. Talking Is the Best Method of Communication We Have

There are many different ways of communicating: kissing, touching, laughing, frowning, even "not talking." (You may have heard the story of the man who wanted to know why his wife hadn't spoken to him for three days, and his psychotherapist replied, "Perhaps she's trying to tell you something.") Talking is, however, the most efficient and the most *specific* way that we have of communicating. Other methods of communication—hugging, touching, and all nonverbal communications—are very important, but for them to be of use we usually have to talk first.

2. Simply Talking about Distress Helps Relieve It

There are many things that a conversation can achieve. In other words, there are many reasons for us to talk. There are obvious ones, such as telling the children not to stick their fingers in the fan, telling a joke, asking about the results of the game or the horse race, and so on. There are also less obvious reasons for talking, one of which is the simple desire to be listened to. In many circumstances, particularly when things go wrong, people talk in order to get what is bothering them off their chest and to be heard. You can see this quite often in the behavior of children. If you have an argument with your child, you may often hear your child later grumbling to his or her teddy bear or even telling the bear off in the way you told the child off. Although this is not exactly dialogue or conversation (since it's one-way), it serves a useful function in releasing a bit of pressure. Human beings can stand only so much pressure. There is relief to be found in talking, which means that there is a relief that *you* can provide for a sick person by listening and by simply *allowing* him or her to talk. That, in turn, means you can help your friend, even if you don't have all the answers.

In fact, simply doing "good listening" is known to be effective *in itself.* In an interesting research study done in the United States, a number of totally untrained people were taught the simple techniques of good listening, and volunteer patients came to see them to talk about their problems. The listeners in this study were not allowed to say or do anything at all. They just nodded and said "I see" or "Tell me more." They weren't allowed to ask questions of the patients or say anything at all about the problems that the patients described. At the end of the hour, almost all the patients thought they had got very good therapy; some of them called the "therapists" to ask if they could see them again, and to thank them for the therapy. Remember, then: **You don't have to have the answers. Just listening to the questions will help a bit.**

3. Thoughts That a Person Tries to Shut Out Will Do Harm Eventually

One of the arguments friends and family put forward in order to *avoid* talking to the patient is that talking about a fear or an anxiety might create that anxiety, even if it didn't exist before the conversation. In other words, a friend might say to herself: *"If I ask my friend whether he's worried about radiotherapy and he wasn't worried about it, I might make him worried about it."* Well, that doesn't happen. There is very good evidence from studies done by psychiatrists talking to patients with terminal illnesses (in Britain in the 1960s) that conversations between the patients and their relatives and friends did not create new fears and anxieties. In fact, the opposite was true: *not* talking about a fear makes it bigger. Those patients who have nobody to talk to have a higher incidence of anxiety and depression. Several other researchers have shown that when people are seriously ill, one of their biggest problems is that people won't talk to them. The resulting feelings of isolation add a great deal to their burden. In practice, a major anxiety occupying a patient's mind frequently makes it difficult for that patient to talk about anything at all.

One reason why bottled-up feelings may cause damage has to do with shame. Many people are ashamed of some of their feelings, particularly of their fears and anxieties. They may be afraid of something but feel they aren't "supposed" to be, and so they feel ashamed of themselves. One of the greatest services you can do for your friend is to hear his or her fears and stay close when you've heard them. By not backing away or withdrawing, you show that you accept and understand them. That in turn will reduce the fear and the shame and help the patient get back a sense of perspective.

In short, you have everything to gain and nothing to lose by trying to talk and listen to someone who's just been told that she or he has cancer.

Obstacles to Talking

Starting such a conversation can be difficult, however. Table 10.4 outlines some of the obstacles to free communication.

Although these seem like major obstacles to communication, don't let that alarm you too much. There are ways of making yourself available for listening and talking without thrusting your offer down the patient's throat, just as there are ways for you to work out whether the patient needs to talk or does not. The next section looks at some basic listening techniques that will help communication along.

How to Be a Good Listener

Let's start with the assumption that you want to be of help and support but don't know how.

You can encourage free conversation and avoid awkward communication gaps by following a few simple rules or techniques of good listening. Both physical and mental techniques are important.

TABLE 10.4: OBSTACLES TO TALKING

PATIENT	FRIEND OR RELATIVE
The patient wants to talk.	You don't.
The patient doesn't want to talk.	You do.
The patient wants to talk but feels he or she ought not to.	You don't know how to encourage him or her.
The patient *appears* not to want to talk but really needs to.	You don't know what is best and do not want to intervene to make things worse.

TABLE 10.5: EFFECTIVE LISTENING: THE S-C-A-N-S MNEMONIC

S — Setting
Get the setting right. Sit down with your eyes on the same level as the other person. Look as "at ease" as you can (for example, drop your shoulders).

C — Communication skills
Don't talk over the other person (that is, keep quiet while he or she is talking). Use simple techniques such as nodding, smiling, and using one word from the person's last sentence in your first sentence (to demonstrate that you were listening).

A — Acknowledgement
Always acknowledge the existence of the other person's emotion (for example, *"It must be very frustrating having to wait for the results. . . ."*).

N — Negotiating
Clarify what it is that the other person wants (for example, practical help, information, emotional support). Then clarify what it is that you can do and are good at. Then do the things on your list that seem to fit the other person's list.

S — Summary
Always end a discussion summarizing the main two or three points that you've been talking about together. Ask if there are other important issues. End with a clear "contract," which can be as simple as *"I'll see you on Friday"* or *"I'll phone you next week."*

The most important components of good listening are summarized in Table 10.5 with a mnemonic (S-C-A-N-S) that makes them easier to remember.

1. Get the Setting Right

The **physical context** is important. Get comfortable, sit down, try to look relaxed (even if you don't feel it), and signal the fact that you are there to spend some time (for instance, take your coat off!).

Keep your **eyes on the same level** as the person you're talking to. This almost always means sitting down. As a general rule, if the patient is in the hospital and chairs are unavailable or too low, sitting on the bed is preferable to standing. All kinds of things conspire against us in circumstances like that. I've sometimes found, on ward rounds, that if I can't sit on the bed because of obstacles, the only available chair is a commode. It causes minor embarrassment, but as long as you acknowledge the circumstances, it's better than trying to talk to someone while towering above the person. In other circumstances, you should try to keep as "private" an atmosphere as possible: don't try to talk in a corridor or on a staircase. That seems obvious, but actually conversations often go wrong because of these simple things. So do try to create the right space. Of course, no matter how hard you try, there will always be interruptions: phones and doorbells ringing, children coming in, and so on. But do your best to keep the atmosphere as intimate as possible.

Keep within a comfortable distance of the patient. Generally there should be one to two feet of space between you. A longer distance makes dialogue feel awkward and formal, and a shorter distance can make the patient feel hemmed in, particularly if he or she is in bed and unable to back away. Try to make sure there are no physical obstacles (desks, bedside tables, and so on) between you. Again, that may not be easy, but if you say something (like, *"It's not very easy to talk across this table; may I move it aside for a moment?"*), it helps both of you.

Keep looking at the person while he or she is talking and while you talk: eye contact tells the other person that the conversation is solely between the two of you. If, during a painful moment, you can't look directly at each other, at least stay close and hold the person's hand or touch the person if you can.

2. Find Out Whether the Patient Wants to Talk

The other person simply may not be in the mood to talk or even may not want to talk to you that day. Try not to be offended if that's the case. If you're not sure what the patient wants, you can always ask (*"Do you feel like talking?"*). Asking is always better than trying to start a deep conversation (*"Tell me about your feelings."*) when the person may be tired or be "talked out" from a previous visit.

3. Listen and Show You're Listening

When the patient is talking, try to do two things. First, listen to the person instead of thinking about what you're going to say next. Second, *show* that you're listening.

To listen properly, you must be thinking about what the patient is saying. You should not be rehearsing your reply (doing so would mean that you're anticipating what you think the patient is *about* to say and not listening to what he or she *is* saying). Try not to interrupt the patient. While the patient is talking, don't talk yourself but wait for him or her to stop speaking before you start. If the patient interrupts you while *you're* talking, with a *"But . . ."* or an *"I thought . . ."* or something similar, stop and let the patient speak.

4. Encourage the Other Person to Talk

Good listening doesn't mean just sitting there like a running tape recorder. You can actually help the patient talk about what's on his or her mind by **encouragement**. Simple things work very well. Try nodding or saying affirmative things like *"Yes," "I see,"* or *"Tell me more."* These all sound simple, but at times of maximum stress it's the simple things you need to help things along.

You can also show that you're listening—and hearing—by **repeating** two or three words from the patient's last sentence. This really does help the talker to feel that his or her words are being taken in. When medical students are shown this technique, they invariably report that using it at home with their friends and family members always moves the conversation along and makes the listener suddenly appear more interested and involved.

You can also **reflect** back to the talker what you've heard, partly to check that you've got it right and partly to show that you're listening and trying to understand. (You can say things like, *"So you mean that . . ."* or, *"If I've got that straight, you feel . . ."* or even, *"I hear you,"* although that last one might sound a bit self-conscious if it isn't your usual style.)

5. Don't Forget Silence and Nonverbal Communication

If someone stops talking, it usually means that she or he is thinking about something painful or sensitive. Wait with your friend for a moment—hold the person's hand or rest your hand on his or her arm if you feel like it—and then ask what he or she was thinking about. Don't rush it, although silences at emotional moments do seem to last for years.

When there's a silence, you may find yourself thinking, *"I have no idea what to say."* On occasion, this may be because there isn't anything *to* say. If that's the case, don't be afraid to say nothing and just stay close. At times like that, a touch or an arm around the patient's shoulder can be of greater value than anything you say.

Sometimes nonverbal communication tells you much more about the other person than you might have expected. Here's one example from a doctor's experience.

Recently I was looking after a middle-aged woman named Gladys who seemed at first to be very angry and uncommunicative. I tried encouraging her to talk, but she kept very "wrapped up." During one interview, while I was talking I put my hand out to hers, rather tentatively because I wasn't sure it was the right thing. To my surprise, she seized it, held it tightly, and wouldn't let go. The atmosphere changed instantly, and she instantly started talking about her fears of further surgery and of being abandoned by her family. The message with nonverbal contact is "try it and see." If, for example, Gladys had not responded so positively, I would have been able to take my hand away, and neither of us would have suffered any setback as a result of it.

6. Don't Be Afraid of Describing Your Own Feelings

You are allowed to say things like, *"I find this difficult to talk about"* or, *"I'm not very good at talking about . . ."* or even, *"I don't know what to say."* Students are often taught this when they learn communication skills. One of them said to me later, *"I tried what you told me — telling the patient that I found it awkward — and it **really worked**."* The student was pleasantly surprised, and so will you be.

7. Make Sure You Haven't Misunderstood

If you are sure you understand what the patient means, you can say so. Responses such as, *"You sound very low"* or, *"That must have made you very angry"* tell the person that you've picked up the emotions he or she has been talking about or showing. But if you're not sure what the patient means, then ask, *"What did that feel like?" "What do you think of it?" "How do you feel now?"* Misunderstandings can arise if you make assumptions and are wrong.

It's certainly advantageous when you instinctively pick up what the patient is feeling, but if you don't happen to do that, don't hesitate to ask. Something like *"Help me a bit more to understand what you mean"* is quite useful.

8. Don't Change the Subject

If your friend wants to talk about how rotten she or he feels, let the person do exactly that. It may be difficult for you to hear some of the things being said, but if you can manage it, stay with the person while he or she talks. If you find it too uncomfortable and think you just can't handle the conversation at that moment, then you should say so and offer to try to discuss it again later (you can even say very simple and obvious things like, *"This is making me feel very uncomfortable at the moment. Can we come back to it later?"*). Don't simply change the subject without acknowledging the fact that your friend has raised it.

9. Don't Give Advice Early

Ideally no one should give advice to anyone else unless it's asked for. Nevertheless, this isn't an ideal world, and quite often we find ourselves giving advice when we haven't quite been asked. Try not to give advice early in the conversation because doing so stops dialogue. If you're bursting to give advice, it's often easier to use phrases like *"Have you thought about trying . . ."* or (if you're a born diplomat), *"A friend of mine once tried. . . ."* Those are both less bald than *"If I were you, I'd . . . ,"* which makes the patient think (or even say), *"But you're not me,"* which really is a conversation stopper.

10. Respond to Humor

Many people imagine that there can't possibly be anything to laugh about if you are seriously ill or dying, but that is to miss an extremely important point about humor. Humor performs an essential function in helping us cope with major threats and fears: it allows us to *ventilate,* to get rid of intense feelings and put things in perspective. Humor is one of the ways human beings deal with things that seem to be impossible to deal with. If you think for a moment about the most common subjects of jokes, they include mothers-in-law, fear of flying, hospitals and doctors, sex, and so on. None of those subjects is intrinsically funny. An argument with a mother-in-law, for instance, can be very distressing for all concerned; but an argument with the mother-in-law has been an easy laugh for the stand-up comedian for centuries, because we often laugh most easily at the things we cope with least easily. We laugh at things to get them in perspective, to reduce the size of the threat they represent.

One patient I particularly remember was a woman in her early sixties who had had a mastectomy for breast cancer many years before I met her. She had an external prosthesis (the kind that is worn under a brassiere or bathing suit). She told me (proudly) that she was swimming with her friend when the prosthesis fell out of her bathing suit and floated off toward the shallow end while she was headed for the deep end. Her friend saw it first and pointed out the loss. Whereupon my patient, to her everlasting credit, covered the embarrassment by saying, *"Oh there it goes, doing the breast stroke on its own."* In telling me the story, she was justifiably proud of the way she had coped with potential embarrassment, and it demonstrated, I think, her true bravery and desire to rise above her physical problems. For her, it was very much in character.

From this experience and many others that I have shared with patients, I have become convinced that laughter helps patients get a different handle on their situation. If the patient wants to use humor—even humor that to an outsider might seem black humor—you should certainly encourage and go along with it. It's helping him or her to cope. This does not mean that you should try to cheer the patient up with a supply of jokes. That simply doesn't work. You can best help your friend by responding sensitively. That means responding to his or her humor rather than trying to set the mood with your own.

Understanding What Your Friend Is Facing

The objective of sensitive listening is to understand as completely as you can what the other person is feeling. You can never achieve complete understanding, of course, but the closer you get, the better the communication between you and your friend will be. *The more you try to understand your friend's feelings, the more support you are giving.* There are, of course, dozens—if not hundreds—of different aspects that induce fear with any illness, and when the diagnosis is cancer, those fears may be more numerous and may loom larger. Understanding some of the most common concerns can help you encourage your friend to talk about her or his feelings.

The Threat to Health

When we are in good health, the threat of serious illness seems remote, and very few of us think about it before it happens. When it happens to us, we are shocked and confused and often angry or even embittered.

Uncertainty

A state of uncertainty may be even harder to tolerate than either good news or bad news. Not knowing where you are and not knowing what to prepare for is a very painful state in itself. You can help your friend a lot by simply acknowledging the unpleasantness of uncertainty.

Unfamiliarity

With cancer therapy there are often many different disciplines involved in the treatment, each with its own expertise and rules or regulations. Often the patient feels, however mistakenly, unskilled and foolish among the skilled and busy staff. You can help by reinforcing the fact that nobody is "supposed" to know all the details in advance. You can also help by getting some of the patient's questions answered.

Physical Symptoms

Physical symptoms are of paramount importance. The patient may, at various stages in the treatment, have a variety of symptoms (including pain or nausea). Don't hesitate to allow the patient to talk about the symptoms.

Visible Stigmata of Treatment or Disease

The same is true of outward signs of cancer or its treatment. The most obvious is hair loss due to chemotherapy (or radiotherapy to the head). You can help the patient feel less self-conscious by being matter-of-fact about the selection of wigs or scarves.

Social Isolation

Most serious diseases, particularly cancer, seem to put up a social barrier between the patient and the rest of society. Visiting the patient and encouraging mutual friends to do the same are good ways to help reduce that barrier.

The Threat of Death

Many patients are cured of cancer, but the threat of dying of it is always present (and sometimes haunts even those who are truly cured). Naturally you can't abolish that fear, but you can allow the patient to talk about it and, by listening, reduce the impact and pain of that threat. Remember: *"You don't have to have all the answers. Simply listening to the questions will help a lot."*

This is only a partial list, but it will at least give you a glimpse of what may be going through your friend's mind. All of these fears and concerns are normal and natural; what is "wrong" or "unnatural" is not having anybody to talk to about them. That is why you can be so important to your friend.

TABLE 10.6: CHECKLIST FOR CAREGIVERS
Make your offer. Do not just say, *"Call me if you need anything."*
Become informed about your friend's medical situation, but don't try to become a world expert on it.
Assess the needs. A good way is to go through an imaginary typical day that your friend is likely to experience.
Decide what you can do and want to do.
Start with small practical things. You can always cook and bring some frozen meals, take the children out for an afternoon, and so on.
Avoid excesses. Inappropriately generous or excessive gifts or gestures are almost worse than doing nothing.
You can always sit and listen (see Table 10.5).
Accept that you have limitations and try to involve other people.

How to Help: A Practical Checklist

One of the most common problems in trying to help a person with cancer is that the friends and relatives simply don't know where to start. They want to help but don't know what to do first. In this section, I outline a logical trail that you can follow (also summarized in Table 10.6), which will help you decide where your help will be most useful and where you can start.

1. Make Your Offer

You must first find out whether or not your help is wanted. If there are other people involved in support, you should find out whether your help is needed and then, if it is, make your offer. Your initial offer should be specific rather than a vague *"Let me know if there's anything I can do,"* and you should say clearly that you'll check back to see if there are things you can help with. Obviously, if you are the parent of a sick child or the spouse of a patient, you don't need to ask; but in most other circumstances it is important to know whether you personally are in the right position to help. Sometimes a distant acquaintance or colleague is *more* welcome than a close relative, so don't prejudge your usefulness. Do not be upset if the patient does not seem to want your support. Do not take it personally. If you are still keen to help, see if there are other family members who need assistance. After you have made your initial offer, do not wait to be called but check back with a few preliminary suggestions.

2. Become Informed (but Not a World Expert)

If you are to be useful to your friend, you will need some information about what the medical situation is, but only enough to make sensible plans. You do not need to—and should not try to—become a world expert on the subject. Many helpers are drawn to acquire more and more details that are not necessarily relevant to their friend's situation. Sometimes their motive is curiosity; sometimes it is a desire to be in control.

3. Assess the Needs

This means assessing the needs of the patient and of the rest of the family. Naturally any assessment is going to be full of uncertainties because the future is often unpredictable, but you should try to think about the patient's needs. These will vary, depending on how disabling the disease is at that time (it may not be disabling at all, of course). If the patient is seriously inconvenienced, here are some of the questions you might ask yourself: Who is going to look after him during the day? Can he get from bed to toilet? Can he prepare his own meals? Does he need medications that he cannot take himself? And of the other family members: Are there children that need to be taken to and from school? Is the spouse medically fit, or are there things she needs? Is the home suitable for the patient's medical condition or are there things that need to be done there? The list could be long and almost certainly will be incomplete, but it is a start. Check your list by going through a day in the life of your friend and thinking about what he will need at each stage.

4. Decide What You Can Do and Want to Do

What are you good at? Can you cook for the patient? (For instance, bringing precooked frozen meals is always welcome.) Can you prepare meals for other family members? Are you handy around the house? Could you put up handrails or wheelchair ramps if required? Could you house-sit, so that the spouse can visit the patient? Could you take the kids out to the zoo for the day to give the couple some time together? If you aren't good at any of these things, would you be prepared to pay for, say, a cleaner for a half-day a week to help out? Could you get hold of relevant booklets for the patient? Can you find videos that the patient likes? Does the patient need the furniture rearranged? (For instance, the patient may need to sleep on the ground floor because he or she cannot manage the stairs.) If so, could you help do it? Will there be flowers at home when the patient gets out of the hospital?

5. Start with Small Practical Things

Look at the list of the things you can do and are prepared to do, and start by offering a few of them. Do not offer all of them—this will overwhelm the patient. Pick some small items that are practical that the patient *might not be able to do easily.* Making a small contract and meeting your target is far better than aiming too high and failing. It may require a little thought and some "inside knowledge." For instance, one patient, David, used to get his hair cut every week. It wasn't a big thing, but it was part of his regular routine. When he was in the hospital, his friend Joseph arranged for the hospital barber to call weekly. It was a nice and thoughtful touch. There are lots of things like that, even doing things like mowing the patient's lawn when he or she is unable to, preparing meals, house-sitting and so on. Another patient, Dora, was a schoolteacher. Her colleagues at the school got the children to draw cards for her. Again, these were little tasks but thoughtful and highly valued by the patients.

6. Avoid Excesses

Don't give huge gifts that overwhelm and embarrass. Don't buy the patient a new car unless you know specifically that this is wanted and will not cause embarrassment. Most large gifts spring from a sense of guilt on the part of the donor and create guilt in the recipient. Similarly, your offers of help should be modest and suited to the patient and family. Be sensitive.

7. Listen

Time is a present you can always give. If you haven't already done so, have a look at the suggestions above on sensitive listening and try to spend regular time with your friend. Don't spend two hours once a month (unless you cannot do anything else). It's better to spend ten or fifteen minutes once a day or every two days if you can. Be reliable and visit your friend when you say you will. As the saying goes, *"Half of Being There for someone is simply being there."*

8. Involve Other People

Be fair to yourself and recognize your own limitations. Every helper and supporter wants to do his or her best, and you may be very tempted to undertake heroic tasks out of a sense of anger and rage against your friend's situation and the injustice of it. But if you make heroic gestures and then fail, you will become part of the problem instead of helping with the solution. You owe it to yourself and to your friend to undertake reasonable tasks so that you succeed. This means you should always be realistic about what you can do and get other people to help with what you can't.

Going through this list in your mind is valuable because it offers a genuinely practical approach to something that is probably unfamiliar to you and because it quells your own sense of panic and not knowing where to start. Whatever plans you make will certainly change with time as conditions change. Be prepared to be flexible and learn on the job.

Conclusion

Of course, it's frightening when your friend has been told she or he has cancer. As has been said, the only people who aren't frightened are those who have no imagination at all! But you can help in the ways discussed so far. And do remember that facts reduce fears. You can help your friend by helping him or her get the facts in perspective: many patients will be cured, and there are many others who will be helped. By listening to what your friend is most concerned about and by helping him or her obtain the right information and understand it, you can be a vital part of your friend's support system, and that is one of the most important things that one human being can do for another.

SPIRITUAL ASPECTS

More than almost any other aspect of daily life, religion and spirituality are deeply personal matters. In fact, some people might be more comfortable about discussing their sexuality with other people than their spirituality. So when discussing religion—and this applies equally to patients and to friends and family—make no assumptions. A useful rule of thumb is, *"The only safe assumption is that there are no safe assumptions."*

A couple of points are worth stressing.

First, be aware that religion and spirituality, as I have said, are personal matters and as much a part of your friend's personality as sexual proclivities or humor. Hence you need to be sensitive to the importance of spiritual issues in that person's life. If spiritual matters have always been important, then a discussion about them now might be very valuable. But you need to try to find out. Of course you can and should ask. But do be aware of and sensitive to the fact that the issues might or might not be important, and your friend might or might not want to discuss them with you.

Second, serious illness creates vulnerability: do not take advantage of it. Surprisingly, a few friends and family members may feel that if a friend is seriously ill, it is a good time to try to bring about a religious conversion. It is not. No matter how certain you are that you know the true path or have a certain way of achieving salvation, if your friend does not want to hear about it, don't persist.

Having given those two cautions, I also stress that religion and spirituality provide many people with a great deal of support and comfort. You can help them even if you do not share their religious views. Serious illness is a good time to practice tolerance, particularly about spiritual matters. If you are able to do that, you will be able to become part of the solution rather than part of the problem.

WHEN THINGS ARE GOING BADLY

This part of the book concerns the most awkward topic of all. It has been called "the final taboo" and, rather unhelpfully, "the ultimate obscenity." Even so, it is a topic that every one of us will benefit from thinking through: the subject is the end of life, in other words, dying.

Very few people actually want to die, and most of us do not think about the subject at all, or, if we do, we think about it as briefly as possible. Nevertheless, many people do die of or with cancer, and I have found that having some idea of how to handle it, and making plans, always helps both patients and family cope better. I want to emphasize that making a plan for what to do if the end is imminent is not the same as wanting to die. As I have often said (and firmly believe), the human mind seems quite capable of planning for the worst while continuing to hope for the best. If things are going badly for you at present, you may well find that making *"What if . . ."* plans actually helps you. Almost all of my patients have found it very helpful to learn about their local palliative care or hospice facilities and to discuss all arrangements with their family and friends. Once they have done that, many of them do not feel the need to talk about it again. When something is settled and everyone knows what you, as patient and person, want, there is often no particular need for further discussion on that subject. Friends and family feel a lot easier and less embarrassed because they all know what you want, and they know that you know they know.

Do You Wish to Read On? Although it is almost always valuable for all of us to think about our own attitudes to dying (whether we are ill or not) and to make plans that reflect what we really want, you may not want to start that thinking process right now. Also you might be more inclined to start the process after a conversation with a friend or your doctor rather than as a result of reading a book. So take a moment now to think about how you would like to approach the subject and to decide whether or not you want to read on.

There is nothing frightening or gruesome in the pages that follow, but the subject matter itself is often difficult for some people. So you may not want to think about the topic at this particular moment. If you feel that you don't want to approach this subject right now, or that you don't want to approach it via a book, you need not continue reading the rest of this section. The book will always be available for you to read later on, and the hints may be of greater value to you if they come at the right moment for you. If that is the case, then you can, if you wish, simply turn to the Conclusion of this book, following this chapter.

For those who do wish to read on, I have divided the rest of this section into three parts. The first, "Issues and Decisions about Dying," explains what palliative care is all about, and then deals with two topics that are very much under discussion at the moment, Living Wills and the debate over euthanasia. The second part, "How to Give Help and Support," is primarily for the friends and family. It is basically a very brief summary of material in my previous book on this subject. I have divided the text in this way only because it is simpler and easier to understand suggestions if the reader knows clearly for whom they are intended. There are no "secrets" in either section that one party should know and the other should not. Familiarity with both sections could help make communication easier. The third section is a brief, personal view that may be of some use to anyone tussling with these very difficult subjects.

Take your time about deciding whether you want to read the rest of this section. You certainly don't need to feel guilty if you don't want to read it right now. The information is there to help you, but only if you want it.

Issues and Decisions about Dying

Decisions about Palliative Care

If your condition is deteriorating, you may need an increasing amount of nursing attention and time. Depending on your family and the resources that can be provided at your home, there may come a time when you need admission to a hospice or palliative care unit so that you can be looked after as an inpatient. The question of making such a change and of when to do so requires careful consideration and usually discussion with your medical team and your family. Some important considerations affecting such a decision are outlined below.

A palliative care unit or a hospice (the names mean the same thing) is a place where doctors and nurses look after patients at the end of life. The objective is to provide effective relief of symptoms, particularly of pain but also of the psychological stress of dying. The personnel in hospices have special training in the relief of pain and other symptoms, and usually hospices have a higher number of nurses per patient than general medical floors in hospitals. Generally speaking, if the unit is located in its own building, it is usually called a hospice; if it is a specially designated ward in a hospital, it is usually called a palliative care unit.

Nowadays many palliative care units have home care teams that provide further and valuable support of the patient in her or his home. In fact, in some communities, home care teams are the sole providers of palliative care services. Teams like these are of tremendous value. The team may come to your home and assess your needs and give important support and help before, after, or even instead of your admission to a palliative care unit. If there is such a team in your region, then you may find that their advice and support are very helpful. In particular, the team may help you think through some of the issues that follow.

For many people, perhaps the most important decision is whether you should continue to be looked after at home or whether you should be an inpatient in a hospice (or palliative care unit). In thinking about the issue, you may find it helpful to consider the following questions.

How Much Nursing Assistance Do I Need? Think about what you actually need at the moment. Are you freely mobile at home or do you need help to get around? Can you get to and from the bathroom?

What Are Social Services and My Family and Friends Able to Do? How are you managing for daily needs such as meals, drinks, shopping, cleaning, making the beds, and so on? If all your physical needs for assistance can be met easily by outside services or by your friends and family (or some combination of both) and those involved are willing to continue to help, then you are basically coping. If your friends and family are providing what you need but are near breaking point and are getting exhausted and worn out, you may need to think about a change in the future. This may be done either by getting increased social services (if that is possible) or by admission to a hospice.

How Comfortable Am I Now? In some respects, this is the crucial question. The word "comfortable" should be understood in both its physical and psychological sense. Are you coping at home, in the sense that you are able to enjoy some aspects of being at home? Are you physically and psychologically comfortable enough to communicate easily and freely with your friends and family? Or are things getting tough for you, so that most of your time is preoccupied with physical and nursing problems?

These questions may help you assess whether you are coping at home or near the point of not coping. Of course, most people who enjoy living at home will generally prefer to be ill and even to die at home if their family can support that. There is a very considerable comfort in being at home, surrounded by your own things, able to do what you want to do, with no concerns about other patients in the same room, the need to call for the nurse, and so on. If your physical and nursing needs are extensive, however, and if you are not able to enjoy your home surroundings, it may be time to think of a hospice.

There are two things about hospices that most people do not realize. First, most hospices will allow you (or a friend) to visit and look around the unit before you decide. That is one reason for thinking about this decision early: if you see the place, you will feel much better about it, because hospices are generally very friendly, well-designed, comfortable places to be in. Second, if your nursing needs decrease and you are able to leave the hospice and go home, you are free to do so! Most people think that admission to a hospice is a one-way ticket, but that is not the case. Most hospices have up to half of their patients going home for visits, for weekends or for long-term stays if their medical condition allows. So don't feel that the decision to be admitted to a hospice means an irrevocable absence from home.

I have visited many of my patients after they have been admitted to a hospice, and all of them said one thing: *Why didn't I do this earlier?* Of course, being at home is the first choice for most people, but if it is no longer enjoyable or feasible, hospice care may be just what is needed.

The Living Will

A Living Will is simply a written record of what you want done in terms of end-of-life medical support. Living Wills can be obtained from varius agencies (contact your local services to locate the nearest; see Appendix D). Many Living Wills ask doctors and medical personnel to refrain from taking heroic measures to prolong life when the situation is hopeless.

Even if you decide not to make a Living Will, you should nevertheless discuss what you want with your friends and family, and you should seriously consider signing a Durable Power of Attorney for Health Care form designating someone to make decisions for you if necessary.

The Controversy over Euthanasia

The word "euthanasia" is used nowadays to mean the action of ending a person's life at the person's own request. The word is used to include all actions that are clearly intended to end the person's life, and it therefore encompasses the phrase "assisted suicide." A case in which a physician might give a prescription that the patient can later use for suicide would be an example of assisted suicide.

At present there is only one part of the world where euthanasia is a legal action, and that is the Northern Territory in Australia where in May 1995 a bill was passed permitting assisted suicide under stringent controls. Other states in Australia are considering whether they might follow suit.

The situation in Holland is one that has evolved over a long time. After medical practitioners, the general public, lawyers, and the government spent many years in careful and wide-ranging discussions, a set of guidelines for the medical act of euthanasia has been provided. Those guidelines include the patient's extreme suffering (physical or mental), the patient's clear understanding of all the options, including further medical treatment, and his or her rejection of those other choices, the patient's repeated request for euthanasia, and so on. Under the law in Holland, if all those guidelines have been met (and a long and detailed questionnaire is filled in afterward by the physician), it is possible for the public prosecutor (the equivalent of the district attorney) to decide not to prosecute the doctor. In the early days, when cases of euthanasia did come to court, if the guidelines had been met, the judges (there is no jury system in Holland) had the ability to pass noncustodial suspended sentences. Hence, although euthanasia is not legally recognized in Holland, it is tolerated.

In Oregon a recent referendum allowed physicians to write prescriptions that would be lethal to the patient. The act of taking the medications, therefore, is still the responsibility of the patient. At the present time, that referendum is being reviewed in the Oregon courts, so it has not yet been implemented.

In Canada the Senate Special Committee on Euthanasia and Assisted Suicide published its conclusions in June 1995 after extensive interviews and discussions. The committee was unable to find a consensus to recommend any change in law (perhaps accurately reflecting the current state of social opinion). Hence the act of euthanasia in Canada is not legally different from murder.

There are several extremely important issues here. Clearly some patients would like to know that they could end their life when they choose rather than go through the last few weeks or months of a terminal illness. Equally, many people are concerned that any change in legislation would be abused and that the elderly and infirm might be killed against their will by overzealous physicians prompted, for example, by the family or the financial costs of health care. Others believe that any change in legislation will adversely affect public attitudes and the funding of palliative care. Yet others believe that all killing is wrong and that all human life, no matter what the suffering (physical or psychological) that it entails, must be preserved, even if the person living that life says it is not worth living.

Although this issue is highly controversial, you can certainly discuss euthanasia with your doctor. There is a very important reason for my suggesting this. In discussing your own feelings you will start discussing what you are really worried about and frightened of. In many cases, that discussion in itself will reduce your concern. For example, you might be frightened of pain, and your doctor may be able to reassure you that good pain control is achievable in the vast majority of cases. Or if you are frightened of becoming dependent, plans for palliative care or a hospice might help. Even more important, if you are strongly opposed to the idea of euthanasia, it is essential for your doctor to know that.

Thus, even though euthanasia remains an illegal act, the discussion of it will genuinely help you and help your doctor to provide the kind of assistance you prefer.

In my own experience, although many people do want to discuss euthanasia, very few would actually choose it if it were legal. In a sense, euthanasia seems to me rather like the life jackets that are under every seat in airplanes. Few people use them, but everyone is glad that they are there. Most people's end-of-life needs can be met without resorting to suicide.

For Friends and Family Members: How to Give Help and Support

What's in This Section

In one of my previous books (*I Don't Know What to Say: How to Help and Support Someone Who Is Dying* [New York: Vintage Books, 1989]), I give a practical approach to understanding the process of dying and to listening to and supporting someone who is threatened by dying or is actually facing it. Without wanting to sound self-serving, I do think it might be worth your having a look at that book, because it goes into some detail about how you, as a friend or family member, can respond to what seem at first to be impossible situations or unanswerable questions. In the next few paragraphs, I summarize very briefly some of the major areas and topics dealt with in the book.

The Transition

The process of dying is a transition—a journey, really—that we each make. And although we each make that transition in our own individual way, certain aspects of the transition are universal. Understanding them can help you support your friend more effectively.

Any attempt to propose a way of understanding the process of dying will be to some extent a matter of personal viewpoint and philosophy. Nevertheless, the framework that I describe in the next few paragraphs has now been used by many thousands of people (health care professionals and patients' relatives and friends) and has been found to be workable and practical. I outline briefly some of the problems with the widely accepted Kübler-Ross stages of dying and then explain why a simpler framework might be more useful.

For more than thirty years, the five stages outlined by Dr. Elisabeth Kübler-Ross have been taken as the best model for the process of dying. She felt that the five significant stages of the dying process were these: denial, anger, bargaining, depression, and acceptance. Although her work was undoubtedly a major contribution to the understanding and hence the care of those facing death, there are some problems with using this framework in practice.

To begin with, many people react to the threat of dying with responses and reactions that are not encompassed in the five stages. For example, almost everyone feels some degree of fear: in fact, most people would regard fear of dying as a normal and appropriate reaction. There is also guilt: a very large number of people experience some feelings of guilt. There are also shock and disbelief, hope and despair. There is (often) humor and so on. So there are a number of responses to the situation that are not included in the five stages.

Second, in the five-stage system, it is implicit that there is a progression through the stages (although, as Dr. Kübler-Ross says, patients may well move back and forth between stages and may also skip some stages). In other words, the five-stage system basically views human beings as moving or progressing from one stage to another, changing from one type of response to the next as they move through the stages.

In my view, this is not the way human beings actually react. In general, people react to a major threat such as dying in the way that they have reacted to all stress and adversity in the past: people who usually get angry will get angry now; people who face adversity by using denial will use denial now; people who feel a lot of guilt will feel guilt now, and so on. When each of us faces the threat of death, we react in a manner characteristic of our own personality and not of the stage of the process.

Third, most people react with several emotions at the same time, some of which might at first seem contradictory. For example, people quite commonly show denial and anger at the same time (I do, for example!). Yet intellectually this does not make sense, for in theory it is not possible both to be angry about something and at the same time deny its existence. Yet we are all capable of that because what probably happens is that one part of our mind does the denying while another part of our mind starts the anger response. I think it is highly likely that we are all capable of simultaneously experiencing and exhibiting several emotions.

I therefore feel that it is more useful and practical to view the process of dying as having not five stages but simply a beginning, a middle, and an end. I have called those three phases of this simpler system "facing the threat," "being ill," and "acceptance."

In the first of these stages ("facing the threat," or the acute stage), the person will experience and show the emotions and responses that he or she has used in facing threats in the past. In the first stage the person will show his or her own individual mixture of emotions and responses. If one can compare emotions to colors, then I am saying that we are all mosaics, with palettes made up of different emotions and reactions in different amounts, rather than chameleons passing from one emotion to another.

In the second stage, which I have called "being ill" (or the chronic stage), what happens is a process of resolution of those reactions that are resolvable. So, to pursue the color analogy, the mixture of the colors is basically the same, but the intensity of the colors becomes muted as we adjust to our new situation. Our anger diminishes as parts of it are resolved (with or without help); our shock and disbelief diminish; we decrease the amount and intensity of our denial (usually); we feel less guilty, and so on. It is at this stage, after the acute reactions have faded, that depression is particularly likely.

The third and last stage is the time when the person accepts that he or she is dying. In many people, that acceptance might not be overt. People may not want to say directly, *"Yes, I realize that I am dying,"*

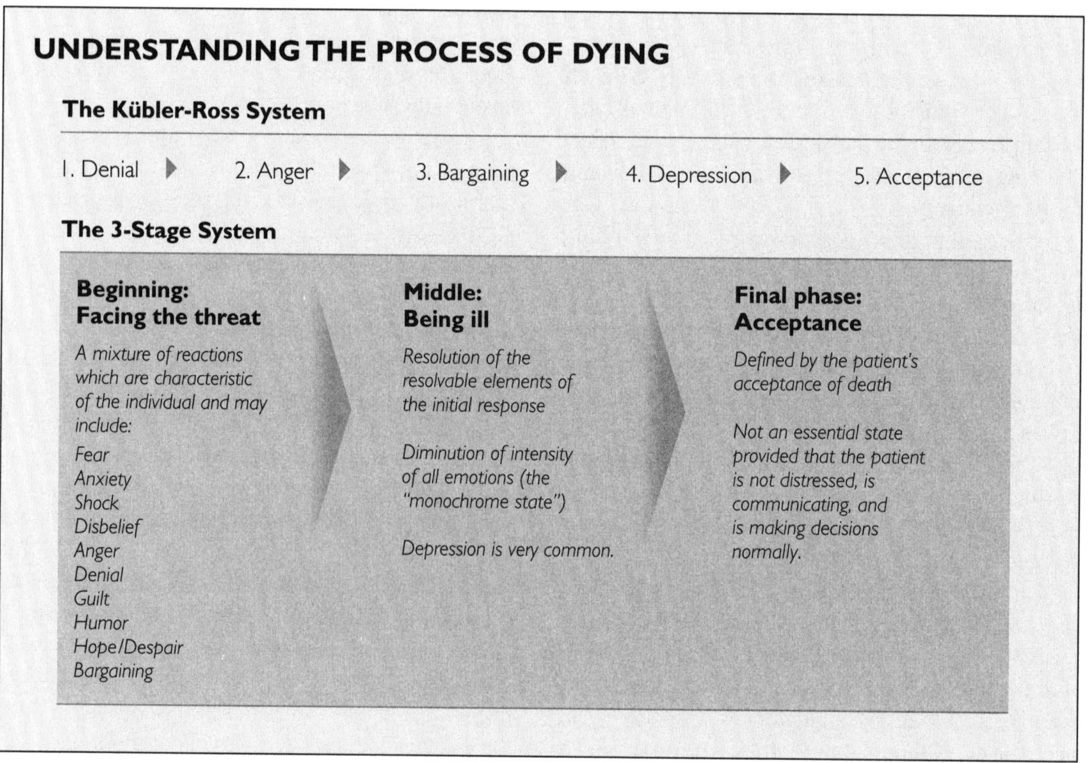

and they may not need to. If your friend does not want or need to acknowledge the situation directly and openly, that fact should not pose a problem for you. If the person is quite comfortable with the situation and is able to communicate freely and normally, then you do not need to do anything.

A few people, however, will not only not acknowledge their situation openly but will refuse to accept the likelihood of their dying at all. Sometimes this stance may increase the stress and distress that they are going through, and it may cause problems in communicating (with you and with other people) and with decision making. This situation is much more tricky and may need some expert assistance.

Practicalities

Understanding the transition that your friend is making will make it much easier for you to listen to and understand what your friend is experiencing. In addition, you will need some guidelines to help you organize the assistance.

There are two ways for you to make more effective plans. First, there are general ways in which you can tailor what you want to do and what you are able to do to what the other person wants and needs. These are dealt with in some detail in *I Don't Know What to Say,* but I have summarized them in Table 10.6.

Second, the nature of the help you can give and the nature of what is expected or wanted varies to some extent with the relationship that you have with the person. In other words, people have different expectations of a spouse than they would have of a parent, a child, a friend, and so on. Obviously a lot also depends on how close the relationship is. Some people have very close relationships with, say, their parents, and others do not. Nevertheless, there are certain aspects that you need to be aware of in the particular relationship that you are in, and again there is a considerable amount of practical detail on the various relationships in *I Don't Know What to Say.*

It's worth pointing out that the book also contains specific suggestions for ways of responding to your friend's feelings and reactions, a discussion of spiritual issues, a section on AIDS, a section on talking to children about dying, and several other topics that may be of use.

What Dying Means: A Personal View

Our society places a very high value on youth, health, and wealth. I do not necessarily think there is anything wrong with that in itself (things may not have been much better in societies that revered old age, for instance), but our current social values do make it harder for anyone who has to face old age, poverty, or sickness. It is almost as if our society has been pretending for the last three or four decades that death did not exist. Therefore, as a society we have (until recently) regarded people who are dying as marginalized, out of the mainstream. As a result, there is currently a large psychological and social gap between the business of living and the process of dying. And that makes it very hard for anyone who is facing the prospect of dying, because, as one approaches the process of dying, one seems to be losing social standing, credibility, and status, and one becomes almost tainted (by the bad luck of ill health) and even shunned.

It is true that things have been changing over the last few years, and the taboos are slowly but steadily being removed. Nevertheless, it is still very difficult to resist or shrug off society's opinion that dying is one of the worst things you can do.

Most of us who have been looking after people at the end of life have an entirely different view. What I am about to say is not unique (although it doesn't usually get included in books about cancer treatment). It is a relatively simple view, although to hold onto it when things are going badly is not necessarily easy. It is this: death ends a life but does not rob that life of meaning. Perhaps the clearest illustration of what I mean comes not from the great philosophers or writers but from an old movie. It is a classic that is screened many times each Christmas: Frank Capra's *It's a Wonderful Life.* In the movie, George Bailey, an honest and principled man (played unforgettably by James Stewart) faces financial ruin and decides to kill himself. An angel (called Clarence) comes down and shows him how life in his town would have been without him: his brother would have drowned, the local pharmacist would have been ruined, a decent housing project would never have happened, and, most important, he would not have had the love of his wife, family, and friends.

I almost feel that I should apologize for using a movie as an allegory, but in fact the story is an important statement about the value of personal contact and how the meaning of our own life should be assessed by the effect we have on other people. Most of us at the end of life will find, probably, that we are not as rich as we had dreamed once, we never did some of the things we had aimed for, and we never made quite as big a splash as we once hoped we would. However—like George Bailey—while those things may be the facts, they are not the truth. The truth is—and we all need a Clarence to tell us this—that the value of our life is contained in the way we have altered the people we have made contact with. Each one of us has been subtly altered by the people who have made contact with us, people whom we have chosen to be influenced by. And we have done the same to others. While we live, we give a sort of immortality to the people who have touched us. When we die we achieve that same sort of immortality in the lives of the people we have touched. So, as the movie said, it *is* a wonderful life, and dying does not obliterate the wonder of it.

Conclusion

I realize that, as Juliette said in the focus group quoted at the start of this book, everyone who is threatened by cancer wants a happy ending. Like all physicians working in the field, I wish I could grant happy endings for everyone. But even when those are not in sight, we can all do something to decrease the feelings of fear and dread that almost always accompany the diagnosis of cancer. Part of the cure for fear is knowledge, and this book was written to help meet the need for more knowledge.

I hope that most of the basic background facts about the cancers have been provided in an accessible way and that the information helps you understand the reasoning behind the treatment decisions in your own case. I know that this book did not offer any quick solutions. That may be because, in most cases, there are no instant solutions; anybody who promises cancer patients that such solutions exist at present or are almost within reach may do more harm than good by encouraging artificially high expectations.

Perhaps in twenty years' time there will be a wonder drug that dramatically changes the treatment of all or most cancers. On the other hand, perhaps there will not be such a drug. Perhaps the impact that cancer has on our society will be changed not by a wonder cure but by understanding more about prevention, by predicting precisely who is at the highest risk of getting which cancer and concentrating preventive methods on those people. Or perhaps in the future surgery for cancer will be followed by lifelong treatments to prevent metastases. Or perhaps there will be a battery or combination of tests and methods that will reduce the incidence and the mortality of the cancers. At the moment it is impossible to be certain which route is going to be the most successful, even in the short term.

Of one thing we can be certain: whatever your treatment, a major part of that therapy is the relationship between you and your doctor. A basic understanding of your own medical situation will help you understand what your doctor is saying. That understanding will reinforce the relationship between you, not replace it. Thus, if this book suggests questions about your own treatment, or about the future, or about any other aspect of your own care, do not hesitate to discuss them openly and honestly with your doctor. That is what doctors are there for.

There is no doubt that cancer has earned its title of "the dread disease." But the antidote to dread is understanding and support. I hope that this book helps you gain that understanding and makes you better able to draw on the support of those around you.

Some Commonly Used Medical Terms and What They Mean

A

abdomen and abdominal cavity The abdomen is the area of the body below the ribs and above the pelvis. Inside the abdomen are the organs of the digestive tract (stomach, bowel, and so on) as well as the liver, spleen, kidneys, and several other organs. All these organs are covered with a lining membrane called the **peritoneum**, which also lines the inside of the wall of the abdomen. The phrase "abdominal cavity" (the medical term is peritoneal cavity) is used to mean the space enclosed by the peritoneum, that is, the abdominal cavity is the space outside the bowel but inside the abdomen. Thus the food that is inside the stomach (or the stool that is inside the bowel) is inside the abdomen but not inside the abdominal cavity. By contrast, if fluid (ascites) forms, it forms inside the abdominal cavity and is not inside the stomach or the bowel. In the same way, cancers (for example, of the ovary) may spread around this cavity, which means they may form metastases that are outside the bowel and stomach but inside the abdominal cavity. I apologize for the length of this definition, but many patients find this a very confusing area.

adenocarcinoma The word means "a cancer that starts inside a gland." There are glands in many areas of the body (for example, breast, lung, uterus, bowel, stomach), and quite often a cancer in an organ begins inside a gland within that organ. Glands are particularly likely to develop a cancer for two main reasons. First, glands are subjected to influences from the *outside* environment (for example, cigarette smoke affects the glands in the lungs) and also from the *inside* environment (for example, glands in the breast and the uterus are under the influence of the body's hormones). Second, the cells in glands multiply very frequently, so that faults in their growth control may appear more quickly than in other tissues. Hence adenocarcinomas are a relatively common type of cancer.

adjuvant therapy Therapy given after surgery to reduce the chance that the cancer will come back. By definition, adjuvant therapy is given when there is no evidence of any cancer left behind at the time—in other words, the patient appears cancer free—but there is a risk that the cancer will come back. The objective of adjuvant therapy is to reduce that risk. As a patient once expressed it, *"The idea is to make me sick temporarily so that I will be well permanently."*

barium enema A procedure in which a liquid containing barium, which shows up white on an X ray, is given into the rectum after which X rays are taken.

biopsy A biopsy is a specimen or piece of tissue. If a doctor looks at, say, a wart on your skin and takes a piece of it for analysis, that is a biopsy (see illustration below).

bone scan A procedure in which the patient is given a small injection of a substance that emits gamma rays (similar to low doses of X rays). The substance is taken up by the bone in the body, and a scan (using a special camera that detects gamma rays) can then show the bones but not most of the other tissues.

brachytherapy The word used to describe a particular type of radiotherapy. Instead of using standard radiotherapy machines and delivering the radiation from outside the patient, small seeds of radioactive material are mounted in special tubes and put inside the patient, thus giving radiotherapy directly to the area of the cancer. Brachytherapy is particularly useful in certain sites of cancer, such as the cervix, the endometrium, the mouth, and some other sites.

CROSS SECTION TO SHOW THE PERITONEAL CAVITY

Spleen

Left kidney

Pancreas

Stomach

Peritoneum

This is the peritoneal cavity, between—but outside—the abdominal organs. Some cancers can create fluid that fills and expands this cavity.

Area of cross section

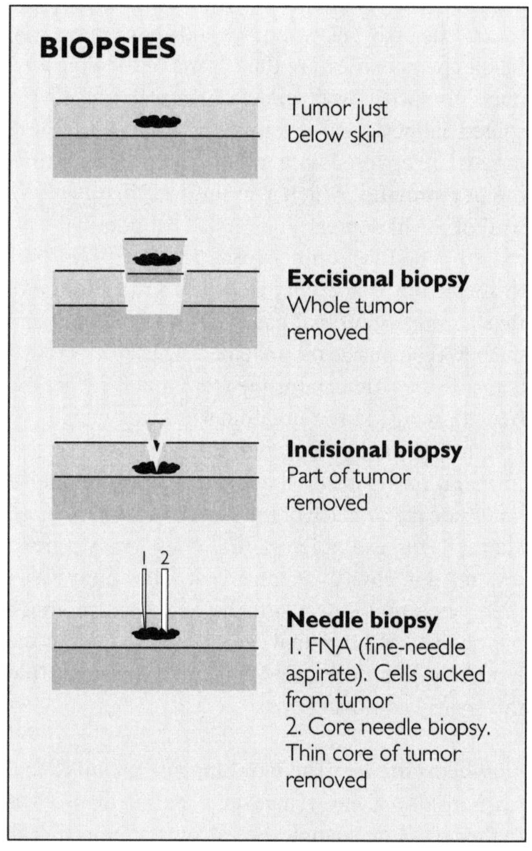

cachexia Becoming abnormally thin or wasting. The term is used to describe what happens when the body is unable to grow and maintain the normal bulk of muscle and fat. There is thinning of the arms, legs, buttocks, and face and a general thin and sallow appearance. Cachexia can be caused if a cancer interferes with absorption or handling of food (for example, if it affects the digestive tract or the liver), but many cancers also cause cachexia without directly affecting the body's ability to handle food.

carcinogen, carcinogenic Capable of causing cancer. Carcinogens are chemicals or substances that may cause cancer in certain circumstances, and **carcinogenesis** means the process by which cancer develops.

cautery Using an electric current to heat up a specially designed piece of wire that can then cut or remove tissue. The advantage of cautery is that because the wire is hot as it does the cutting, it also seals the tissues underneath so there is no bleeding. It is only used in places and situations where there will be no pain.

colonoscopy A procedure in which the doctor can examine (and take small specimens of) the lining of the rectum and the whole colon using an instrument that is like a long, thin, flexible telescope.

colposcopy A procedure in which the doctor can examine (and take small specimens of) the lining of the vagina and the cervix using an instrument that is like a thin telescope.

constitutional symptoms This rather old-fashioned phrase is used to describe the general symptoms of cancer (as opposed to the symptoms caused in one area or part of the body). Constitutional symptoms, therefore, include problems such as weight loss, loss of appetite, tiredness, loss of energy, fevers, and night sweats. These problems are very common in the general population, so do not think you have cancer if you occasionally experience any of these. If they accompany a diagnosed cancer, however (particularly tumors such as Hodgkin's disease or lymphoma), they may provide useful information.

CT or CAT scan The initials "CT" stand for Computerized Tomography (and "CAT" for Computerized Axial Tomography). The CT scan is really an X ray with a very sophisticated computer system that analyzes the way the X rays are altered as they pass through the body. This allows the CT scanner to produce images that are just like visual slices of the body and far superior to ordinary X rays in what they can show. The procedure is quite simple. The patient lies on a special table that is slowly and steadily moved through what looks like a large metal doughnut. In many CT procedures, some dye may be given intravenously before the scan, or you may be asked to drink some white fluid or to have some of the same fluid given as an enema. These procedures allow the radiologist to distinguish normal from abnormal structures.

cystoscopy A cystoscopy is a procedure in which a thin telescope is passed into the bladder, allowing the specialist to see the inside of the bladder and to take biopsies of any areas that look suspicious.

cytology The process in which cells (taken, for example, from the cervix, the mouth, or the stomach) are examined by a specialist to see if there is any sign of cancer or some other problem.

distant spread The same thing as metastasis, the process by which a primary cancer gives rise to secondary cancers elsewhere in the body (for example, a primary cancer in the bowel may give rise to secondary tumors in the liver). In contrast to distant spread, local recurrence means recurrence of the cancer in the area in which it first appeared (for example, in the scar of the original operation or in the lymph nodes nearby).

endoscopy Any procedure in which a specialist uses a thin tube to look inside a part of the body is an endoscopy (which therefore includes bronchoscopy, gastroscopy, laryngoscopy, and so on).

hormone A hormone is a substance produced by one part of the body (a gland) and released into the bloodstream. It then produces a change in some other part or parts of the body. Thus the hormone insulin is produced by the pancreas and alters the handling of glucose by various parts of the body such as the liver and the muscles; the hormone adrenalin is produced by the adrenal glands on top of the kidneys and speeds up the pulse rate and increases the blood pressure.

incidence Incidence means the number of new cases that occur per year. As many conditions occur more frequently in one age group than another (say, in late adulthood as opposed to childhood), we use the phrase "**peak incidence**" to mean the age at which the condition occurs most commonly, that is, has its highest incidence.

IVP The initials stand for **intravenous pyelogram**, which is an X-ray test of your kidneys and urinary system. A dye is given as an intravenous injection, and then X-ray pictures are taken as the dye comes out through the kidneys, down the ureters, and into the bladder (see page 109). The IVP can show several types of problems that affect the kidneys or ureters and is also very useful in showing exactly where they are (their position varies somewhat from person to person), so that treatment can be planned accurately.

laser Laser light is basically light produced in a way that creates a beam of high energy that can be focused and controlled very accurately and that is capable of causing permanent changes in tissues.

lesion A problem area where something abnormal is going on. A lump, a nodule, and a wart are all lesions. A lesion means *"Something is happening here"*; it does not mean *"This is definitely cancer."*

local recurrence The reappearance (recurrence) of a tumor in the area in which it was originally diagnosed. Hence, if there is a local recurrence of a breast cancer, that would mean that the cancer has recurred in the scar of the mastectomy, or in the breast if only part of the breast was removed, or in the armpit.

lymphogram (or lymphangiogram) An X ray in which some dye is injected between the toes and then X rays are taken as the dye flows upward along the lymph channels in the pelvis and abdomen. It is very useful for showing the shape of lymph nodes in the pelvis and abdomen. If they are enlarged, ordinary X rays can be taken later on to show how the lymph nodes are shrinking during treatment.

markers Substances produced by a number of cancers that can be detected in the bloodstream and can be useful in both the diagnosis of the particular cancer and in following progress during treatment. For example, in testicular cancers, germ-cell cancers of the ovary, and choriocarcinoma, there are very useful markers called the **AFP** (alpha-fetoprotein) and **βHCG** (beta human chorionic gonadotrophin). In myeloma the malignant cells produce a monoclonal protein usually called the **M band**. Ovarian cancers produce a marker called the **CA-125**. In bowel cancer and in breast cancer, the **CEA** (carcinoembryonic antigen) may be useful in some circumstances. Prostate cancer produces the **PSA** (prostate-specific antigen). In many other cancers, there are markers that are currently being investigated and that may provide useful information in the future.

mediastinoscopy A procedure in which a thin telescope is introduced, under general anesthetic, into the space between the lungs in the center of the chest. The space is called the **mediastinum**, hence the name of the procedure. It is very useful for assessing and taking biopsies of lymph nodes in that area. It is therefore often used in cases of lung cancer for determining the stage of the condition and in cases of Hodgkin's disease or other lymphomas where there is evidence that lymph nodes in that area are enlarged.

metastasis A metastasis is a secondary tumor, a further cancer that has grown when a fragment of the primary tumor detached itself and made its way to some distant part of the body (the process is called metastasizing). A metastasis almost always has all or most of the characteristics of the primary tumor. Hence, if a person has breast cancer and it metastasizes to the liver, the secondary metastases will behave like cancer of the breast (and have a high chance of responding to chemotherapy, for example) rather than like primary cancer of the liver.

MRI scan The initials stand for magnetic resonance imaging. A method of visualizing tissues of the body not with X rays (as in CT scans) but with magnetic fields. A strong magnet gives the magnetic equivalent of a "push" to many types of molecules in human tissues, and as they relax after the "push" they emit a small magnetic signal of their own. These signals can be analyzed by a computer system and can give images of extremely high clarity and definition. MRI scans are particularly useful in looking at the brain and spinal cord. An MRI scan may not be needed if a CT scan shows the problem clearly.

neoadjuvant therapy Neoadjuvant therapy means giving therapy before surgery to reduce the size of the cancer and make the surgery technically easier and perhaps more effective. Also, giving therapy (say, chemotherapy) before the surgery can show whether or not the cancer does actually respond to those drugs. If so, they may be useful after the operation as well.

prognosis Prediction of the future course of the patient's life. *"A good prognosis"* means that the future looks good, that is, the chance of cure or of long life is high. *"A guarded prognosis"* means that there is a high chance of serious deterioration in the foreseeable future.

sigmoidoscopy A procedure by which a physician can examine the lining of the rectum using a tube inserted via the anus.

speculum An instrument that allows the doctor to see a little bit farther into an area of the body such as the vagina. It simply consists of a tube made into two parts that can be inserted closed together, and then gently opened so that, for example, the walls of the vagina are held apart and there is a clear view of the cervix.

squamous The type of lining of an organ in which the cells are flattish and, when seen under the microscope, resemble skin. There is a squamous lining to the mouth, the upper parts of the airways, the lower part of the cervix, the upper part of the esophagus, the anus, and several other organs. If a cancer develops in such a lining, it is called a squamous cancer. Squamous cancers are the most common types of cancer in the cervix, lung, mouth, throat, and several other areas and are relatively common cancers of the skin and some other organs.

systemic Spread around the body or having the potential to do that. If a tumor has a high tendency to spread to distant parts of the body, we may say "This tumor should be regarded as a systemic condition."

thoracotomy An operation done under a general anesthetic in which an incision is made so that the surgeon can look directly into the chest cavity (and at the lungs and the heart). The incision may be made between the ribs or through the breastbone, depending on which part of the chest cavity needs to be investigated. A thoracotomy is required for any removal of a lobe of the lung or if a biopsy of lymph nodes in the middle of the chest is required and mediastinoscopy is not feasible.

ultrasound A method of imaging the inside of the body using a microphone-type device that generates high-frequency waves and produces an image from the reflections of those waves.

Commonly Asked Questions

B

Most of the information in this section appears elsewhere in the book. This summary is intended as a quick reference guide. The questions dealt with here are those that patients and family have asked me most frequently. The answers are based on the main text. The answers to some of the more controversial questions, particularly in the ethical sphere, represent my own personal opinions only.

- ***What is cancer?***

Cancer is what happens when a group of cells grows uncontrollably and in an abnormal and disorderly way. It is really a result of what happens when, for reasons that are only partly understood, the normal growth-control mechanisms fail. Cancer cells have two properties that make them dangerous: they can invade into neighboring tissues; and they can spread to distant areas of the body, forming secondary tumors or metastases.

- ***What causes cancer?***

There are basically two types of factors that contribute to the cause of cancer. One is a tendency or predisposition to develop cancer; the other is exposure to the triggers that start it off (such as cigarettes, sun exposure, liver damage, and so on).

- ***Why do some people get cancer and not others?***

In a few cancers (such as retinoblastoma) and in a small proportion of the more common cancers (such as a small proportion of breast and ovarian cancers), there seems to be an inherited factor that we can (partly) identify. In most cancers we assume that a person's cells have a low threshold for becoming malignant, and thus that he or she will develop a cancer with relatively less prompting by a trigger (such as cigarettes or sun) than another person whose cells have a higher threshold and who may be able to tolerate more exposure to a trigger without developing a cancer.

- ***Do we get cancer from what we eat?***

Yes and no! The high-fat, low-fiber diet common in the developed countries may play a role in about a third of all cancers (though we do not know this for certain yet). There are, however, no toxins or chemicals in modern foods that cause cancer; in fact, the opposite is true. For example, the fact that cancer of the stomach is becoming less common may be due to the way we preserve foods and prevent bacterial decomposition of what we eat.

• ***Are chemicals and pollutants causing cancer?***

In a very small proportion of special cases only. In certain occupations, prolonged exposure to a few identified chemicals may cause certain (rare) kinds of cancers. Nowadays almost all these substances have been identified and are regulated. Chemical exposure, whether at work or at home, probably accounts for less than 3 or 4 percent of all cancers.

• ***Does cigarette smoking really cause cancer?***

Yes. Cigarettes cause approximately 95 percent of cancer of the lung and are a major factor in cancers of the bladder, pancreas, mouth, larynx, esophagus, and kidney.

• ***Why does the diagnosis seem to be so delayed in so many cases?***

Cancer cells can multiply to produce literally billions of cells before a tumor becomes big enough to detect. That is why prevention and some methods of screening are so important.

• ***Why do people with the same cancer get different treatment and have different problems?***

A lot depends on the stage of the disease and on the particular individual. For instance, in breast cancer with involved lymph nodes, if you are postmenopausal the best treatment may be a hormone tablet; if you are premenopausal it may be chemotherapy.

• ***Is there an epidemic of cancer?***

Not really. An epidemic means a very rapid increase in the amount of the disease, and in most cancers there is no real change. In some cancers (such as stomach) there is a decrease, and in some cancers (such as breast) there is a small, steady increase, which may be partly accounted for by better diagnosis. There is an epidemic of discussion and awareness (thank goodness), so that at last people are talking about cancer, whereas until recently it had been a taboo subject.

• ***Why are we all so frightened of cancer?***

Probably because the other major threats to our health have faded somewhat. Until the 1940s we used to be afraid of syphilis and tuberculosis; before that it was cholera and smallpox. Currently cancer and the infectious disease AIDS are occupying the roles of humankind's bogeyman diseases. Cancer has not changed very much, but our perception of it has.

• ***Does conventional treatment work?***

About half of all people with cancer will be cured, and the majority of those cures will be achieved by surgery. The other cures will be achieved by radiotherapy (after or instead of surgery) and (with a few cancers) chemotherapy. In addition, conventional treatment *can produce remissions in a proportion of cases* when cure is not possible. So in some cases it works, and in other cases it does not—and your doctor will be able to explain whether the chance of it working in your own case is high or low or in between. That is why the discussions you have with your doctor about your own particular case are so important.

• ***Why is the treatment so awful?***

Treatment is so awful mostly because cancer cells are only slightly different from normal cells. In this respect, cancers are totally different from, say, bacterial infections such as pneumonia or tuberculosis. Because bacteria are completely different from our body's cells, antibiotics can kill them and not affect us very much. But because cancer cells are very like our normal cells, in order to kill them we (usually) risk doing considerable damage to normal cells or tissues.

• ***With so many advances, how come there's no progress?***

There is tremendous—and increasing—progress in our understanding of cancer, but the gap between understanding and treatment (between laboratory and bedside) is a wide one. Because stories about cancer research are often reported in the media as if that gap were small, people tend to expect big changes in treatment. This tendency is partly responsible for the widespread feeling of disappointment with the impact of cancer research.

• ***Do complementary remedies work against cancer?***

The brief answer is: not as far as we know. As you will see from the cases in Chapter 6, many reported anecdotes may have alternative explanations, and there are very few studies that have genuinely investigated the effects of complementary medicines against cancer. The studies that have been done show no effect. On the other hand, complementary medicines make almost everyone feel better, and the chance of serious harm is relatively small.

• ***Can a change in diet alter the course of cancer?***

Again, not as far as we know. Many cancer centers are currently involved in finding out whether a low-fat diet can alter the course of breast cancer in some selected early cases. There is no evidence, however, that diet supplements, vitamins, minerals, or special diets actually change the course of a cancer once it has developed.

• ***Should a cancer patient try complementary remedies anyway?***

If you want to, and it isn't a big deal for you, yes. If it involves a major investment of time or money or both and you are pinning all your hopes and plans on a successful outcome, then it is worth pausing and thinking and perhaps discussing it with a friend.

• ***Why are there so many conspiracy theories?***

Humans are good at thinking up conspiracy theories to explain anything that is really frightening or threatening. Somehow it comforts us—although it scares and angers us as well—to think that a disaster was brought about, or is being manipulated, by some human agency. Of course, with cancer it is true in some cases. For instance, the increase in smoking among women is a direct result of trends in social attitudes and values exploited to the full by changes in advertising.

• ***How do I know what to believe?***

Anecdotes and stories do not, unfortunately, tell you what to believe. It is only when the results of many similar cases are added together that a picture begins to emerge. And those cases do have to be genuinely similar. The best criterion for believing something is if it has been tested in a properly conducted, randomized, controlled trial so that bias and prejudice are ruled out.

• ***Will there ever be a cure for cancer?***

Probably not *a* cure. It is quite likely that we will make some further advances in some cancers. The biggest changes in cancer may come from prevention or from other directions, such as treatments or vaccines to prevent spread after the primary cancer has been removed. Obviously nobody knows what is going to happen, but a single, sudden breakthrough that produces a universal miracle cure is very unlikely.

• ***Why isn't there a simple, universal test for cancer?***

Because cancer cells are very similar to normal cells, and a cancer begins with a very small number of cells. In a small number of cancers, certain tests can detect early changes: the best example is cancer of the cervix (the Pap test).

• ***Can cancer be prevented?***

We think a lot of it can. The established preventive methods (including refraining from smoking, avoiding sun damage, sensible sexual behavior, eating a high-fiber, low-fat diet, having regular Pap tests) would reduce the incidence of cancer dramatically. We could probably prevent more if we knew more, so research is very active in this field.

• ***Can attitudes or stress cause cancer?***

Not as far as we know. In fact, the idea that the cancer "personality" or a bad attitude contributes to the cause of cancer may be part of the ancient human habit of blaming the patient for the disease.

- ***Does positive thinking change the course of cancer?***

Positive thinking does not, as Bernie Siegel's own research showed. On the other hand, group support for people dealing with the possibility of progressive disease or dying—in other words, a specific form of stress management—may prolong survival. Dr. David Spiegel's study investigated this approach (in which patients confront the situation rather than trying to pretend it doesn't exist) and showed that it prolonged survival in breast cancer. This important research is now being repeated in several places, and if the results confirm the initial findings, the use of support groups may be a useful adjunct to the treatment of cancer.

- ***How can I get the best from my doctor?***

Doctor-patient relationships are similar in some respects to marriages: some are good and some are bad, and a lot depends on the people involved. The key to getting the best from your medical team is to present your problems as clearly and accurately as you can and to clarify exactly what it is you want to know and what you need.

- ***Can our species ever be free of cancer?***

Probably not. It is likely that our human species evolved with a design that was quite satisfactory if the individual lived for three, four, or perhaps five decades. Our problem, so to speak, is that we are now quite good at dealing with the forces that, centuries ago, used to kill us off before we were sixty. Now that many more of us are living into our sixties, seventies, and beyond, cancer is a flaw that appears with increasing frequency as cells do more and more multiplying and get older. It is possible that we can devise ways of stopping this flaw from appearing, but it is equally possible that cancer is not eradicable in the way smallpox was.

Further Readings and References

C

This is not a textbook, so I have not included a complete bibliography or a comprehensive list of the references. However, some readers might be interested in a few of the more unusual or hard-to-locate references relating to topics in Chapters 5, 6, 7, and 9, so I list a few of them below.

Chapter 5: The Main Types of Conventional Treatment

The first published report of the use of autologous marrow transplant (as it would be called now) was in 1961: P. Clifford, R. A. Clift, and J. K. Duff, "Nitrogen Mustard Therapy Combined with Autologous Marrow Infusion," *Lancet* i(1961):687–89.

Chapter 6: Complementary, Alternative, or Unconventional Treatments

Eczema The trial that compared a tea made from Chinese herbs to a tea made of other herbs (ones not used for eczema) was published in 1992: M. P. Sheehan and D. J. Atherton, "A Controlled Trial of Traditional Medicinal Plants in Widespread Non-Exudative Atopic Eczema," *British Journal of Dermatology* 126(1961):179–84.

Chiropractic manipulation for back pain The two randomized studies of chiropractic manipulation/osteopathic treatment for back pain (when there was no serious disease present) were published in 1990 and 1992: T. W. Meade, S. Dyer, W. Browne, J. Townsend, and A. O. Frank, "Low Back Pain of Mechanical Origin: Randomised Comparison of Chiropractic and Hospital Outpatient Treatment," *British Medical Journal* 300(1990):1431–37; B. W. Koes et al., "Randomised Clinical Trial of Manipulative Therapy and Physiotherapy for Persistent Back and Neck Complaints: Results of One-Year Follow-Up," *British Medical Journal* 304(1992):601–5.

Chapter 7: Cancer, Attitudes, and the Mind

Social Attitudes

A brilliant and highly readable description of the many major breakthroughs (real and imagined) in cancer treatment since the turn of the century is *The Dread Disease* by James T. Patterson (Cambridge, Mass.: Harvard University Press, 1987).

Can the Mind Cause Cancer?

Life events One of the biggest and most definitive studies on the effects of life events and life stress was a survey of 4,905 people who were widowed or widowered under the age of sixty. Over the four years after their bereavement, there was no discernible increase in the diagnosis of cancer. In the researchers' view, these findings provided "little support for the hypothesis that stress is implicated in the etiology [causation] of cancer": D. R. Jones, P. O. Goldblatt, and D. A. Leon, "Bereavement and Cancer: Some Data on Deaths of Spouses from the Longitudinal Study of Office of Population Censuses and Surveys," *British Medical Journal* 289(1984):461–64.

A similar study from Israel showed the same thing—no increase in cancer—among parents whose children had died: I. Levar, Y. Friedlander, J. Kark, and E. Peritz, "An Epidemiologic Study of Mortality among Bereaved Parents," *New England Journal of Medicine* 319(1988):457–61.

Depression Another study was published in 1989 and concluded that people who had depression did not have an increased chance of getting cancer. The study was of 6,403 people, of whom 1,002 had self-reported depressive symptoms. The incidence of cancer was the same in both depressed and nondepressed people: A. B. Zonderman, P. T. Costa, and R. R. McRae, "Depression as a Risk for Cancer Morbidity and Mortality in a Nationally Representative Sample," *Journal of the American Medical Association* 262(1989):1191–95.

Stress and breast cancer Many studies have been done, but one early and straightforward one presented the results of stress questionnaires completed by 100 women with breast cancer, 100 women with benign breast lumps, and 100 women with no apparent medical problems. There were no differences in stress levels between women with malignant and benign diseases, though the healthy volunteers appeared to have more stress than either of the other two groups: T. J. Priestman, S. G. Priestman, and C. Bradshaw, "Stress and Breast Cancer," *British Journal of Cancer* 51(1981):493–96.

Effects of radiation One of the most detailed studies of the effects on survivors of the Hiroshima and Nagasaki atomic bombs was published in 1975: review of "Thirty Years Study of Hiroshima and Nagasaki Atomic Bomb Survivors" in the supplement to the *Journal of Radiation Research* 1975.

Review of the subject An excellent overview of this subject was published by Dr. Bernard H. Fox, "Psychogenic Factors in Cancer, Especially Its Incidence," in *Topics in Health Psychology,* cd. S. Macs, C. D. Spielberger, P. B. Defares, and I. G. Sarason (New York: J. Wiley and Sons, 1988, pp. 37–54), Fox reviewed more than eighty papers and studies. His review is detailed and careful and worth reading if you are interested in the subject. In brief, he found that there were serious flaws in many of the studies and conflicting results from other studies. He felt that there was no reliable and reproducible basis to support the hypothesis that psychological or life-event factors were implicated in causing cancer or in changing the outcome.

Stress and the common cold The best-known study showing an effect of stress on infections with common-cold viruses was published in 1991: S. Cohen, D.A.J. Tyrell, and A. P. Smyth, "Psychological Stress and Susceptibility to the Common Cold," *New England Journal of Medicine* 325(1991): 606–12. In this study, volunteers were given various doses of three varieties of common-cold viruses (via their nostrils). Stress events in the previous two weeks were recorded carefully and were found to correlate with the number of people who actually developed colds after getting the viruses. In other words, stresses increased the susceptibility to catching a cold but not by very much. On average, the number of infections in the "low-stress" group was about 20 percent, and the rate in the "high-stress" group was about 28 percent. This shows that there may be some effect on susceptibility to infections related to stress, as many people have also believed, but it is a small effect.

The Mind and the Outcome of Cancer

British study in 1979 S. Greer, T. Morris, and K. W. Pettingale, "Psychological Response to Breast

Cancer: Effect on Outcome," *Lancet* ii(1979): 785–87.

Bristol The study that precipitated so much debate was published in 1990: F. S. Bagenal, D. F. Easton, E. Harris, et al., "Survival of Patients with Breast Cancer Attending Bristol Cancer Help Centre," *Lancet* 336(1990):606–10. A study designed on the same lines, carried out by Dr. Barrie Cassileth, compared survival (among other things) of patients at a conventional center with those at a complementary medicine center in California. This study showed that patients at the complementary center did not live longer than those at the conventional center, and the complementary center later expressed satisfaction with the way the study had been carried out: B. R. Cassileth, E. J. Lusk, D. J. Miller, et al., "Survival and Quality of Life among Patients Receiving Unproven as Compared with Conventional Cancer Therapy," *New England Journal of Medicine* 324(1991):1180–85.

Stress and relapse of breast cancer A study that suggested that severe life stressors might have an effect on the recurrence of breast cancer was published in 1989: A. J. Ramirez, T.J.K. Craig, J. P. Watson, and I. A. Fentiman, "Stress and Relapse of Breast Cancer," *British Medical Journal* 298(1989): 292–93. However, the data on the patients (50 women with recurrence and 50 with no recurrence) were collected at the time of recurrence and not prospectively (that is, not in advance). A better study collected data on a group of 204 women and then followed their progress for about four years: J. Barraclough, P. Pinder, and M. Cruddas, "Life Events and Breast Cancer Prognosis," *British Medical Journal* 304(1992):1078–81. The results gave "no support to the theory that psychosocial stress contributes to relapse in breast cancer." These researchers reported later follow-up on the same group of patients at five years, and the results were the same—stress did not affect the chance of relapse: J. Barraclough, C. Osmond, and I. Taylor, "Life Events and Breast Cancer Prognosis," *British Medical Journal* 307(1993):325. The authors concluded that the results of the 1989 study (Ramirez et al.) might have been caused by women recalling events and stresses differently if they had had relapse, in other words, that the results might have been caused by the way that study was designed.

Dr. Bernie Siegel Bernie Siegel was involved in two research studies, looking for an effect of attending ECaP groups on the survival of women with breast cancer. The first (and smaller) study was published in 1984: H. Morganstern, G. A. Gellert, S. D. Walter, A. M. Ostfeld, and B. S. Siegel, "The Impact of a Psychosocial Support Program on Survival with Breast Cancer: The Importance of Selection Bias in Program Evaluation," *Journal of Chronic Disease* 37(1984): 273–282. The second, larger study was published in 1993: G. A. Gellert, R. M. Maxwell, and B. S. Siegel, "Survival of Breast Cancer Patients Receiving Adjunctive Psychosocial Support Therapy: A 10-Year Follow-Up Study," *Journal of Clinical Oncology* 11(1993): 66–69. The reference on "EPHO" and "HOPE" was in W. M. Buchholtz, "The Medical Uses of Hope," *Western Journal of Medicine* 1(1988): 148.

Group support and survival with breast cancer The important study was published by Dr. David Spiegel in 1991: D. Spiegel, J. R. Bloom, H. C. Kraemer, and E. Gottheil, "Effect of Psychosocial Treatment on Survival of Patients with Metastatic Breast Cancer," *Lancet* ii(1991):888–91. It was a follow-up on the patients enrolled into his group-support program described in an earlier paper: D. Spiegel, J. R. Bloom, and I. Yalom, "Group Support for Patients with Metastatic Cancer," *Archives of General Psychiatry* 36(1981):527–33. Another book that is recommended is Bob Stone's *Where the Buffaloes Roam: Building a Team for Life Challenges* (Atlanta: Lapidum Press, 1993).

Chapter 9: With So Many Breakthroughs, Why's There No Progress?

Marrow clean-up The work that identified breast cancer cells in bone marrow was led by Drs. Dearnaley, Ormerod, and Sloane: D. P. Dearnaley, J. P. Sloane, M. D. Ormerod, K. Steele, R. C. Coombes, et al., "Increased Detection of Mammary Carcinoma Cells in Marrow Smears Using Antisera to Epithelial Membrane Antigen," *British Journal of Cancer* 44(1981):85–90. The technique that our group devised to eliminate them was described in 1982: R. Buckman, R.A.J. McIlhinney, V. Shepherd, S. Patel, R. C. Coombes, and A. M. Neville, "The Elimination of Carcinoma Cells from Human Bone Marrow," *Lancet* ii(1982):1428–30. The early results of using that technique in the treatment of women with breast cancer were published in 1986: R. C. Coombes, R. Buckman, J. A. Forrester, et al., "In Vitro and In Vivo Effects of a Monoclonal Antibody-Conjugate for Use in Autologous Bone Marrow Transplantation for Patients with Breast Cancer," *Cancer Research* 46(1986):4217–20.

Magic bullets Our work was designed to try to reproduce the early results reported by Dr. Agamemnon Epenetos in 1982: A. A. Epenetos, K. E. Britton, S. E. Mather, et al., "Targeting of Iodine-123 Labelled Tumour-Associated Monoclonal Antibodies to Ovarian, Breast and Gastro-Intestinal Tumours," *Lancet* ii(1982):999–1002. The monoclonal antibody we tested and characterized was described in 1989: P. Shaw, R. Buckman, J. Law, R. Baumal, and A. Marks, "Reactivity of Tumor Cells in Malignant Effusions with a Panel of Monoclonal and Polyclonal Antibodies," *Tumour Biology* 9(1989):101–9. The results of testing the antibody "armed" with radioactive iodine were described later: A. Marks, R. Buckman, C.-S. Kwok, et al. "Preclinical and Clinical Studies of Radioiodinated Monoclonal Antibody 2G3 for Therapy of Intraperitoneal Effusions Associated with Carcinoma of Breast and Ovary," *Antibody, Immunoconjugate and Radiopharmaceuticals* 2(1989):83–92.

Information available on videotape

The *What You Really Need to Know about . . .* videotapes, which cover a wide range of diagnoses and medical problems, are designed specifically to help patients understand their own medical conditions. Each videotape explains clearly the basic facts about the condition, how it causes symptoms, how the diagnosis is made, and the types of treatment used, together with any other important topics. Each video is introduced by John Cleese and presented by Robert Buckman, and makes full use of graphics and models as illustrations.

The series is projected to cover 120 medical conditions; 45 titles are available now. The four titles that deal with types of cancer or aspects of cancer are *Breast Cancer, Prostate Cancer, Chronic Lymphocytic Leukemia*, and *Cancer Pain.* Another video that may be of particular interest to anyone who has a stoma is called *Colostomies, Ileostomies, and Urinary Stomas.*

The videotapes are produced in the United Kingdom by Videos for Patients Ltd. and are available in the United States from

Medical Audio-Visual Communications
2601 Matheson Boulevard, Suite 41
Mississauga ON L5W 5A, Canada
Toll-free telephone: 1-800-757-4868

Other Sources of Help

D

AMERICAN CANCER SOCIETY, NATIONAL HEADQUARTERS

American Cancer Society
National Headquarters
1599 Clifton Road NE
Atlanta, GA 30329-4251
1-800-227-2345

AMERICAN CANCER SOCIETY, STATE OFFICES

Alabama Division, Inc.
504 Brookwood Boulevard
Homewood, AL 35209
(205) 879-2242

Alaska Division, Inc.
1057 West Fireweed Lane, #204
Anchorage, AK 99503
(907) 277-8696
1-800-478-9355 statewide
Internet: cancer@anc.ak.net

Arizona Division, Inc.
2929 East Thomas Road
Phoenix, AZ 85016
(602) 224-0524

Arkansas Division, Inc.
901 North University Avenue
P.O. Box 3822
Little Rock, AR 72203
(501) 664-3480

California Division, Inc.
1710 Webster Street
Oakland, CA 94612
(510) 893-7900

CALIFORNIA REGIONAL OFFICES

Border Region
8880 Rio San Diego Drive, Suite 100
San Diego, CA 92108
(619) 299-4200

Central Valley Region
4191 North Blackstone Avenue, #204
Fresno, CA 93726
(209) 225-8018

Desert Sierra Region
7130 Magnolia Avenue, Suite T
Riverside, CA 92504
(909) 320-7142

East Bay Region
1700 Webster Street
Oakland, CA 94612
(510) 452-5229

CALIFORNIA REGIONAL OFFICES
(continued)

Gold Coast Region
426 E. Barcellus, Suite 304
Santa Maria, CA 93454
(805) 925-8190

Los Angeles Region
3255 Wilshire Boulevard, #701
Los Angeles, CA 90010-1110
(213) 386-7660

North Valley Region
350 Alhambra Boulevard
Sacramento, CA 95816
(916) 446-7933

Orange Region
Alton Deere Plaza
1940 E. Deere Avenue, Suite 100
Santa Ana, CA 92705
(714) 261-9446

Redwood Empire Region
1451 Guerneville Road, Suite 220
Santa Rosa, CA 95403
(707) 545-6720

Silicon Valley/Central Region
1715 South Bascom Avenue, #100
Campbell, CA 95008
(408) 287-5973

West Bay Region
235 Montgomery Street, #320
San Francisco, CA 94104
(415) 394-7100

Colorado Division, Inc.
2255 South Oneida
Denver, CO 80224
(303) 758-2030

Connecticut Division, Inc.
Barnes Park South
14 Village Lane
P.O. Box 410
Wallingford, CT 06492
(203) 265-7161

Delaware Division, Inc.
92 Read's Way, Suite 205
New Castle, DE 19720
(302) 324-4227

District of Columbia Division, Inc.
1875 Connecticut Avenue NW, Suite 730
Washington, DC 20009
(202) 483-2600

Florida Division, Inc.
3709 West Jetton Avenue
Tampa, FL 33629
(813) 253-0541

Georgia Division, Inc.
2200 Lake Boulevard
P.O. Box 190429
Atlanta, GA 30319
(404) 816-7800

Hawaii Pacific Division, Inc.
2370 Nuuanu Avenue
Honolulu, HI 96817-1714
(808) 595-7500

Idaho Division, Inc.
2676 Vista Avenue
P.O. Box 5386
Boise, ID 83705
(208) 343-4609

Illinois Division, Inc.
77 East Monroe Street, 13th Floor
Chicago, IL 60603-5795
(312) 641-6150

Indiana Division, Inc.
8730 Commerce Park Place
Indianapolis, IN 46268
(317) 872-4432

Iowa Division, Inc.
8364 Hickman Road, Suite D
Des Moines, IA 50325
(515) 253-0147

Kansas Division, Inc.
1315 S.W. Arrowhead Road
Topeka, KS 66604
(913) 273-4114

Kentucky Division, Inc.
701 West Muhammad Ali Boulevard
P.O. Box 1807
Louisville, KY 40201
(502) 584-6782

Louisiana Division, Inc.
2200 Veterans Memorial Boulevard, Suite 214
Kenner, LA 70062
(504) 469-0021

Maine Division, Inc.
52 Federal Street
Brunswick, ME 04011
(207) 729-3339

Maryland Division, Inc.
8219 Town Center Drive
P.O. Box 43026
Baltimore, MD 21236-0026
(410) 931-6850

Massachusetts Division, Inc.
247 Commonwealth Avenue
Boston, MA 02116
(617) 267-2650

Michigan Division, Inc.
1205 East Saginaw Street
Lansing, MI 48906
(517) 371-2920
Internet: http://www.mi.cancer.org

Minnesota Division, Inc.
3316 West 66th Street
Minneapolis, MN 55435
(612) 925-2772

Mississippi Division, Inc.
1380 Livingston Lane
Lakeover Park
Jackson, MS 39213
(601) 362-8874

Missouri Division, Inc.
3322 American Avenue
P.O. Box 1066
Jefferson City, MO 65102
(314) 893-4800

Montana Division, Inc.
17 North 26th Street
P.O. Box 1080
Billings, MT 59103-1080
(406) 252-7111

Nebraska Division, Inc.
8502 West Center Road
P.O. Box 241255
Omaha, NE 68124-5255
(402) 393-5800

Nevada Division, Inc.
1325 East Harmon
Las Vegas, NV 89119
(702) 798-6857

New Hampshire Division, Inc.
360 Route 101, Unit 501
Bedford, NH 03110
(603) 472-8899

New Jersey Division, Inc.
U.S. Highway 1
P.O. Box 6001
North Brunswick, NJ 08902
(908) 297-8000

New Mexico Division, Inc.
5800 Lomas Boulevard NE
Albuquerque, NM 87110
(505) 260-2105

New York State Division, Inc.
6725 Lyons Street
P.O. Box 7
East Syracuse, NY 13057
(315) 437-7025

New York City
19 West 56th Street
New York, NY 10019
(212) 586-8700

North Carolina Division, Inc.
11 South Boylan Avenue, Suite 22
Raleigh, NC 27603
(919) 834-8463

North Dakota Division, Inc.
123 Roberts Street
P.O. Box 426
Fargo, ND 58102
(701) 232-1385

Ohio Division, Inc.
5555 Frantz Road
Dublin, OH 43017
(614) 889-9565

Oklahoma Division, Inc.
4323 N.W. 63rd, Suite 110
Oklahoma City, OK 73116
(405) 843-9888

Oregon Division, Inc.
0330 S.W. Curry Street
Portland, OR 97201
(503) 295-6422

Pennsylvania Division, Inc.
Route 422 and Sipe Avenue
Hershey, PA 17033
(717) 533-6144

Philadelphia Division, Inc.
1626 Locust Street
Philadelphia, PA 19103
(215) 985-5400

Rhode Island Division, Inc.
400 Main Street
Pawtucket, RI 02860
(401) 722-8480

South Carolina Division, Inc.
128 Stonemark Lane
Westpark Plaza
Columbia, SC 29210
(803) 750-1693

South Dakota Division, Inc.
4101 Carnegie Place
Sioux Falls, SD 57106
(605) 361-8277

Tennessee Division, Inc.
1315 8th Avenue South
Nashville, TN 37203
(615) 255-1227
Internet: acstndiv@usit.net

Texas Division, Inc.
2433 Ridgepoint Drive, A
Austin, TX 78754
(512) 928-2262

Utah Division, Inc.
941 East, 3300 South
Salt Lake City, UT 84106
(801) 483-1500

Vermont Division, Inc.
13 Loomis Street
Montpelier, VT 05602
(802) 223-2348

Virginia Division, Inc.
4240 Park Place Court
P.O. Box 6359
Glen Allen, VA 23058-6359
(804) 527-3700

Washington Division, Inc.
2120 First Avenue North
P.O. Box 19140
Seattle, WA 98109
(206) 283-1152
1-800-729-1151

WASHINGTON REGIONAL OFFICES

Eastern Area Office
900 North Maple, Suite 200
Spokane, WA 99201
(509) 326-5802

Northwest Area Office
14450 N.E. 29th Place, Suite 220
Bellevue, WA 98007
(206) 869-5588

Southwest Area Office
1551 Broadway, Suite 200
Tacoma, WA 98402
(206) 272-5767

West Virginia Division, Inc.
2428 Kanawha Boulevard East
Charleston, WV 25311
(304) 344-3611

Wisconsin Division, Inc.
N19 W24350 Riverwood Drive
Waukesha, WI 53188
(414) 523-5500

Wyoming Division, Inc.
4202 Ridge Road
Cheyenne, WY 82001
(307) 638-3331

CANCER HOSPITALS

The following hospitals were ranked as the top twenty cancer hospitals by *U.S. News and World Report* in August 1996. They are listed here in alphabetical order by state, with the actual ranking number appearing within parentheses following the name.

UCLA Medical Center (University of California, Los Angeles) (16)
10833 Le Conte Avenue
Los Angeles, CA 90024
(310) 825-9111

University of California, San Francisco Medical Center (10)
500 Parnassus Avenue
San Francisco, CA 94143
(415) 476-1000

Stanford University Hospital (6)
300 Pasteur Drive
Stanford, CA 94305
(415) 723-4000

University of Chicago Hospitals (9)
5841 South Maryland
Chicago, IL 60637
(312) 702-1000

Indiana University Medical Center (13)
550 North University Boulevard
Indianapolis, IN 46202
(317) 274-5000

University of Iowa Hospitals and Clinics (20)
200 Hawkins Drive
Iowa City, IA 52242
(319) 356-1616

Johns Hopkins Hospital (4)
Oncology Center
600 North Wolfe Street
Baltimore, MD 21287-8985
(410) 955-5000

Dana-Farber Cancer Institute (3)
375 Longwood Avenue
Boston, MA 02215
(617) 632-3300

Massachusetts General Hospital (11)
32 Fruit Street
Boston, MA 02114
(617) 726-2000

University of Michigan Medical Center (15)
1500 East Medical Center Drive
Ann Arbor, MI 48109
(313) 936-4000

Mayo Clinic (5)
200 S.W. First Street
Rochester, MN 55905
(507) 284-8540

Barnes-Jewish Hospital (17)
216 South Kingshighway Boulevard
St. Louis, MO 63110
(314) 747-3000

Mary Hitchcock Memorial Hospital (19)
One Medical Center Drive
Lebanon, NH 03756
(603) 650-7422

Memorial Sloan-Kettering Cancer Center (1)
1275 York Avenue
New York, NY 10021
(212) 639-2000

Roswell Park Cancer Institute (12)
Elm and Carlton Streets
Buffalo, NY 15263
(716) 845-2300

Duke University Medical Center (8)
Box 3708
Durham, NC 27710
(919) 684-5414

Fox Chase Cancer Center (14)
7701 Burholme Avenue
Philadelphia, PA 19111
(215) 728-3633

Hospital of the University of Pennsylvania (18)
3400 Spruce Street
Philadelphia, PA 19104
(215) 662-4000

University of Texas M.D. Anderson Cancer Center (2)
1515 Holcombe Boulevard
Houston, TX 77030
(713) 792-2121

University of Washington Medical Center (7)
1959 N.E. Pacific Street
Seattle, WA 98195
(206) 548-3300

INDEX

Page numbers in **boldface** type refer to definitions, main discussions, or medical emergencies. The sites of cancer are also set in **boldface** when they appear as main entries. Page numbers for figures are followed by an *f*; those for tables are followed by a *t*.

abdomen/abdominal cavity, **327**, 328f. *See also* ascites; bloating
  lymph nodes, 16f, 103f, 121f
  mesotheliomas, 210–11
abdominal pain, 32, 277
  emergencies and their management, 289t
  with endometrial cancer, 95
  gallbladder tumors and, 209–10
  with prostatic cancer, 179t
abdominoperineal resection, 54
ABVD, 105
acetaminophen, **279**
achalasia, **99**
acid production in stomach, 193
acne, 123
acral melanoma, **153**
actinomycin D
  choriocarcinoma or molar pregnancy, 91
  side effects, 224t, 226t, 229t
  soft tissue sarcomas, 186
  Wilms' tumor, 204
acupuncture, 283
acute leukemias
  granulocytic-myelocytic, **119**, **129–32**
  lymphocytic, 32, **119**, **127–29**
  nonlymphoblastic (ANLL), **129–32**
adaptation. *See* coping/adjustment/adaptation; quality of life
adenocarcinoma, **327**
  cervical, 87
  esophageal, 100
  kidney, 109
  lung, 139
  stomach, 194
adhesion molecules, 270
adjustment. *See* coping/adjustment/adaptation; quality of life
adjuvant therapy, **327**
  bile duct cancer, 208
  bowel cancer, 54
  breast cancer, **63**, **73–74**
  melanoma, 155
adolescents
  bone cancer incidence in, 42, 45
  sexual activity of, 83
Adriamycin
  bladder cancer, 41
  breast cancer, 74
  carcinoid tumors, 209
  choriocarcinoma or molar pregnancy, 91
  Kaposi's sarcoma, 108
  leukemias, acute lymphoblastic, 129
  leukemias, acute myelocytic, 131
  leukemias, chronic lymphocytic, 125
  lung cancer, 142
  lymphoma, 146
  lymphoma, AIDS-related, 108
  mesotheliomas, 211
  myeloma, 164
  prostate cancer, 182
  side effects, 224t, 226t, 227, 229t
  soft tissue sarcomas, 186
  stomach cancer, 195
AFP (alpha-fetoprotein), **330**
  with liver cancer, 135, 136
  ovarian cancer screening, 173
  testicular cancer, 197
  tumors of unknown primary, 79, 80
AIDS/HIV, 246
  anal cancer risk, 206
  Kaposi's sarcoma, 29t, **106–8**, 232, 240–41, 244, 258t
  preventive actions, 258t
  skin cancer, 188
AIDS-related lymphoma, 29t, **108**, 144
airway
  carcinoid tumors, 208
  extramedullary plasmacytomas, 164
  as primary site of carcinomas of unknown primary, 77
alcohol
  epidemiological factors, 28
  and esophageal cancer, 97, 98, 99
  Hodgkin's disease symptoms, 102
  and laryngeal cancer, 115
  and liver cancer, 134
  and oral cancer, 158
allogeneic bone marrow transplantation, 228, 230
all-trans retinoic acid, and leukemias, 132
American Cancer Society offices, 341–45
ampulla of Vater, 175f
anal fissures, 51, 56, 206
analgesics
  emergencies and their management, 289t
  pain control, **279–82**, 279f
anaplastic thyroid carcinoma, 201
Anatomy of an Illness, 300
anemia, **120**
  chemotherapy side effects, 124, 227, 228
  colony-stimulating factors, 232
  with leukemia, acute granulocytic, 131
  with leukemia, acute lymphoblastic, 128
  with leukemia, chronic lymphocytic, 123
  myeloma and, 162
  pernicious, 193
angiogenesis (blood supply of tumor), **17–18f**, 269–70

angioinfarction, **113**
anthracyclines, 129
antibodies
  monoclonal, 136, 148, 231–32, 263, 267, 268
  plasma cells, **161–62**
antibody-guided therapy, 268
anticancer drugs. *See* chemotherapy
anticipatory nausea, **224**
antidepressants, 285, 286
antigen, tumor. *See* markers
antigrowth factors, 270
anti-inflammatory drugs, 282
antinausea agents, 225–26, 225t
antioncogene products, 270–71
antitelomerase, 269, 270f
anus
  cancer of, 78f, **205–7**, 206f
  melanomas, 154
  surgical management of bowel cancer, 54
anxiety, 295
apoptosis, **11**
appendix, 208
appetite
  loss of. *See* constitutional symptoms
  steroid hormones and, 123
arsenic, 188
arterial route, chemotherapy administration, 221–22
arteriography, 111
asbestos, 137, 210
ascending colon, 47f
ascites, 268
  with carcinomas of unknown primary, 78f, 79
  intraperitoneal therapy, 172
  with liver cancer, 135
  with mesotheliomas, 210
  with ovarian cancer, 167–68, 169f, 172
  with stomach cancer, 193
Asia
  liver cancer incidence, 134
  stomach cancer incidence, 191
Asians
  esophageal cancer incidence, 98–99
  prostatic cancer incidence, 178
  skin pigment, 150
asparaginase, 244
  in leukemias, acute lymphoblastic, 128, 129
  side effects, 224t
aspiration curettage, 95
astrocytomas, **60**
attitudes, **245–54**, 335, 337
  alternative medicine, **235–44**, 237t
  perceptions and misperceptions of cancer, 1–3
  public perception of cancer research, 261–74
  and talking about cancer, 296–97
atypical hyperplasia, breast lumps, 65t, 66
autologous bone marrow transplantation (ABMT), 148, 230f, 231, 231f, 266–68
automatic brain, **57**
awkwardness, 296

back pain, 32, 337
  with pancreatic cancer, 175
  soft tissue sarcomas, 185
bacteria
  bowel flora, **46, 48**
  Helicobacter pylori, 193
bacterial infection. *See* infection
barium enema, **327**
barium studies, 218
  in esophageal cancer, 99
  large bowel, 52
Barrett's esophagus, **99**
basal-cell carcinoma, 187–90, 188f
basal layer, skin, 148f, **150**
basement membrane, **14**
BCG, 40
B complex vitamins, 99
Bence Jones protein, **162**
benign prostatic hypertrophy (BPH), 178
benign tumors and lesions, 14
  of brain, 58, 61, 63
  breast, 65t, 66, 68
  liver, 134
  thyroid, 201
benzene, 130
bereavement, 249
beta-carotene, 48
bias, research data, 250, 335
bile, 46, **175**
bile ducts/biliary system, 134
  blockage by lymphoma, 147
  cancer of, **207f–8**
  gallbladder cancer, **209–10**, 208f
  pancreatic cancer and, 174, 175f, 176
biologic therapy, 33, 213, 214, **231–33**
  in Kaposi's sarcoma, 108
  in kidney cancers, 109, 112
  in leukemias, chronic granulocytic, 127
  in leukemias, hairy-cell, 132
  in lymphoma, 148
  in melanoma, 155
  in myeloma, 164
  in skin cancer, 190
biology of cancer. *See* tumor biology
biopsy, **328f**
  anal cancer, 206f
  bile duct cancer, 207
  with bone cancer, 44
  bone marrow sample, **120**
  brain, 59–60
  breast, 68–69
  cervix, 84, 85, 86f, 87
  colon, 51–52
  endometrial, 95
  Hodgkin's disease diagnosis, 102, 104
  larynx, 116
  liver, 135
  lymph node, **122**, 145
  in lymphomas, 102, 104, 145
  melanoma, 153
  oral cancer assessment, 159
  ovarian tumor management, 171
  prostate, 179, 180f
  screening tests, 256t
  stomach, 194
  thyroid, 201–2
birth control pills
  breast cancer risk factors, 66
  endometrial cancer risk factors, 94
  and liver changes, 134
  and ovarian cancer incidence, 166
blacks
  esophageal cancer incidence, 98
  and leukemias, acute lymphoblastic, 128
  melanoma location, 151
  and prostatic cancer, 178
  skin pigmentation, 150
bladder
  hysterectomy complications, 88
  prostate and, 177f, 180f
  after prostate surgery, 181
bladder cancer, 29t, **36–41**, 37f, 39f, 254
  preventive actions, 258t
  sexual problems after surgery, 287, 294
blast cells, **131**
bleeding. *See also* blood
  anal lesions and, 206
  blood clotting problems and, **120**, 124, 128, 137, **227–28**
  chemotherapy side effects, 124
  digestive tract, 51, 55t, 56, 124, 288t
  emergencies and their management, 288t
  with esophageal cancer, 99
  with leukemias, acute granulocytic, 131
  with leukemias, acute lymphoblastic, 128
  with leukemias, chronic granulocytic, 126
  with lung cancer, 139, 141
  mole, 155
  myeloma and, 162
  from nipple, 67, 68t
  with oral cancer, 159
  rectal/occult blood in stool, 32, 51, 55t, 56, 256t
  steroid hormone side effects, 123
  with stomach cancer, 194
  urinary tract (hematuria), **37**, 111, 179t
  vaginal, 88, 90, 92, 93, 94, 95, 97
bleomycin, 222
  choriocarcinoma or molar pregnancy, 91
  Kaposi's sarcoma, 108
  lymphoma, AIDS-related, 108
  ovarian cancer, 173
  side effects, 224t, 226t, 229t
  testicular cancer, 198

bloating
with bowel cancer, 51
chemotherapy and, 229t
with endometrial cancer, 95
ovarian cancer and, 167, 168
blockage/obstruction
bile duct, 147
intestinal, 168, 194
mediastinal blood vessels, 138, 141
blood
coughing up, 99, 115, 139, 141, 288t
in stools, 51, 55t, 56, 288t
in urine (hematuria), 37, 111, 179t
vomiting, 124, 288t
blood cells, **120**, 213, 232. *See also* anemia; bone marrow; leukemias
blood clots, 288t
blood clotting, **120**. *See also* bleeding; platelets; petechiae (purple spots)
blood markers. *See* markers
blood pressure, endometrial cancer risk factors, 94, 97
bloodstream, cancer spread via
bone cancer, 43
kidney cancer, 109, 110
myeloma, 162
stomach cancer spread via, 193
tumor cell delivery to distant site, 17, 17f, 18f
tumor cell invasion, 11, 11f, 15, 15f
blood supply, tumor
angiogenesis, **17–18f**
angioinfarction, therapeutic, **113**
blood tests. *See also* markers
in Hodgkin's disease, 104
in leukemias, acute lymphoblastic, 128
tumors of unknown primary, 80
blood transfusions, 227
blood vessels
carcinoid tumors and, 208
chemotherapeutic drug administration routes, 221, 222f–23
chemotherapy and, 229t
mediastinal, tumor blockage of, 138, 141
therapeutic embolization, 209
boils, 125, 227
bone
myeloma and, 161, 162
osteoporosis, 172
bone cancer, primary (osteosarcoma), **41–45**, 42f, 184
bone cancer, secondary
bladder cancer and, 38
breast cancer and, 67
endometrial cancer and, 95
esophageal cancer and, 99
kidney cancer and, 112
lung cancer and, 138, 142
bone marrow, **120**, 121f, 213. *See also* leukemias
biologic therapy, 232
chemotherapy side effects, 124, 221, 227–28
colony-stimulating factors, 232
Hodgkin's disease, 102
leukemias, acute lymphoblastic, 128, 129
lymphomas, non-Hodgkin's, 142, 144
myeloma, **161–64**
bone marrow cleanup, 266–68, 340
bone marrow rescue, 230, 231f
bone marrow sampling, **120**
in Hodgkin's disease, 104
in leukemias, acute granulocytic, 131
in leukemias, acute lymphoblastic, 128, 129
in leukemias, chronic lymphocytic, 123
in lung cancer, 141
lymphoma staging, 145
in myeloma, 163
bone marrow transplantation, 132, 228, **230f–31f**, 232, 244
in leukemias, acute lymphoblastic, 128–29
in leukemias, chronic granulocytic, 127
in lymphoma, 148
marrow clean-up, 266–68
in myeloma, 164
bone pain, 277
in leukemias, acute lymphoblastic, 129
in prostate cancer, 182
bone scans, 112, **328**
prostatic cancer, 179
radiation therapy planning, 218
bowel
anal cancer localization, 206f
anatomy of digestive tract, 47f, 192f
hysterectomy complications, 88
ileal neobladder, 40
lymphomas, 143, 145
pancreatic cancer and, 175
radiosensitivity, 216
bowel cancer, 23, 24, 28, **46–56**, 47f, 50f, 53f, 55t
brain metastasis, 60
contributing factors, 29t
markers, 80, **330**
preventive actions, 258t
as primary site of carcinomas of unknown primary, 78f, 79, 80
screening tests, 256t
bowel flora, **46**, **48**
bowel function. *See also* stool
analgesic side effects, 282
carcinoid and, 208
chemotherapy and, 229t
normal, 46, 38
ovarian cancer and, 167, 168
after prostate surgery, 181
radiation therapy and, 88, 221
bowel habits. *See also* stool
bowel cancer prevention, 55t
bowel cancer risk factors, 48–49
bowel cancer symptoms, 51
after gastrectomy, 195
myeloma and, 163
stoma management issues, 292–93
bowel obstruction
with ovarian cancer, 168
with pancreatic cancer, 174
with stomach cancer, 194
brachytherapy, 73, **87**, **217**, **328**
in endometrial cancer, 96
in esophageal cancer, 100
brain
prophylactic treatment in lymphoma management, 147–48
tumor cell products affecting, 18
brain cancer, primary, **56–63**, 57f, 277
intrathecal drug administration, 222
lymphoma, AIDS-related, 108
brain cancer, secondary
breast cancer and, 67
carcinomas of unknown primary, 78f
lung cancer and, 138, 142
melanoma and, 153
nonseminoma-like tumors, 199
prophylactic treatment in lymphoma management, 147–48
testicular cancer and, 197
brain scans, 141
brainstem, **57f**
BRCA1 and BRCA2 genes, 26–27, 65t, 66, 167, 272
breakthrough doses of analgesics, 280
breast cancer, 28, 32, **63–76**, 215, 239, 240, 249–50, 338
age and incidence, 64
attitudes and, 249
biologic therapy, 232
contributing factors, 29t
definition of cure, 19
diagnosis and tests, 68–69
early detection, 257t
genetic factors, 26–27
HER2/*neu* oncogene, 271
incidence, 32
inflammatory, **68**, 70t
markers, 80, **330**
metastasis of, 17–18, 60
preventive actions, 258t
as primary site of carcinomas of unknown primary, 78f, 79, 80
prognosis, 70
risk factors, 64–66, 65t
screening tests, 256t
social support groups, 252
spread of, 63–64, 66–67
symptoms, 67f–68t
tamoxifen in, 94
treatment objectives, 70–71
types of cancer, 69
types of treatment, 71–75

breast feeding, 65t
breast self-examination, 76, 257t
breathlessness
  anemia and, 120
  chemotherapy and radiation therapy effects, 106
  emergencies and their management, 288t, 289t
  with Hodgkin's disease, 102
  with leukemias, acute granulocytic, 131
  with leukemias, acute lymphoblastic, 128
  with lung cancer and, 138–39, 141
  with mesotheliomas, 210
  with myeloma, 162
  with ovarian cancer, 168
  with testicular cancer, 197
Bristol Cancer Help Centre, 249–50
bronchoscopy, **139**, 140, 141, 159
bruising
  blood clotting problems and, **120**
  chemotherapy side effects, 124, 227–28
  emergencies and their management, 288t
  with leukemia, acute lymphoblastic, 128
  with leukemia, chronic granulocytic, 126
  with leukemia, chronic lymphocytic, 123
  with myeloma, 162
B symptoms, Hodgkin's disease, 102, 105
burns, 188
busulfan, 127, 224t
bypass
  bile duct, 176, 207
  esophageal obstruction, 100
  stomach cancer management, 195

CA-125, 80, 168, 172, 183, **330**
cachexia, **18**, **329**. *See also* constitutional symptoms
  with bowel cancer, 51
  with esophageal cancer, 99
  with Hodgkin's disease, 102
  with myeloma, 163
calcitonin test, 202
calcium, 18, 55t
  emergencies and their management, 289t
  lung cancer and, 139, 141
  myeloma and, 161, 163
  protective effect on bowel cancer, 48, 55t
calcium deposits, gallbladder, 209
cancer biology. *See* tumor biology
cancer cells, 333
cancer centers and hospitals, 345–46
cancer of unknown primary (CUP), **77–81**
cancer(s). *See also* tumor biology
  attitudes toward, 245
  carcinogenesis, **21–30**
  as group of diseases, 1–2
  living with. *See* quality of life
  perceptions and misperceptions of, 1–3
  variability of disease course, 240
carboplatinum
  ovarian cancer, 171
  side effects, 224t
  stomach cancer, 195
carcinogenesis. *See* causes of cancer/carcinogenesis
carcinogens, **24–25**, **329**
  and esophageal cancer, 99
  and sarcomas, soft tissue, 184
carcinoid tumors, **208–9**
carcinoma in situ, breast, 69
carmustine, 224t
cartilage tumors (chondrosarcomas), 42
castration, surgical, 182
cathepsin D, 70t
catheters, urinary, 40, 181, 287
causes of cancer/carcinogenesis, 6, **21–30**, 32, 329, 333
  epidemiology, 27–30, 29t
  mind-body question, 246–49
  oncogenes and tumor suppressor genes, 25–27
  tumor biology, 24–25f
  types of factors, 21–24, 22f, 23f
cautery, 86, **329**
CEA (carcinoembryonic antigen), 52, 55–56, 80, 330
cell adhesion molecules, 270
cell death, programmed, **11**
cell growth
  abnormal, 11f–12
  carcinogenesis, **21–30**
  normal, 9–11, 10f
cells. *See also* tumor biology
  cancer as process, 1–2
  carcinogenesis, **21–30**
  of central nervous system, 58
  myeloma, 161
  skin, **150**
central nervous system
  anatomy, **57f**
  tumor cell products affecting, 18
central nervous system prophylaxis, lymphoma management, 147–48
central nervous system tumors. *See* brain cancer, primary; brain cancer, secondary
cerebellum, 57f
cerebral cortex, 57f
cerebral hemispheres, **57**
cerebrospinal fluid (CSF), **57**
  intrathecal drug administration, 222
  methotrexate injection into, 128
cervical cancer, 23, **81–89**
  age and incidence, 82
  anatomy, 82, 83f
  causes and risk factors, 82–83
  contributing factors, 29t
  definition of cure, 19
  invasive, 86–89
  precancerous changes and screening, 84f, 85f, 86f
  preventive actions, 258t
  as primary site of carcinomas of unknown primary, 78f, 79
  radiotherapy, 217
  risk reduction and prevention, 88t, 89
  screening tests, 256t
cervical smear (Pap) test, 34, 82, 83f, 84, 85f–86f, 88t, 256t, 335
cervix, 93f
  anatomy, 82, 83f
  choriocarcinoma spread to, 90
chemical carcinogens, 334
  and bladder cancer, 37
  and leukemias, chronic granulocytic, 130
  lymphomas, non-Hodgkin's, 143–44
  and sarcomas, soft tissue, 184
  skin cancer, 188
chemotactic trigger zone (CTZ), 223
chemotherapy, 33, 213–14, **221–33**, 222f, 224t, 225t, 226t, 229t. *See also specific tumor sites*
  bone marrow transplantation, 228, 230f–31f
  breast cancer, 74
  carcinoma of unknown primary, 80–81
  delivery routes and systems, 221–23, 222f
  fatigue and exhaustion, 283–84
  leukemia caused by, 130
  leukemias, chronic lymphocytic, 123
  rate of progress of research in, 261–62
  second cancer caused by, 106, 130, 144
  side effects, 223–28, 224t, 225t, 226t, 229t
chest pain
  lung cancer and, 139, 141
  mesotheliomas, 210
chest X-rays, 102, 257–58
  with bone cancer, 44
  carcinomas of unknown primary, 79, 80
  lymphoma staging, 145
  mesotheliomas, 210, 211
  testicular cancer, 198–99
chicken pox virus, 125
childhood cancers, 21, 214
  advances in treatment of, 262
  bone, **41–45**, 42f
  of brain and spinal cord, 56–57, 58, 60, 61, 62
  intrathecal drug administration, 222
  leukemias, acute lymphoblastic, 127–29
  rare, **203–5**
  sarcomas, soft tissue, 184, 185, 186
  Wilms' tumor, 109

children, talking about cancer with, 305–6
China
 esophageal cancer incidence, 98
 liver cancer incidence, 134
chiropractic manipulation for back pain, 337
chlorambucil
 leukemia, chronic lymphocytic, 124, 125
 lymphoma, 146
 side effects, 224t
2-chloro-deoxyadenosine (2-CDA), 132
choking, 159
cholangiography, 207
cholecystitis, 209, 210
chondrosarcoma, **45**
choriocarcinomas, **89–92**, 214, 262
 carcinomas of unknown primary, 79
 spontaneous remissions, 112, 242
chromosomes
 antitelomerase, 269, 270f
 leukemic cells, 131
 Philadelphia, 126
 translocations, **26**
chronic irritation
 and oral cancer, 158
 and skin cancer, 188
chronic leukemias
 granulocytic-myelocytic, **119**, **126–27**, 232
 lymphocytic, **119**, **122–26**, 125f
chronobiology, 269
cigarette smoking. *See* smoking
cirrhosis, 134
cis-platinum
 bladder cancer, 41
 esophageal cancer, 100
 laryngeal and pharyngeal cancer, 117
Clark levels, melanoma, 154
clinical nurse specialists, 40, 278
clinical trials, 54, **233–34**, 236, 272, 335
clone, **161**
cobalt therapy, 216
codeine, **279**
coffee grounds, vomiting, 124, 288t
colic, 51, 168, 277
collagen, **14**
collagenase, **14**
colon. *See* bowel
colon cancer. *See* bowel cancer
colonoscopy, 51–52, 256t, **329**
colony-stimulating factors (CSFs), 232
colostomy, 52–54, 53f, 206–7, 215, 290
 stoma management, 291–93f, 292f, 294
colposcopy, 84, 85, 87, **329**
columnar epithelium, cervix, 82, 83f
coma/confusion, 135, 141, 163
combination chemotherapy
 breast cancer, 74
 choriocarcinoma or molar pregnancy, 91
 Hodgkin's disease, 105
 lymphoma, AIDS-related, 108
communication, family/friends with patient, 307–16
 help checklist, 314t, 315–16
 listening and understanding, 307–8, 313–14
 obstacles and barriers to, 309t–13
 reasons for listening and talking, 308–9
communication, patient with doctor, 303–5
 depression, therapeutic dialogue, 285–86
 interpretation of survival figures and prognosis, 34–35
 misinterpretations, 241–42
 pain, describing, 277–78
 reporting symptoms, 32–33
communication, patient with family/friends, 295–307
 benefits of, 297–98
 with children, 305–6
 choosing support person/confidant(e), 298, 299t
 conflict resolution, 306–7
 feelings and reactions of family and friends, 296–97
 feelings and reactions of patient, 295–96
 how to "break the news" about illness, 302–3
 how to talk about feelings, 300–301
 intimacy issues, 290
 needs, 298, 300
 responding to reactions, 301–2
complementary medicine, **235–44**, 237t, 335, 337
complete debulking, **170**
complete remission, **19**
cone biopsy, cervix, 86f, 87
confidant(e), choosing, 298, 299t
conflict resolution, 306–7
confusion/disorientation/coma, 135, 141, 163
congenital abnormalities
 with Wilms' tumor, 203–4
 and sarcomas, soft tissue, 184–85
conization, 86f, 87
Connecticut study, 251–52
connective tissue, **14**
consipiracy theories, 335
consolidation therapy, 128
constipation
 analgesic side effects, 282
 bowel cancer risk factors, 48–49
 myeloma and, 163
constitutional symptoms, **329**
 anemia and, 120
 chemotherapy side effects, 227–28, 229t
 with Hodgkin's disease, 102
 with leukemia, acute granulocytic, 131
 with leukemia, acute lymphoblastic, 128
 with leukemia, chronic granulocytic, 126
 with leukemia, chronic lymphocytic, 123
 with liver cancer, 134, 135
 with lung cancer, 139, 141
 with lymphomas, non-Hodgkin's, 144
 with mesotheliomas, 210
 with myeloma, 162, 163
 with pancreatic cancer, 175
 steroid hormones and, 124
 with stomach cancer, 193
contact inhibition, **10**
continent diversions, 40
control issues, 297–98, 237
controlled clinical trials, 54, **233–34**, 236, 272, 335
conventional treatments. *See* treatments, conventional
coping/adjustment/adaptation, 245, 246, 249, 250, 254, 336. *See also* communication; quality of life
 arranging social support system, 299t
 denial and, 295–96
 understanding of disease process, 3, 5–6
core needle biopsy, 328f
corpus, uterus, **93**
cosmetic considerations, 159, 160, 314
cosmetic surgery
 after mastectomy, 73
 reconstruction, 215
cough
 with Hodgkin's disease, 102
 with lung cancer, 139, 141
 with ovarian cancer, 168
coughing up blood, 99, 115, 139, 141, 288t
counseling, 215
 with depression, 285–86
 after prostate surgery, 181
 sexual problems, 291
Cousins, Norman, 251, 300
craniotomy, **60**
criticism, 305
crying, 301
cryosurgery
 cervix, 86
 skin cancer, 189
cryotherapy, liver cancer, 136
CT scans, 213, **329**
 anal cancer, 206
 biliary system, 207, 210
 bladder cancer, 38
 bone cancer, 44
 brain tumors, 59, 60
 carcinoma of unknown primary, 80
 endometrial cancer diagnosis, **95**
 esophageal cancer, 99

CT scans (*continued*)
Hodgkin's disease, 104
kidney cancer, 111, 112
large bowel, 52
laryngeal cancer, 116
leukemia, chronic granulocytic, 126
liver cancer, 135
lung cancer, 141
lymphoma staging, 145
mesotheliomas, 211
oral cancer assessment, 159
ovarian cancer, 168
pancreatic cancer, 175
prostatic cancer, 179
radiation therapy planning, 218
soft tissue sarcomas, 185
stomach cancer, 194
testicular cancer, 197
thyroid, 202
CTZ (chemotactic trigger zone), 223
cure/curability, defined, 6, **19**, **335**
curette/curettage, **95**
cyclophosphamide
breast cancer, 74
choriocarcinoma or molar pregnancy, 91
leukemia, acute lymphoblastic, 129
leukemia, chronic lymphocytic, 124
lung cancer, 142
lymphoma, 146
lymphoma, AIDS-related, 108
mesotheliomas, 211
ovarian cancer, 171
side effects, 224t, 226t, 227
soft tissue sarcomas, 186
Wilms' tumor, 204
cyproterone, 182
cystectomy, 40
cystoscopy, **38**, 39–40, **329**
cysts, 14
breast, 67, 68–69
breast cancer risk factors, 65t
thyroid, 201
cytogenetic testing, **131**
cytology, **329**
cervical, 34, 82, 83f, 84, 85f–86f, 88t, 256t, 335
cytosine arabinoside
leukemias, acute granulocytic, 131
leukemias, acute lymphoblastic, 128, 129
lymphoma, AIDS-related, 108
side effects, 224t

dacarbazine, 209, 224t, 229t
dactinomyin. *See* actinomycin D
dark-skinned people, melanoma sites, 153
daunorubicin, 128, 129, 131, 224t
death and dying, 303, 314, **317–24**
death of cells, programmed (apoptosis), **11**
debulking, surgical, 170–71
decision making, 298
arranging social support system, 299t
about dying, 318–20
denial, 249, 295–96, 322f
dentists, 159
depression, 249, 284–87, 285t, 338
dermis, 149f, **150**
descending colon, 47f
detection (screening and early diagnosis), 34, **255**
dexamethasone, 62
diabetes, 94
diagnosis, 33, 334, 335
early, 34, **255**
size of tumor and, 12, 13f, 14
diarrhea
bowel cancer symptoms, 51
with carcinoid, 208
chemotherapy and, 229t
after prostate surgery, 181
radiation therapy and, 88, 221
diary, pain, 278f
diet, 23, 29t, 249, 333, 335
and bowel cancer, 48
bowel cancer prevention, 55t
and breast cancer, 64
with chemotherapy, 228
epidemiological factors, 28
and esophageal cancer, 99
foods to avoid when taking MAOI antidepressants, 287
preventive actions, 258t
and prostatic cancer, 178
and stomach cancer, 191, 193
stoma management issues, 292–93, 294
diethylstilbestrol, 29t
digestive system
chemotherapy and, 229t
lymphomas, 145
digestive tract
anatomy of, 47f, 98f, 192f
bowel cancer, **46–56**, 47f, 50f, 53f, 55t
carcinoid tumors, 208–9
chemotherapy effects, 221
pancreatic cancer and, 174, 175f
radiation therapy and, 221
radiosensitivity, 216
digestive tract cancer. *See specific primary sites*
dilatation and curettage (D&C), 95
disability
oral cancer treatment considerations, 159, 160
speech rehabilitation after laryngectomy, 117f–18
disbelief, 295
distant spread, **329**. *See also* secondary tumors; *specific sites*
dizziness, emergencies and their management, 288t
DNA
damage to, 22–23, 24f
oncogenes and tumor suppressor genes, 25–27
DNA technology, 263–64
doctor. *See* communication, patient with doctor; health care professionals; patient-physician relationship
domperdone, 225t
dosage, radiation, 218, 219
dose-limiting organ, 228
double vision, 59
Down's syndrome, 127, 129, 130, 254
dread, 246, 295, 334
perceptions and misperceptions of cancer, 1–3
talking about cancer, 295–316
dronabinol, 225t
drowsiness
analgesic side effects, 282
antidepressant side effects, 286–87
brain tumor symptoms, 59
with liver cancer, 135
myeloma and, 163
DTIC, 209, 224t, 229t
duodenum, 207f
anatomy of digestive tract, 47f, 192f
pancreatic cancer and, 174, 175f, 176
durable power of attorney, 303
dyspepsia, 175
dysplastic nevus, 151–52f

early diagnosis, **255**
early stomach cancers, 194
economic anxieties, 295, 299t
electrocautery, cervix, 86
electrodessication, skin cancer, 189
electroencephalography, 59
electrolarynx, 118
electron microscopy, 79
embarrassment, 304
embolization, therapeutic, **113**, 209
embryonal cells, 199
embryonal tumors
brain, **58**
testis, 196
emergencies, 287, 288–89t
emotions
of children, 305
death and dying, 303, 314, **317–324**
talking about cancer, 295–316
encouragement, communcation techniques, 311
endometrial cancer, **92–97**, 93f
definition of cure, 19
preventive actions, 258t
as primary site of carcinomas of unknown primary, 78f, 79
radiotherapy, 217
endometrium, **93f**
endoscopic retrograde cholangiopancreatography (ERCP), 175–76

endoscopy, **330**
in bile duct cancer, 207
in carcinoma of unknown primary, 80
colonoscopy and sigmoidoscopy, 51–52, 256t, **329**
esophagoscopy, 99, 159
gastroscopy, 159, 194
hysteroscopy, 80, **95**
laparoscopy, 168, 171, 172
laryngoscopy, **115**
in lung cancer, 139, 141
mediastinoscopy, 102, **139**, 141, **331**
oral cancer assessment, 159
with ovarian cancer, 168, 171, 172
in pancreatic cancer, **175**
screening tests, 256t
energy loss. *See* constitutional symptoms
enzymes
cathepsin D, 70t
estrogen production in fatty tissue, 94
pancreatic, 174
tumor cell invasion, 14f–15
ependymomas, **60**, 61
epidemic of cancer, 64, 334
epidemiology, 24–25, **24**
epidermis, 149f, **150**
epidural analgesia, 283
epiglottis, **114f**, 115f
epirubicin, 224t, 226t
epithelial cancer of ovary, 165–72
epithelium, cervix, 82, 83f
ERCP (endoscopic retrograde cholangiopancreatography), 175–76
erythroplakia (red patches), 158
erythropoietin, 232
esophageal cancer, **97–100**, 98f
preventive actions, 258t
as primary of carcinomas of unknown primary, 78f, 80
radiotherapy, 217
esophageal reflux, **98**
esophageal speech, 118
esophagitis, **98**
esophagoscopy, 99, 159
esophagus
anatomy of digestive tract, 47f, 192f
endoscopic examination, 99, 159
radiosensitivity, 216
tracheoesophageal fistula, 117f, 118
estrogen
birth control pills, 66, 94, 134, 166
and endometrium, 93, 94
fatty tissue and, 94
estrogen receptors, breast cancer, 70t, 73–74
estrogen therapy
breast cancer risk factors, 66
prostate cancer therapy, 182
ethics, 233–34
etoposide
choriocarcinoma or molar pregnancy, 91
Kaposi's sarcoma, 107
leukemias, acute lymphoblastic, 128
lung cancer, 140, 142
lymphoma, 146
lymphoma, AIDS-related, 108
oral cancer, 160
ovarian cancer, 173
side effects, 224t, 226t
soft tissue sarcomas, 186
stomach cancer, 195
testicular cancer, 198
Wilms' tumor, 204
euthanasia, 319–20
Ewing's sarcoma, **42**, **45**
examination under anesthesia (EUA), **115–16**
exceptional cancer patients (ECPs), 250, 251
excisional biopsy, **153**, 328f
exercise, 55t, 138–39
external beam radiation, **87**, 96, **217**
extramedullary plasmacytomas, 164
extranodal lymphomas, **145**, 148
eye
melanoma of, 151, 154
retinoblastoma, **204–5**

facial flushing, 208
facial swelling, as steroid hormone side effect, 123
fainting, 288t, 289t
Fallopian tube, 166f
false positives, 257
familial disorder of immunity, 144
familial polyposis coli, 50
family. *See* friends and family
family history, 21, 333
bowel cancer, 49, 50
breast cancer, 64, 65t
carcinoid tumors, 208
mammography recommendations, 76
melanoma, 152
ovarian cancer, 167, 172
retinoblastoma, **204–5**
testicular cancer, 197
thyroid cancer, medullary, 202
Wilms' tumor, 203–4
fat, dietary, 23, 258t
and bowel cancer, 48, 49, 55t
and breast cancer, 64
pancreatic cancer and, 175
and prostatic cancer, 178
fatigue. *See* constitutional symptoms
fatty tissue
estrogen production in, 94
liposarcomas, 183, 185
fear, 246, 334
perceptions and misperceptions of cancer, 1–3
talking about cancer, 295–316
feces. *See* stool
feeling better, 243, 245, 254
feelings
breast cancer treatment options, 74, 75
symptoms of depression, 285t
talking about cancer, 295–316
fertility
chemotherapy and, 229t
after testicular cancer treatment, 199
after trophoblastic tumor treatment, 92
fetal development
brain tumor causes, 58
chemotherapy and, 229t
testicular cancer causes, 196
fever
chemotherapy side effects, 227
emergencies and their management, 288t
with gallbladder tumors, 209–10
with Hodgkin's disease, 102
with leukemias, chronic lymphocytic, 123
with mesotheliomas, 210
with myeloma, 163
fiber, dietary, 48, 55t
fibroadenomas, breast, 65t, 68
fibrosarcoma, 173, 183, 185
field, radiation, **218**, 219
fine-needle aspirate, 201
fine-needle aspirate biopsy, 328f
fistula, tracheoesophageal (speech), 117f, **118**
flange, colostomy bag, 293
flank pain, **111f**
flat-type melanoma, **153**
flatulence, 167, 168
flu, 125
fludarabine, 125
fluid buildup
abdomen (ascites). *See* ascites
chest (pleural effusion), 139, 141, 167, 169f, 288t
hormone therapy side effects, 96
fluids. *See* ascites; pleural effusion
5-fluorouracil
anal cancer, 207
bowel cancer, 54
breast cancer, 74
carcinoid tumors, 209
esophageal cancer, 100
laryngeal and pharyngeal cancer, 117
mesotheliomas, 211
oral cancer, 160
side effects, 224t, 226t, 229t
stomach cancer, 195
flushing, as hormone therapy side effect, 96
flutamide, 182
folinic acid, 195
follicular thyroid carcinoma, 201
foreign travel, 125
fractionated radiation, 218, 219

fractures, 162, 277
Frankl, Viktor, 254
freckles, **151**
frequency, urinary, **38**
friends and family
  dying process, 321–23, 322f
  listening to and talking with patient, 307–16
  talking with about having cancer, 295–307
future prospects, patient, 6

gallbladder, 47f, 192f, 207f
gallbladder cancer, 209f–10
gallium scans, 104
gallstones, 134
gamma rays, 216, 328
gastrectomy, 195
gastroscopy, 159, 194
gastrostomy, 100
gemcytobine, ovarian cancer, 176
gender differences in incidence of tumors
  bladder cancer, 37
  brain tumor, 58
  Hodgkin's disease, 101
  kidney cancer, 110
  leukemias, acute lymphoblastic, 128
  lung cancer, 137
  melanomas, 153
  myeloma, 162
  oral cancer, 157–58
generalized effects of tumors, 11, 18. *See also* constitutional symptoms
gene therapy, 270–71
genetic factors. *See also* family history
  in breast cancers, 65t, 66
  in ovarian cancer, 167
  in skin cancer, 188
genetic identification of high-risk individuals, 272
genetic material
  damage to, 22–23, 24f
  oncogenes and tumor suppressor genes, 25–27
  Philadelphia chromosome, 126
genital herpes, 82
geographic comparisons
  epidemiology, 28
  stomach cancer incidence, 191
germ cells
  ovary, 167f
  testis, 196
germ-cell tumors, 135
  carcinomas of unknown primary, 79
  markers, 80, **330**
  ovary, 32, 165, 172–73
  testis, 196
glioma multiblastiforme, **61**
gliomas, **60**, 61
global survival figures, 34
goserelin, 182
grade of cancer (microscopic appearance). *See* staging and grading
granisetron, 225t, 226
granulocytes, **120**
granulocytic/myelocytic leukemias
  acute, **119**, **129–32**
  chronic, **119**, **126–27**
gray (unit of radiation dosage), 107, 218
growth factor antagonists, 270
growth factors, **10–11**. *See also* biologic therapy
growth of cells, 1–2
  abnormal, 11–12, 13f, **21–30**
  normal, 9–11, 10f
growth of tumors
  grade and, 60
  melanoma, 152–53
  primary, 12–14, 13f
  prostatic cancer, 179–80, 182, 183
  secondary (metastatic), 18
guilt, 296, 322f
gums, 116f, 157f
  bleeding, 131
  oral cancer, 159, 160

hair loss, 290, 314
  breast cancer, 74
  chemotherapy and, 226t–27
  radiation therapy and, 219, 221
hairy-cell leukemia, 132
hairy cell leukemia, 232
hard palate, 116f, 157f
βHCG, **330**
  choriocarcinoma and hydatidiform mole, **89**, 91
  ovarian cancer screening, 173
  testicular cancer, 197
  tumors of unknown primary, 79
headache, 32, 277
  brain tumor symptoms, 58
  with leukemias, acute lymphoblastic, 129
healing
  appeal of complementary medicine, 237
  normal tissue growth and repair, 10f–11
healing ceremony, 243
health care agent, 303
health care professionals, 298. *See also* communication, patient with doctor; patient-physician relationship
  multidisciplinary care, 214–15
  nursing assistance, 318
  palliative care, 318
  social services, 319
  stoma management issues, 293
  support team, 278
  talking with children, 305
hearing, and side effects of chemotherapy, 229t
heart, and chemotherapy and radiation therapy effects, 106
Helicobacter pylorii, 193, 254
helplessness, 6, 249
hematuria (blood in urine), **37**, 111, 179t
hemorrhoids, 32, 51, 55t, 56, 206
hepatitis B or C, 133, 134, 135, 136, 258t
hepatocellular carcinoma/hepatoma, **133f–36**, 258t
hereditary nonpolyposis coli (HNPC), 50
herpes simplex virus, 82
herpes zoster, 125f–26
Hickman catheter, **223**
high-grade astrocytoma, **60**
high-risk individuals, genetic identification of, 272
high-voltage radiation, 217, 217f
history. *See* family history; lifestyle factors
HIV, 29t. *See also* AIDS/HIV
hoarseness, 99, 115
Hodgkin's disease, **101–6**, 103f, 143, 214, 262
  chemotherapy, 228
  as primary site of carcinomas of unknown primary, 78f, 79
hope, 237–38, 250–51
hopelessness, 249
hormonal markers. *See* markers; *specific markers*
hormone receptors
  breast cancer, **63**, 70t, 73–74
  male breast cancer, 76
  prostatic cancer, 180
hormone replacement therapy (estrogen), 172
  breast cancer risk factors, 66
  after cervical cancer treatment, 89
  endometrial cancer risk, 94
  for radiation-induced menopause, 89
hormone replacement therapy (thyroid), 202
hormones, **330**
  carcinoid production, 208
  and endometrium, 93, 94
  lung tumor production, 141
  ovarian cancer and, 166, 167
  prostate sensitivity, 178, 180
  psychoneuroimmunology, 253
  steroid. *See* steroid hormones
  thyroid, 200–201, 202
  tumor production of, 18, 141, 208
hormone therapy, 214
  breast cancer, 74, 75
  dexamethasone, 62
  endometrial bleeding, premalignant, 92
  endometrial cancer, 96
  estrogen replacement therapy. *See* hormone replacement therapy (estrogen)
  kidney cancer, 112
  prostate cancer, 182
hospitals and cancer centers, 345–46
H3 blockers, 225t, 226

Huber needle, **223**
human papilloma virus (HPV), 29t, 82, 206
humor, 300
hydatidiform mole, **89–92**
hydromorphone, **279**
5-hydroxytryptamine, 208
hydroxyurea, 127, 224t
hygiene, 24, 25
hypernephroma, 109, 110
hyperplasia, endometrial, 93
hypertension, 94, 97
hyperthermia, 155
hypopharynx, **114**
hysterectomy, 88
hysterography, **95**
hysteroscopy, **95**

idarubicin, 131
ifosfamide
  oral cancer, 160
  side effects, 224t
  soft tissue sarcomas, 186
  Wilms' tumor, 204
ileal neobladder, 40
ileostomy, 215, 290, 291, 293
illness, historical attitudes, 246
Illness as Metaphor, 246
imaging studies. *See* CT scans; MRI scans; ultrasound; *specific primary sites*
immune system, 338
  AIDs lymphomas and Kaposi's sarcoma, 107
  chemotherapy side effects, 227
  inherited disorders of, 144
  leukemias, chronic lymphocytic, 123, 125–26
  myeloma and, 161, 162
  plasma cells, 161–62
  psychoneuroimmunology, 253
  and skin cancer, 188
  steroid hormones and, 124
immunization
  with leukemias, 125
  preventive actions, 258t
immunohistochemistry, **79**
incidence rates, 31–32, **330**
incisional biopsy, 328f
indigestion, 175, 193
Indonesia, 98, 99, 134
induction chemotherapy, 128, **131–32**
infection. *See also* viruses
  anal cancer risk, 206
  and bladder cancer, 37
  chemotherapy side effects, 227, 228
  cholecystitis, 209
  defense system, **120**
  emergencies and their management, 288t
  and Hodgkin's disease, 101
  with leukemias, acute granulocytic, 131
  with leukemias, acute lymphoblastic, 129
  with leukemias, chronic granulocytic, 126
  with leukemias, chronic lymphocytic, 123, 125–26
  myeloma and, 161, 162
  white blood cell deficiency and, 120
infertility, 172
inflammation, gallbladder, 209
inflammatory bowel disease, 50
inflammatory breast cancer, **68**, 70t
inherited cancers, 21, 333. *See also* genetic factors; family history
inherited disorders of immune system, 144
inhibitory growth factors, **11**
injury-repair processes, normal, 10f
insulin, 174
intercellular matrix, **14**
interferons, 108, 155, 214
  carcinoid tumors, 209
  Kaposi's sarcoma, 108
  kidney cancers, 109, 112
  leukemias, chronic granulocytic, 127
  leukemias, chronic myelocytic, 214
  leukemias, hairy-cell, 132
  lymphoma, 148
  melanoma, 155
  myeloma, 164
  skin cancer, 190
interleukin-2, 214, 244
  kidney cancers, 109, 112
  lymphoma, 148
  melanoma, 155
interleukins, 148, 232
intestinal obstruction. *See* Bowel obstruction
intracavitary administration of chemotherapy, 222
intraductal carcinoma, breast, 69
intraperitoneal therapy, 172
intrathecal chemotherapy, 128, 222
intravenous administration of chemotherapeutic drugs, 222f
intravenous pyelography (IVP), **38**, 111, 198, **330**
intravesical instillation of chemotherapeutic drugs, 40
invasion, 1–2, 14f–15f
invasive cancer
  bladder, 38, 39f
  breast, 69
  cervix, 86–89
  oral, 158
invasive mole, **90**, 91
iodine, 201
iodine, radioactive, 200, 202
ionizing radiation. *See* radiation exposure
iris, eye, 154
isolated limb perfusion, 155
itching
  as Hodgkin's disease symptom, 102
  vulvar cancer and, 211
IVP (intravenous pyelography), **38**, 111, 198, **330**

Japan, stomach cancer incidence, 191
jaundice, **175**
  gallbladder tumors and, 209–10
  with liver cancer, 134, 135
junctional area, skin, **150**

Kaposi's sarcoma, 29t, **106–8**, 232, 240–41, 244, 258t
keratin, **150**
keratoses, **187**, **188f–89**, 190
kidney
  anatomy and function of, 109f–10
  chemotherapeutic drug toxicity, 131
  chemotherapy and, 229t
  IVP (intravenous pyelography, **38**, **330**
  myeloma and, 161, 163
  radiosensitivity, 216
  urinary system anatomy, **36**, 37f
kidney cancers, **109f–13**, 111f, 254
  brain metastasis, 60
  contributing factors, 29t
  interleukins in, 232
  preventive actions, 258t
  Wilms' tumor, **203–4**
Kübler-Ross, Elisabeth, 321–23, 322f

laetrile, 236, 244
LAK cells, 232
language. *See also* speech
  brain centers controlling, **57**
  brain tumor symptoms, 59
laparoscopy, **168**, 171, 172
laparotomy
  with ovarian cancer, 168, 171, 172
  staging, 104
large bowel, 46, 47f. *See also* bowel cancer
large-cell carcinomas of lung, 139
laryngeal cancer, **113–18**, 114f, 115f, 116f, 117f, 215
  carcinomas of unknown primary, 79
  contributing factors, 29t
  preventive actions, 258t
  as primary site of carcinomas of unknown primary, 77, 78f
laryngectomy, 215
  partial, **116**
  total, **117f**
laryngopharynx, **114**, 114f
laryngoscopy, 80, **115**
larynx, 98f, **114f**, 115f
laser therapy, **330**
  laryngeal cancer, **116**

laser therapy (*continued*)
lung cancer, **140**
oral cancer, 160
porphyrin phototherapy, **40**
retinoblastoma, 205
skin cancer, 190, **330**
legal issues
arranging social support system, 299t
health care agent, 303
living will, 219
leiomyosarcoma, 185
lentigo maligna melanoma, **153**
leucovorin, 54
leukemias, 32, 203, 267
acute granulocytic/myelocytic, **119**, **129–32**
acute lymphocytic, **119**, **127–29**
advances in treatment of, 262
biologic therapy, 232
bone marrow and lymph nodes, **120f–22**, 121f
bone marrow transplantation in, 132
chemotherapy, 228
chronic granulocytic/myelocytic, **119**, **126–27**
chronic lymphocytic, **119**, **122–26**, 125f
intrathecal drug administration, 222
leukoplakia (white patches), 158, 211
leuprolide, 182
levamisole, 54
life events, 3, 337–38
lifestyle factors, 28, 254. *See also* alcohol; diet; smoking
and bowel cancer, 48
and breast cancer, 64
and ovarian cancer, 166
linitis plastica, **194**
lip, 116f, 157f
melanoma, 151
oral cancer, 159
liposarcoma, 183, 185
liver
in Hodgkin's disease, 104
in lymphoma, 145
pancreas and, 175
stomach cancer spread to, 195
liver biopsy, 104, 145
liver cancer, primary, 133f–36
biologic therapy, 232
contributing factors, 29t
markers, 80
preventive actions, 258t
as primary site of carcinomas of unknown primary, 78f, 80
liver cancer, secondary
bladder cancer and, 38
bowel cancer and, 52, 54
breast cancer and, 67
carcinoid and, 208
carcinomas of unknown primary, 79
esophageal cancer and, 99
lung cancer and, 138
melanoma and, 153
testicular cancer and, 197
liver damage, 29t
liver scans
with bowel cancer, 52
radiation therapy planning, 218
liver transplantation, 136
living will, 319
living with cancer. *See* quality of life
lobectomy, lung, **140**
lobular carcinoma in situ, breast, 69
local recurrence, **329–30**
breast cancer, 71, 75
local spread of tumor, 14f–15f
lomustine, 224t, 226t
longevity, 246
lorazepam, 225t
Love, Medicine, and Miracles, 250
low-voltage radiation, 217f
lumpectomy, 71, 72f
lung
carcinoid tumors, 208
leukemic cells in, 131
pancreas and, 175
radiosensitivity, 216
lung cancer, primary, 21, 22, 23, 28, 30, **137–42**, 247, 248
brain metastasis, 60–61
contributing factors, 29t
incidence, 32
non–small-cell, **138–40**
preventive actions, 258t
as primary site of carcinomas of unknown primary, 78f, 79
small-cell/oat-cell, **140–42**
lung cancer, secondary
bladder cancer, 38
bone cancer, 43, 44, 45
breast cancer, 67
carcinomas of unknown primary, 78f, 79
cervical cancer, 86
choriocarcinomas, 90, 91
endometrial cancer, 95
esophageal cancer, 99
kidney cancers, 109, 110, 112
melanoma and, 153
skin cancer and, 189
testicular cancer and, 197
lupus erythematosus, 188
lymphangiography, **330**
lymphatics, **15**
lymphatic spread
bladder cancer, 39f
bowel cancer, 50f–51
breast cancer, 66–67
laryngeal cancer, 116
liver cancer, 134–35
tumor cell invasion, 15f
lymph nodes, **15**, 16f
anatomy, 103f, 121f, 122
breast cancer, 70t, 71, 72f, 73, 74
cancer with unknown primary site (CUP), 77–81, 78f
cervical cancer, 86
endometrial cancer, 94
esophageal cancer, 99
Hodgkin's disease, 101–6, 103f
leukemias, acute lymphoblastic, 129
leukemias, chronic lymphocytic, 123
lymphomas, non-Hodgkin's, 142–48
mastectomy procedures, 71, 72f, 73
mediastinal, **138f**
mediastinoscopy, **331**
melanoma, sentinel node sampling, **153**
ovarian cancer, 169f
pancreatic cancer, 175
radical hysterectomy, 88
stomach cancer, 193
lymphocytes, 107, **120**, **122**
lymphocytic leukemias
acute, **119**, **127–29**
chronic, **119**, **122–26**, 125f
lymphography
in cervical cancer, 87
in Hodgkin's disease, 104
testicular cancer, 197
lymphomas, 240, 268
advances in treatment of, 262
AIDS-related, **108**
biologic therapy, 232
of bone, 45
brain or spinal cord, 60, 62–63
chemotherapy, 228
contributing factors, 29t
esophageal, 100
Hodgkin's disease, **101–6**, 103f
intrathecal drug administration, 222
non-Hodgkin's, **142–48**
as primary site of carcinomas of unknown primary, 78f, 79
stomach, 143, 144, 145, 194
Waldenström's macroglobulinemia, 164

McQueen, Steve, 239
macroglobulinemia, Waldenström's, 164
magical thinking, 306
magic bullets, 340
maintenance therapy, 128
male breast cancer, 75–76
male-female differences in incidence. *See* gender differences in incidence of tumors
malignant fibrous histiocytoma (MFH), 185
malignant transformation, **24–25**
mammography, 34, **68**, 76, 272
in carcinoma of unknown primary, 80
screening tests, 256t, 257
Man's Search for Meaning, 254
markers, **330**
Bence Jones protein, **162**

bowel cancer, 52, 55–56
breast cancer, 69
choriocarcinoma and hydatidiform mole, 89
leukemic cells, 131
liver cancer, 135, 136
ovarian cancer, 168, 172–73
prostatic cancer, 179, 182, 183
testicular cancer, 197
tumors of unknown primary, 79
marrow cleanup, 266–68, 340
massage, 283
mastectomy, 71, 72f, 75, 215
M band, **162**, 163, **330**
mediastinoscopy, 102, **139**, 141, **331**
mediastinum, **138**
nonseminoma-like tumors, 199
obstruction, emergencies and their management, 289t
medical checkups
bowel cancer prevention, 55t
cervical cancer risk reduction, 88t
early detection, 257t
endometrial cancer risk reduction, 97
ovarian cancer screening, 172
medical professionals. *See* health care professionals
medroxyprogesterone, 96
medullary cancer of thyroid, 202
medulloblastoma, **60**, 62
megestrol, 96
melanin, **150**
melanocytes, 149f, **150**
melanoma, **149f–56t**, 152f, 244
acral, **153**
biologic therapy, 232
brain metastasis, 60
contributing factors, 29t
early detection, 257t
esophageal, 100
as primary site of carcinomas of unknown primary, 78f, 79
spontaneous remissions, 112, 242, 243
melodysplasias, **130**
melphalan
leukemia caused by, 130
lymphoma, 146
myeloma, 163, 164
side effects, 224t, 226t
menarche, 65t
meninges, 277
meningiomas, 58, 61, 63
menopausal status, 334
and breast cancer treatment options, 73–74, 75
and endometrial cancer, 93
menopause
breast cancer risk factors, 65t
after cervical cancer treatment, 89
and ovarian cancer incidence, 166
surgical, 172
menstrual cycle, 94, 165
breast cancer risk factors, 65t
breast changes, 68
endometrial changes, 92
ovarian cancer and, 167, 173
mental function
symptoms of depression, 285t
confusion, disorientation, coma, 135, 141, 163
mercaptopurine
leukemias, acute lymphoblastic, 128, 129
side effects, 224t
mesothelioma, 239
metastasis, **329**, **331**
defined, **15**
distant, 15–18f, 16f, 17f. *See also* secondary tumors; *specific sites*
invasion and local spread, 14f–15f
methotrexate, 214
bladder cancer, 41
breast cancer, 74
choriocarcinoma or molar pregnancy, 91
leukemias, acute lymphoblastic, 128, 129
lymphoma, AIDS-related, 108
mesotheliomas, 211
oral cancer, 160
prostate cancer, 186
side effects, 224t, 226t
stomach cancer, 195
metoclopramide, 225t
MFH (malignant fibrous histicytoma), 185
microscopic appearance. *See* staging and grading
mind-body relationship, 335, 337–39
alternative medicine, **235–44**, 237t
attitudes, **245–54**
feeling better versus getting better, 243
mitomycin, 207, 224t, 226t
mitoxantrone, 224t, 226t
mixed germ-cell tumors, 196
modified radical mastectomy, 71, 72f
Moh's surgery, 189
molar pregnancy, **89–92**
moles, **151–52f**, 155, 257t
monoamine oxidase inhibitors (MAOIs), 286
monoclonal antibodies, 231–32, 263, 267, 268
liver cancer treatment, 136
lymphoma treatment, 148
monoclonal protein, **162**, 163
mood
psychoneuroimmunology, 253
symptoms of depression, 285t
moon-shaped face, as steroid hormone side effect, 124
MOPP, 105
Mormons, 28, 48
morphine, **279**, 280, 281
mouth. *See also* oral cancer
anatomy of digestive tract, 47f, 98f, **114f**, 116f, 192f
bleeding from, 56, 288t
melanomas, 154
M protein, **162**, 163, **330**
MRI scans, **331**
bladder cancer, 38
bone cancer, 44
brain tumors, 59, 60
endometrial cancer, **95**
liver cancer, 135
lymphoma staging, 145
ovarian cancer, 168
pancreatic cancer, 175
radiation therapy planning, 218
soft tissue sarcomas, 185
stomach cancer, 194
mucosa, stomach, 191, 191f
mucus in stools, 51
multidisciplinary care, 214–15
multiple myeloma, 32, **161–64**
muscle
sarcomas, 185
tumor cell products affecting, 11, 18
mutations, 27
myeloblasts, **131**
myelocytic/granulocytic leukemias
acute, **119**, **129–32**
chronic, **119**, **126–27**
myelomas, 45, **161–64**, **330**
myometrium, **93f**

nabilone, 225t
nailbeds, melanoma lesions, 151, 153
nasopharyngoscopy, 159
nasopharynx, **114f**, 115, 118
nausea and vomiting (constitutional symptoms), 290
blood in, 124
with bowel cancer, 51
with choriocarcinoma or molar pregnancy, 90
emergencies and their management, 288t
with liver cancer, 135
with myeloma, 163
with ovarian cancer, 168
nausea and vomiting (side effects of treatment)
analgesics, 282
chemotherapy, 74, 223–26, 224t, 225t
hormone therapy, 96
medications for management of, 225t–26
radiation therapy, 88, 219, 221
needle biopsy, 328f
neoadjuvant therapy, 331
nephrectomy, 112

nerve blocks, 283
nerve cells, neurofibrosarcomas, 185
nerve sectioning, 283
nervous system
  brain and spinal cord tumors, **56–63**, 57f
  chemotherapy and, 229t
  myeloma and, 161, 163
  nonanalgesic pain control, 283
  pain mechanisms, 277
  psychoneuroimmunology, 253
  tumor cell products affecting, 11, 18
neuroblastoma, 32, **204**
  spontaneous remissions, 112
  spontaneous remissions in, 242
neurofibromatosis, 184–85
neurofibrosarcoma, 185
neurons, **58**
neutropenia, **120**
neutrophils, **120**
nevus, dysplastic, 151–52, 152f
nicotine patches and gum, 259t, 260
nicotinic acid, 99
night sweats. *See also* constitutional symptoms
  with Hodgkin's disease, 102
  with leukemias, chronic lymphocytic, 123
nilutamide, 182
nipple, inverted, 67f, 68t
nitrates and nitrosamines, 99, 193
nitrogen mustard, 214, 224t, 226t, 229t
nitrosoureas, for brain and spinal cord cancer, 62
nodular melanoma, **153**
nodular sclerosis, **104**
nongestational trophoblastic tumors, **89**, **90**
non-Hodgkin's lymphoma, **142–48**, 262
  after chemotherapy or radiation therapy, 106
  intermediate and high-grade, 147–48
  low-grade, 146–47
noninvasive breast cancer, 69, 75
nonseminomas, 196, 198, 199
non-small cell tumors of lung, 80
nonverbal communication, 308, 311–12
normal cells
  appearance of, 24, 25f
  growth and repair, 9–11, 10f, 21, 22f
  malignant transformation, **24–25**
normal tissue
  cell growth and division in, 221
  radiation therapy planning, 218
  radiosensitivity, 216
nuclear radiation. *See* radiation exposure
numbness
  chemotherapy and, 229t
  emergencies and their management, 288t
  myeloma and, 163
nurses. *See* health care professionals
nutrition
  cervical cancer risk factors, 83
  and oral cancer, 158
  oral cancer management, 160

oat-cell (small-cell) lung cancer, **140–42**
obesity
  endometrial cancer risk factors, 94, 97
  hormone production by lung tumors, 141
obstruction
  bile duct cancer, 207
  biliary, gallbladder tumors and, 209–10
  bowel, emergencies and their management, 289t
  esophagus, 100
  intestinal, with stomach cancer, 194
  pancreatic cancer and, 175, 176
occult blood in stools, 32, 51, 55t, 56, 256t
occupational exposures. *See* workplace exposures
odor, stoma management, 293
oncogenes, **25–26**, 263–64
  anti-oncogene products, 270–71
ondansetron, 225t, 226
one-piece colostomy bag, 293
opioids, **279f**
optimal debulking, **170**
oral cancer, **157f–60**, 254
  contributing factors, 29t
  preventive actions, 258t
  as primary site of carcinomas of unknown primary, 77, 78f, 79, 80
oral cavity, anatomy, 47f, 98f, **114f**, 116f, 192f
orchiectomy, 182, 197
oropharynx, **114f**, 118
osteosarcoma (bone cancer), **41–45**, 42f, 184
ostomies
  with bowel cancer, 52–54, 53f, 206–7, 215, 290
  stoma management, 291–93f, 292f, 294
ovarian cancer, **165–73**, 166f, 167f, 169f, 216, 244, 248, 268, 272–73
  age and incidence, 32
  birth control pills and, 66
  contributing factors, 29t
  epithelial, 165–72
  genetic factors, 26–27, 64, 65t
  germ cell, 172–73
  markers, 80, **330**
  preventive actions, 258t
  as primary site of carcinomas of unknown primary, 78f, 79, 80
  secondary, stomach cancer and, 193
  sex-cord stromal tumors, 173
ovary
  endometrial cancer spread to, 94
  stomach cancer metastasis, 193
  removal of, 171
oxycodone, **279**

Paget's disease, 42, 43
pain, 32
  chemotherapeutic drugs causing irritation of veins, 229t
  during intercourse, 88t
  during urination, 38
pain clinic, 278
pain diary, 278, 278f
pain management, 276–83, 278f, 279f, 280f, 281f, 337
  in prostate cancer, 182
pain symptoms, 314
  with bladder cancer, 30, 38
  with bone cancer, 43
  with bowel cancer, 51
  with cervical cancer, 88, 88t
  with choriocarcinoma or molar pregnancy, 90
  emergencies and their management, 289t
  with endometrial cancer, 95
  with esophageal cancer, 99
  with kidney cancer, 111
  with leukemias, acute lymphoblastic, 129
  with liver cancer, 135
  with lung cancer, 139, 141
  with mesotheliomas, 210
  with myeloma, 162, 163
  with oral cancer, 159
  with ovarian cancer, 168
  with pancreatic cancer, 175
  with prostatic cancer, 179t
  with stomach cancer, 193
palate, 116f, 157f
palliative care, 318
palmar surfaces, melanoma, 153
pancreas
  anatomy of digestive tract, 47f, 192f
  stomach cancer spread to, 193, 195
pancreatic cancer, 29t, **174–76**, 175f, 254, 258t
papillary cancer of bladder, 38, 39f
papillary thyroid carcinoma, 201
Pap test, 34, 82, 84, **85f–86f**, 88t, 256t, 335
paralysis, 59, 163, 289t
parosteal sarcoma, **44**
partial cystectomy, 40
partial gastrectomy, 195
partial mastectomy, 71, 72f, 215
partial remission, **19**
patient. *See also* coping/adjustment/adaptation
  blaming, 253–54
  talking about cancer, 295–316

patient-physician relationship, 7, 336. *See also* communication, patient with doctor
interpretation of survival figures and prognosis, 34–35
reporting symptoms to doctor, 32–33
patient preferences
breast cancer treatment options, 74, 75
cervical cancer treatment options, 88
oral cancer treatment, 159
treatment decisions, 298
peak incidence, **330**
pelvic examination, 84f–85
cervical cancer, **84f–85**
ovarian cancer, 168, 172
screening tests, 84, 85, 172, 256t. *See also* Pap test
pelvic organs
endometrial cancer spread, 94
ovarian cancer spread, 169f
pelvic pain
cervical cancer risk reduction, 88
with choriocarcinoma or molar pregnancy, 90
with endometrial cancer, 95
with myeloma, 162
with prostatic cancer, 179t
pelvis of kidney, 110, 113
periosteal sarcoma, **44**
periosteum, 277
peritoneal cavity, **327**, 328f
mesotheliomas, 210–11
pancreas and, 175
peritoneum, **327**
pernicious anemia, 193
personality changes, brain tumor symptoms, 59
personality traits, 248, 249, 250, 335. *See also* coping/adjustment/adaptation
petechiae (purple spots), **120**
chemotherapy side effects, 124, 227–28
with leukemia, acute lymphoblastic, 128
with leukemias, acute granulocytic, 131
p53, 271
pharyngeal cancer, 77, 80, 113, 118, 215, 258t
pharynx, 98f, **114**, 114f
pheresis, 230
Philadelphia chromosome, 126
photocoagulation, retinoblastoma, 205
photodynamic therapy, for skin cancer, 190
phototherapy, for bladder cancer, 41
physicians. *See* communication, patient with doctor; health care professionals; patient-physician relationship
physiological effects of tumor, 11, 18. *See also* constitutional symptoms
pituitary tumors, 61
placenta, tumors of, **89–92**
plasma cells, myeloma, **161–64**
plasmacytomas, 164
platelets, **120**, 213, 288t
chemotherapy side effects, **120**, 124, 227–28
with leukemia, acute lymphoblastic, 128
with leukemia, chronic granulocytic, 126
myeloma and, 162
transfusions of, 131
platinum drugs, 272
choriocarcinoma or molar pregnancy, 91
lung cancer, 140, 142
mesotheliomas, 211
oral cancer, 160
ovarian cancer, 171, 173
side effects, 224t, 226t, 229t
stomach cancer, 195
testicular cancer, 198
Wilms' tumor, 204
pleura, mesotheliomas, 210–11
pleural effusion, 139
emergencies, 288t
with ovarian cancer, 167, 169f
pneumonectomy, **140**
pneumonia, 139, 288t
polypoid cancers of stomach, 194
polyps, colon, 49, 50, 50f
porcelain gallbladder, 209
porphyrins, **40**
Port-a-Cath system, 222–23
power of attorney, 303
prayer, 243
precancerous changes
bowel, 49, 50f
cervix, 88
endometrium, 92, 93, 95
mouth, 158
skin (keratoses), **187**, **188f–89**
vulva, 211
predisposing factors, 27
prednisolone, 123
prednisone
in leukemias, acute lymphoblastic, 128
in leukemias, chronic lymphocytic, 123
in lymphoma, 146
pregnancy, 82, 165
breast cancer risk factors, 65, 65t
choriocarcinoma and hydatidiform mole, **89–92**
and ovarian cancer incidence, 166
stilbestrol during, 29t
prevention, 34, **255–56**, 258t–60, 335
primary site, **12**
primary tumor. *See also specific sites*
defined, **12**
size and growth, 12–14, 13f
unknown, **77–81**
procarbazine, 224t, 226t
brain and spinal cord cancer, 62
prochlorperazine, 225t
progesterone, 94
prognosis, 33, 34–35, **331**
programmed cell death, **11**
prophylaxis
central nervous system, in lymphoma management, 147–48
in leukemias, acute lymphoblastic, 128
prospective studies, **30**
prostate cancer, 28, **177f–83**, 179t, 180f, 181f
contributing factors, 29t
family history of, 64
markers, 80, 179, 182, 183, 258, **330**
preventive actions, 258t
as primary site of carcinomas of unknown primary, 78f, 79, 80
prostatectomy, 181
prosthetics, 159, 160, 215
proteases, **14**
PSA, 80, 179, 182, 183, 258, **330**
psychiatrist, 285
psychological factors, 248, 249, 250, 335. *See also* attitudes; coping/adjustment/adaptation
psychological intimacy, 297, 307
psychological support
with depression, 285–86
and survival, 252–53
talking about cancer, 294–317
pain management approaches, 283
psychoneuroimmunology, 253
p27, 270
pulmonary embolus, 288t
pumps, pain, 281f, 282
purine analogs
leukemias, acute lymphoblastic, 129
leukemias, chronic lymphocytic, 125
leukemias, hairy-cell, 132
purple spots. *See* petechiae

quality of life
death and dying, 317–24
depression, 284–87, 285t
emergencies, 287, 288–89t
feeling better, 243, 245
pain management, 276–83, 278f, 279f, 280f, 281f
selection of health care agent, 303
sexuality, 287–91
spiritual aspects, 316–17
stoma management, 291–94, 292f, 293f
talking about cancer, 294–317
tiredness, 283–84

race
esophageal cancer incidence, 98
and leukemias, acute lymphoblastic, 128
melanoma location, 151, 153

race (*continued*)
  myeloma incidence, 162
  and prostatic cancer, 178
  skin pigmentation, 150
rad (unit of radiation dosage), 107
radiation exposure, 127, 338
  and bone cancer (osteosarcoma), 43
  and leukemias, acute lymphoblastic, 129
  and leukemias, chronic granulocytic, 126, 130
  and sarcomas, soft tissue, 184
  and thyroid cancer, 201
radiation field, **218**, 219
radiation oncology, **213**
radical hysterectomy, modified, 88
radical mastectomy, 71, 72f
radical nephrectomy, 112
radioactive iodine, 200, 202
radioactive isotopes, monoclonal antibody delivery system, 231–32
radiotherapy, 33, 213, **216f–21**, 217f, 218f, 220f. *See also specific tumor sites*
  anal cancer, 207
  carcinoid tumors, 208–9
  carcinoma of unknown primary, 80
  cervical cancer, 87–88
  fatigue and exhaustion, 283–84
  Kaposi's sarcoma, 107
  leukemias, acute lymphoblastic, 129
  lymphoma, 147
  mastectomy or lumpectomy with, 71, 73
  prostate cancer, 182
  retinoblastoma, 205
  sexual problems after, 287
  skin cancer, 189–90
  skin damage, 188
  testicular cancer, 198, 199
  thyroid cancer, 200, 202
randomized clinical trials, 233
ras oncogene, 270–71
RB1 (retinoblastoma) gene, 26, 27
Recklinghausen's disease, 184
reconstruction, 215
  after mastectomy, 73
  after oral cancer surgery, 159, 160
rectal bleeding, 32
rectal cancer, primary. *See* bowel cancer
rectal cancer, secondary, 193
rectal examination, 34, 55t, 180f, 206, 256t
rectum, 47f
  prostate and, 177, 180f
  surgical management of bowel cancer, 54
recurrence, 216, 248
  of bladder cancer, 39
  of bowel cancer, 54
  of breast cancer, 71
  defined, **19**
  local, **329–30**
  of lymphoma, 148
  of testicular cancer, 199
  of trophoblastic tumor, 92
red cells, **120**, 213. *See also* anemia
  chemotherapy side effects, 227
  colony-stimulating factors, 232
  transfusions of, 131
red patches (erythroplakia), 158
reflection as communication technique, 311
reflux disease, **98**
rehabilitation, 181, 215
relaxation techniques, 283
remission, 6
  defined, **19**
  spontaneous, 112–13, 242–43
renal-cell carcinoma, 109, 110, 232, 242, 244
renal pelvis, 110, 113
repetition as communication technique, 311
research, 334, 336, 340
  laboratory models, 264–65
  mind-body relationship, 249, 250
  overoptimistic reporting, 265–66
  public perception of, 261–74
  social support groups and survival, 252–53
  trial and error process of, 266–68
reservoir systems for drug administration, 222–23
resistance to chemotherapy, 92, 146, 270
retina, 154
retinoblastoma, 21, **204–5**, 333
rhabdomyosarcoma, 185
riboflavin, 99
rib pain, 162
right cerebral hemisphere, **57**
risk factors, **27–30**, 29t, 32. *See also* alcohol; diet; smoking; *specific tumor sites*
rodent ulcer, 188f
rolfing, 283
route of administration, for pain medication, 281–82

salivary gland swelling, 128
salt balance
  emergencies and their management, 289t
  hormone production by lung tumors, 141
  myeloma and, 161
  tumor cell products affecting, 11, 18
salvage therapy, Hodgkin's disease, 105
sarcomas, 215
  bone cancers, **41–45**, 42f
  Kaposi's, **106–8**
  ovary, 172
  as primary site of carcinomas of unknown primary, 78f, 79
  soft tissue, **183–86**
  stomach, 194
  stromal tumor, of ovary, 165, 173
satellite lesions, mole, 152f, 155
scalp cooling, 227
S-C-A-N-S mnemonic for effective listening, 310t–11
scapegoating, 224–25
scars, 11, 188
screening, 34, **255**, **256t–58**
scrotal cancer, 24–25
secondary tumors, **11**, 15–18f, 16f, 17f, 216. *See also specific sites*
  brain or spinal cord, 56, 60–61, 63
  breast, 71
  cancer with unknown primary site (CUP), **77–81**, 78f
  lung cancer, 142
  metastasis, defined, **15**
second cancer after chemotherapy or radiation therapy, 106, 130, 144
second-hand smoke, 137
second-look surgery, ovarian cancer, 172
second opinions, 305
seedlings, ovarian cancer, 167, 169f
segmental mastectomy, 71, 72f
seizures, 58–59, 289t
selectron, **217**
selenium, 48, 55t
self-examination, breast, 76, 257t
seminal fluid, 82–83, 181
seminomas, 196, 197, 198
sensitivity of test, 256–57
sentinel node sampling, **153**
serosa, stomach, 191f
serotonin, 208
serotonin-specific re-uptake inhibitors (SSRIs), 286
set thinking, 247
sex-cord stromal tumors, 165, 173
sexual activity
  in adolescents, 83
  AIDs lymphomas and Kaposi's sarcoma, 107
  anal cancer risk factors, 206
  cervical cancer risk factors, 82–83, 84, 86, 88t, 89
  preventive actions, 258t
  stoma effects, 294
sexuality, 287–91, 302
  after ovary removal, 172
  after prostate surgery, 181–82
shark cartilage, 241, 244
shiatsu massage, 283
shingles, 125f–26
shock and disbelief, 295
shortness of breath. *See* breathlessness
side effects
  of analgesics, 279, 282

of antidepressants, 286–87
of chemotherapy, 223–28, 224t, 225t, 226t, 229t
of radiation therapy, 219
Siegel, Bernie, 250–52, 336, 339
sigmoid colon, 47f
sigmoidoscopy, 51–52, 56, 256t, **331**
single cell death, **11**
size of tumor, primary, 12–14, 13f
skin
breast, dimpling of, 67–68, 68t
chemotherapy side effects, 227–28, 229t
genetic damage, 22, 22f
Kaposi's sarcoma, 29t, **106–8**, 232, 240–41, 244, 258t
keratoses, **187**, **188f–89**, 190
moles, **151–52f**, 155, 257t
normal tissue growth and repair, 10f–11, 22f
purple spots (petechiae). *See* petechiae
radiation penetration, 217f
radiation therapy effects, 219–20
radiation therapy planning, 218
shingles, 125f–26
steroid hormone side effects, 123
structure, 149f, 150–51
warts, 11, 14
skin cancer, 1, 21, **22f–23**, 254
basal-cell and squanous-cell, 187–90, 188f
contributing factors, 29t
melanoma, **149f–56t**, 152f
preventive actions, 258t
skin infections, 125, 227
skin pigmentation, 150, 151
slow-release preparations, analgesics, 280
small bowel, **46**, 49
anatomy of digestive tract, 47f, 192f
carcinoid tumors, 208
pancreas and, 174, 175f
radiosensitivity, 216
small-cell lung cancer, **140–42**
brain metastasis, 60–61
carcinomas of unknown primary, 79
small talk, 300
smell, stoma management, 293
smoking, 21, 22, 23, 30, 247, 248, 254, 334
and bladder cancer, 37, 38
and CEA marker, 56
and cervical cancer, 83, 88t
epidemiology of cancer, 28, 29t
and esophageal cancer, 97, 98, 99
and kidney cancer, 110
and kidney cancer risk, 109
and laryngeal cancer, 114, 115
and lung cancer, 137
and oral cancer, 158
and pancreatic cancer, 174
quitting, 258t, 259t, 260
social isolation, 314
social services, 319
social status, 290
socioeconomic factors
bowel cancer incidence, 48
breast cancer incidence, 64
cervical cancer incidence, 83–84
ovarian cancer, 166
sodium regulation. *See* salt balance
soft palate, 116f, 157f
soft tissue sarcomas, **183–86**
solid cancer of bladder, 38, 39f
somatostatin, 209
Sontag, Susan, 246
soot, 24, 25
specificity of screening test, 257
speculum, **331**
speculum examination, 84f–85, 87
speech
brain centers controlling, **57**
brain tumor symptoms, 59
oral cancers and, 159
oral cancer treatment and, 159, 160
rehabilitation after laryngectomy, 117f–18
speech fistula, 117f, **118**
speech therapy, 215
sperm banks, 199
Spiegel, David, 250, 252–53
spinal cord, **57f**
emergencies and their management, 288t, 289t
epidural nerve blocks, 283
radiosensitivity, 216
spinal cord tumors, **56**, **61**, 63, 67
spirituality, 249, 316–17
spleen, 16f, 103f, 121f
in leukemias, **122**, 126
lymphomas, non-Hodgkin's, 143
pancreas and, 175
stomach cancer spread to, 193, 195
splenectomy
in Hodgkin's disease, 104
in leukemias, hairy-cell, 132
spontaneous remissions, 112–13, 242–43
spread of cancer, 1–2, 11–12, 32
to distant sites, 15–18f, 16f, 17f
local, 14f–15f
melanoma, 152–53
sputum, **139**, 141
squamocolumnar junction, cervix, 82, 83f
squamous cell carcinoma, **331**
of anus, 205–7, 206f
of lung, 139
oral cavity, 159
skin, 187–90, 188f
vulva, 211
squamous epithelium, 82, 83f, **331**
staging and grading, 334
bladder cancer, 39
bowel cancer, 52
endometrial cancer, 96
factors affecting treatment and prognosis, 33
growth rate, 60
Hodgkin's disease, 104, 105
lymphoma, 145–46
melanoma, 154
ovarian cancer, 170
prostatic cancer, 179–80
sarcomas, soft tissue, 185–86
stomach cancer, 194–95
standard deviation, 35
standards of care, 233
statistics
epidemiological studies, 28–30
survival figures, 34–35
stem-cell rescue, 164, 230–31
stereotactic biopsy, **60**
steroid hormones, 225t
dexamethasone, 62
leukemias, acute lymphoblastic, 129
leukemias, chronic lymphocytic, 123
lung tumor production of, 141
lymphoma, AIDS-related, 108
myeloma, 163–64
with painkillers, 282
tumor cell production of, 18, 141
stilbestrol, 29t, 182
stoma, 215, 290
management of, 291–94, 292f, 293f, 340
urinary diversion, 40
stomach, 207f
anatomy of digestive tract, 47f, 98f, 175f
bleeding from, as steroid hormone side effect, 124
stomach cancer, **190–95**, 191f, 192f, 333
carcinoid tumors, 208
lymphomas, 143, 144, 145, 194
as primary site of carcinomas of unknown primary, 78f
stool. *See also* bowel habits
anal cancer symptoms, 206
blood in, 32, 51, 55t, 56, 123, 208t, 256t
bowel cancer symptoms, 51
colostomies, 52, 53f, 54
constipation, 48–49, 163, 282
diarrhea. *See* diarrhea
fatty, 175
normal bowel function, 46, 48
tarry, 288t
streptozotocin, 209, 224t
stress, 3, 253, 254, 290, 336, 337–38, 339
mind-body question, 246–49
psychoneuroimmunology, 253
and sexual problems, 287–88
stroke, 289t
stroma, ovary, 167f
stromal tumors of ovary, 165, 173
strong opioids, **279f**
submucosa, stomach, 191f

substance P, 208
suction curettage, molar pregnancy, 91
suicidal thoughts, 285t
sunblock, 155, 156t
sunlight, 22, 30, 254
  and oral cancer, 158
  sensitization by chemotherapeutic agents, 229t
  and skin cancer, 29t, 149, 151, 188, 190
  skin cancer risk reduction, 155, 156t, 258t
sun protection factor (SPF), 156t
superficial spreading melanoma, **153**
support groups, 252, 283, 298, 336, 339
support system
  alternative medicine, **235–44**, 237t
  talking about cancer, 295–316
support team, 278
surgery, 33, 213, **215–16**. *See also specific tumor sites*
surgical castration, 182
surgical debulking, ovarian cancer, 170–71
survival, 34–35, 336
swallowing, difficulties with
  with esophageal cancer, 99
  with oral cancers, 159
  oral cancer surgery and, 160
sweating. *See also* constitutional symptoms
  with Hodgkin's disease, 102
  hormone therapy side effects, 62, 96, 123
  leukemias, chronic lymphocytic, 123
swelling
  blockage of mediastinal blood vessels and, 138, 141
  with bone cancer, 43
  brain, 62
  emergencies and their management, 289t
  salivary gland, 128
  testes, 128
symptoms, 32–33, 314. *See also* constitutional symptoms
  pain. *See* pain symptoms
  talking about, 299t
systemic effects of tumor, 11, 18. *See also* constitutional symptoms

talking about cancer, 294–317
tamoxifen, 214, 240
  breast cancer, female, 74
  breast cancer, male, 76
  endometrial cancer risk with, 94
Taxol, 75, 244, 272–73
  lung cancer, 140
  oral cancer, 160
  ovarian cancer, 171
  side effects, 224t, 226t, 229t
Taxotere, 75
teeth, 116f, 157f
tendency (causes of cancer), 21, **22f–23f**
TENS (transcutaneous electrical nerve stimulator), 283
teratomas, 196
testes
  with leukemia, acute lymphoblastic, 128
  removal of, 182
  undescended, 197
testicular cancer, **196–99**, 214
  advances in treatment of, 262
  age and incidence, 32
  definition of cure, 19
  markers, **330**
  as primary site of carcinomas of unknown primary, 78f, 79
tetracyclic antidepressants, 286
therapy. *See* treatments, alternative; treatments, conventional
thioguanine, 224t
thiotepa, 224t
thirst, 59, 163
thoracotomy, 102, **332**
threat, 313
throat cancer, 77, 80, 113, 118, 215
thrombocytopenia, **120**, 124. *See also* platelets
thyroid cancer, **200f–202**
  lymphomas, 143, 145
  as primary site of carcinomas of unknown primary, 77, 78f
thyroid gland, chemotherapy and radiation therapy effects on, 106
thyroid hormone, 200–201, 202
thyroid scan, 201
thyroxine, 200–201, 202
tingling
  chemotherapy and, 229t
  myeloma and, 163
tiredness, 283–84. *See also* constitutional symptoms
tongue, 116f, 157f, 159
total cystectomy, 40
total gastrectomy, 195
trachea, **114f**, 115f, 138f
tracheal cancer, 77
tracheoesophageal fistula, 117f, **118**
tracheostomy, **117**
transcutaneous electrical nerve stimulator (TENS), 283
transformation, malignant, **24–25**
transfusions, 131, 227
transitional cell tumors, renal pelvis, 113
transit time, colon, 48–49
translocation of genetic material, **26**
transplantation, liver, 136
transplant patients, skin cancer in, 188
transverse colon, 47f
treatments, alternative, **235–44**, 237t, 335, 337
treatments, conventional, 6, 33, **213–34**, 334, 337. *See also specific cancer sites*
  with alternative therapies, 240–41
  biologic therapy, 213, 214, **231–33**
  bone marrow transplant, 228, **230–31**, 230f, 231f
  chemotherapy, 213–14, **221–33**, 222f, 224t, 225t, 226t, 229t
  clinical trials, **233–34**
  factors affecting, 33
  history of, 213–14
  hormone therapy. *See* hormone therapy
  interpretation of survival data and prognosis, 34–35
  multidisciplinary care, 214–15
  radiotherapy, 213, **216f–21**, 217f, 218f, 220f
  rate of progress of research on, 261–22
  surgery, 213, **215–16**
tricyclic antidepressants, 286
triggers (causes of cancer), 21, **22f–23f**
trophoblastic tumors, **89–92**
tumor biology, **9–19**
  antigenic markers. *See* markers
  carcinogenesis, **21–30**
  cell growth, abnormal, 11f–12
  cell growth, normal, 9–11, 10f
  cure, recurrence, and remission, 19
  effects of tumor on physiology, 18
  growth, spread, and invasion, 1–2, 13f–14
  invasion and spread, 14f–15f
  laboratory models, 264–65
  primary tumor size and growth, 12–14, 13f
  public perception of cancer research, 261–74
  research advances, 263–64
  research in progress, 269–70
  spread to distant sites, 15–18f, 16f, 17f
tumor suppressor genes, **25**, **26–27**, 29t, 65t, 270
tumor vaccines, melanoma, 155
twin studies, 29
two-piece colostomy bag, 293

ulcerative colitis, 50
ulcers
  oral, 158–59
  skin, 188f
  stomach, 193, 194, 254
ultrasound, **333**
  anal cancer, 206
  bile duct cancer, 207
  biliary system, 210
  breast evaluation, 68
  endometrial cancer diagnosis, **95**
  Hodgkin's disease, 104
  kidney cancer, 111
  leukemia, chronic granulocytic, 126

liver cancer, 135, 136
lymphoma staging, 145
ovarian cancer screening, 172
prostatic cancer, 179
screening tests, 256t
testicular cancer, 197
thyroid, 201
ultraviolet light. *See* sunlight
uncertainty, 6, 304–5, 313. *See also* fear
unconventional treatments. *See* treatments, alternative
understanding of disease process, 3, 5–6
undescended testis, 197
unfamiliarity, 313–14
uranium miners, 137
ureteral catheters, 40
ureters, 109f, 110
urethra, **36**, 37f, 177f, 180f
urinary system
anatomy, 36, 37f, 109f, 110, 177f, 180f
intravenous pyelography, **38**, 111, 198, **330**
urination
frequency, **38**, 179t
hesitation, 179t
inability, 288t
myeloma and, 163
prostatic cancer symptoms, 178–79t
urine
blood in (hematuria), **37**, 111
management after cystectomy, 40
urine tests, in kidney cancer, 111
urostomy, 215, 291, 293f–94
uterine cancer
definition of cure, 19
endometrial, 19, **92–97**, 93f
as primary site of carcinomas of unknown primary, 78f
radiotherapy, 217
uterus
anatomy, 166f
cervix, 82, 83f
choriocarcinoma and hydatidiform mole, **89–92**
removal of in ovarian cancer, 171

vaccination
with leukemias, 125
preventive actions, 258t
vaccination, with leukemias, 125
vaccines, anti-cancer, 270–71
vaccines, melanoma, 155
vagina
anatomy, 166f
cervix, 82, 83f
choriocarcinoma spread to, 90
endometrial cancer spread to, 94
melanomas, 154
vaginal bleeding
cervical cancer risk reduction, 88
with choriocarcinoma or molar pregnancy, 90
with endometrial cancer, 92, 93, 94, 95, 97
vaginal cancer, 29t
vaginal discharge, 167
values, 303
variability of disease course, 240
videotape resources, 340
vinblastine
bladder cancer, 41
choriocarcinoma or molar pregnancy, 91
Kaposi's sarcoma, 107
lung cancer, 140
side effects, 224t, 226t, 229t
vincristine
brain and spinal cord cancer, 62
Kaposi's sarcoma, 107
leukemias, acute lymphoblastic, 128, 129
lung cancer, 142
lymphoma, 146
side effects, 224t, 226t, 229t
soft tissue sarcomas, 186
Wilms' tumor, 204
vindesine, 224t
vinorelbine, 224t, 226t
lung cancer, 140
viruses, 23, 29t, 258t
AIDs. *See* AIDS/HIV
anal cancer risk, 206
cervical cancer risk factors, 82–83, 85
and Hodgkin's disease, 101
and liver cancer, 133, 134, 135, 136, 133, 134
shingles, 125–26
vision
blurring, 277
brain tumor symptoms, 59
retinoblastoma and, 205
vitamin B complex, 99
vitamin C, 48, 55t
vitamin D, 151
vitamin deficiencies
and esophageal cancer, 99
and oral cancer, 158
vitamins, protective effect of in bowel cancer, 48
vocal cords, **114f**, 115f
partial laryngectomy and, 116
voice box. *See* laryngeal cancer
vomiting. *See also* nausea and vomiting
coffee grounds, 124
emergencies and their management, 289t
vulva, cancer of, 79

Waldenström's macroglobulinemia, 164
warts, 11, 14
genital, 82
water absorption, bowel function, 46
weakness, 288t. *See also* constitutional symptoms
weak opioids, **279**, 279f
weight
endometrial cancer risk factors, 94, 97
hormone therapy side effects, 96
weight loss. *See* constitutional symptoms
wheezing, 208
white cells, **120**, 213. *See also* leukemias
chemotherapy side effects, 227
colony-stimulating factors, 232
white patches (leukoplakia), 158, 211
wigs, 227, 314
Wilms' tumor, 109, 110, **203–4**
womb. *See* uterus
work, return to, 284
workplace exposures, 24–25
and bladder cancer, 37
and leukemias, chronic granulocytic, 130
and lung cancer, 137
and lymphomas, non-Hodgkin's, 143–44
and mesotheliomas, 210

X-ray radiation. *See* radiation exposure
X-ray studies, 213, 216, 257–58. *See also* barium studies
biliary system, 210
bone cancer, 44
carcinoma of unknown primary, 80
kidney (IVP), **38**, 111, 198
large bowel, 52
mammography, **68**
mesotheliomas, 210, 211
myeloma, 163
ovarian cancer, 168
uterus (hysterography), **95**
X-ray therapy. *See* radiotherapy

zinc, 99

Library of Congress Cataloging-in-Publication Data

Buckman, Robert.
What you really need to know about cancer : a comprehensive guide for patients and their families / Robert Buckman, in collaboration with the specialists at M. D. Anderson Cancer Center ; foreword by Robert C. Bast Jr.
p. cm.
Canadian ed. (Key Porter Books, Toronto, 1995) has same title.
Includes bibliographical references and index.
ISBN 0-8018-5594-2 (alk. paper). ISBN 0-8018-5593-4 (pbk. : alk. paper)
1. Cancer—popular works. I. Title.
RC263.B76 1997 97-5203
616.99'4—dc21 CIP